EIGHTH EDITION

Fitness and Wellness

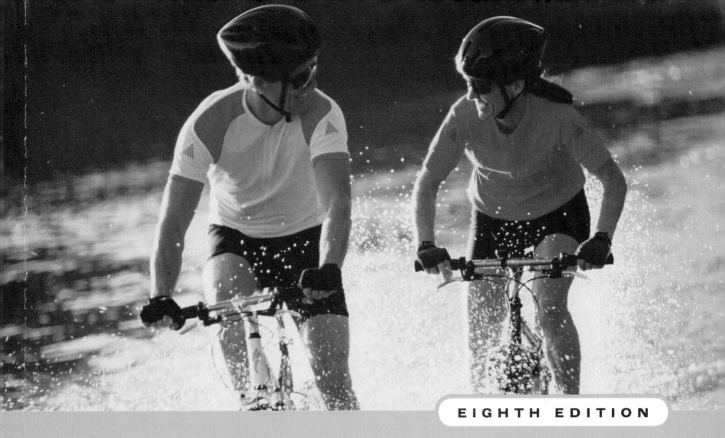

EIGHT EDITION

Fitness and Wellness

WERNER W. K. HOEGER
Boise State University

and **SHARON A. HOEGER**
Fitness & Wellness, Inc.

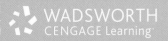

WADSWORTH
CENGAGE Learning

Australia • Brazil • Japan • Korea • Mexico • Singapore • Spain • United Kingdom • United States

WADSWORTH
CENGAGE Learning

Fitness and Wellness, **Eighth Edition**
Werner W. K. Hoeger, Sharon A. Hoeger

Publisher: Yolanda Cossio

Development Editor: Anna Lustig

Associate Development Editor: Elesha Feldman

Editorial Assistant: Elizabeth Momb

Marketing Manager: Jennifer Somerville

Marketing Assistant: Katherine Malatesta

Marketing Communications Manager:
Belinda Krohmer

Project Manager, Editorial Production:
Trudy Brown

Creative Director: Rob Hugel

Art Director: John Walker

Print Buyer: Judy Inouye

Permissions Editor: Mollika Basu

Production Service: Graphic World Inc.

Text Designer: Brian Salisbury

Photo Researcher: Terri Wright

Copy Editor: Graphic World Inc.

Cover Designer: Bill Reuter

Cover Image: Jacob Taposchaner/
The Collection/Getty Images

Compositor: Graphic World Inc.

For product information and technology assistance, contact us at
Cengage Learning Customer & Sales Support, 1-800-354-9706

For permission to use material from this text or product,
submit all requests online at **cengage.com/permissions**

Further permissions questions can be e-mailed to
permissionrequest@cengage.com

Library of Congress Control Number: 2008920617

ISBN-13: 978-0-495-38840-1

ISBN-10: 0-495-38840-8

Wadsworth
10 Davis Drive
Belmont, CA 94002-3098
USA

Cengage Learning is a leading provider of customized learning solutions with office locations around the globe, including Singapore, the United Kingdom, Australia, Mexico, Brazil, and Japan. Locate your local office at **international.cengage.com/region**.

Cengage Learning products are represented in Canada by Nelson Education, Ltd.

For your course and learning solutions, visit **academic.cengage.com**.

Purchase any of our products at your local college store or at our preferred online store **www.ichapters.com**.

Printed in the United States of America
1 2 3 4 5 6 7 12 11 10 09 08

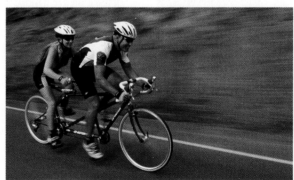

© Mark Johnson/Mira.com/drr.net

4 Evaluating Fitness Activities 99

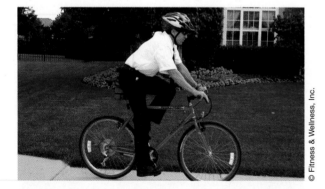

© Fitness & Wellness, Inc.

5 Nutrition for Wellness 119

6 Weight Management 145

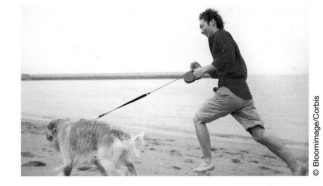

© Bloomimage/Corbis

Appendixes

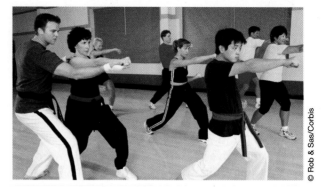

© Rob & Sas/Corbis

Most people go to college to learn how to make a living. Making a good living, however, won't help them unless they live an active lifestyle that will allow them to enjoy what they have.

The good news at the beginning of the 21st century is that health, fitness, and wellness throughout life are within the grasp of most people. Debilitating conditions are largely prevented by living a healthy lifestyle.

The bad news is that the lifestyle of far too many people is unhealthy, primarily because it does not include sufficient physical activity or proper nutrition. As a result, an epidemic of physical inactivity and obesity is sweeping across America and is so harmful to health that it actually increases the deterioration rate of the human body and leads to premature aging, illness, and death.

This book offers you the necessary information to start on your path to fitness and wellness by adhering to a healthy lifestyle. Because fitness and wellness needs vary significantly among individuals, all exercise and wellness prescriptions are personalized to obtain the best possible results.

The information in the following chapters and the subsequent activities at the end of each chapter will enable you to develop a personal lifetime program that promotes fitness, preventive health care, and personal wellness. The activities have been prepared on tear-out sheets so they can be turned in to class instructors.

What the Book Covers

As you study this book and complete the respective activities, you will learn to:

- Determine whether medical clearance is needed for your safe participation in exercise
- Conduct nutrient analyses and follow the recommendations for adequate nutrition
- Develop sound diet and weight-control programs
- Assess the health-related components of fitness (cardiorespiratory endurance, muscular strength and endurance, muscular flexibility, and body composition)

- Write exercise prescriptions for cardiorespiratory endurance, muscular strength and endurance, and muscular flexibility
- Understand stress, lessen your vulnerability to stress, and implement a stress management program, if necessary
- Implement a cardiovascular disease risk-reduction program
- Follow guidelines to reduce your personal risk of developing cancer
- Implement a smoking cessation program, if applicable
- Understand the health consequences of chemical dependency and irresponsible sexual behaviors and learn guidelines for preventing sexually transmitted infections
- Discern between myths and facts of exercise and health-related concepts
- Learn behavior modification techniques to help you adhere to a lifetime fitness and wellness program

New and Enhanced Features of the Eighth Edition

As with previous editions, the chapters in the eighth edition of *Fitness and Wellness* have been updated to include new information reported in the literature and at professional health, physical education, and sports medicine meetings. The following are the most significant updates to the eighth edition:

- In Chapter 1, *Introduction to Physical Fitness and Wellness*, all pertinent statistics related to this chapter, including physical activity participation, life expectancy, and the leading causes of death in the United States, have been brought up-to-date. New information is also included on the importance of increased physical activity and the benefits of vigorous-intensity exercise.
- The contents of Chapter 2, *Assessment of Physical Fitness*, were revised to ensure that these assessments comply with the guidelines for exercise testing by the American College of Sports Medicine and that recommended body weight complies with national body mass index guidelines.

- In Chapter 3, *Exercise Prescription,* the benefits and differences between moderate-intensity and vigorous-intensity physical activity according to the most recent (2007) information available from the American College of Sports Medicine and the American Heart Association have been updated. Using this information, students can make an informed decision as to the best approach to aerobic training. Tips to increase daily physical activity, including pedometer use and the number of steps required to walk or jog a mile at different speeds based on the latest (2008) research in the literature, are included. A new concept of repetition maximum training zone (RM zone), new dietary guidelines for strength development, the effects of flexibility on posture and its relationship to back pain, and an update on the importance of aerobic exercise and spinal stability exercises for the prevention and recurrence of back injury have all been included in the chapter.
- In Chapter 4, *Evaluating Fitness Activities,* the information on several of the aerobic activity choices has been revised and includes safety measures for participation in some of the activities listed.
- Chapter 5, *Nutrition for Wellness,* includes new information on trans fatty acids, vitamin D, probiotics, and fish. Updates on the information on fiber, nutrient supplementation, and antioxidants are also provided.
- The topic of Chapter 6, *Weight Management,* includes an expanded discussion on the role of strength training on resting metabolism. The most recent activity guidelines for weight gain prevention and weight loss maintenance are provided for the reader as well.
- An expanded Chapter 7, *Stress Management,* now addresses the power of the mind over the body, the impact of emotions on health, and visual imagery as a stress management technique.
- In Chapter 8, *A Healthy Lifestyle Approach,* all statistics on the incidence and prevalence of cardiovascular disease, cancer, addictive behavior, and sexually transmitted infections have been updated. Included also are the *2006 Diet and Lifestyle Recommendations* by the American Heart Association to decrease cardiovascular disease risk, new information on trans fats and heart disease, and updates on healthy lifestyle guidelines to prevent cancer. Emphasis is also provided on the ever-increasing role of physical activity on cardiovascular disease risk and cancer risk prevention.

- Chapter 9, *Relevant Fitness and Wellness Issues,* has been extensively revised. Many new frequently asked questions related to "hot" fitness and wellness issues were added to the chapter and previous questions have been brought up-to-date to conform with advancements in the area. Among these changes is a new section on *Wellness Behavior Modification Issues,* including the role of core values and emotions in triggering the process of behavioral change; information on the benefits of physical activity on fitness on disease risk reduction; the difference between "ideal" and "recommended" body weight; the effectiveness of diet versus exercise in weight loss; the role of low-intensity versus vigorous-intensity exercise in weight loss; the benefits of organic foods in the diet; and specific nutrient recommendations for optimal development and recovery following exercise.
- Extensive new photography has also been added throughout the book.

Ancillaries

The following ancillaries are provided free of charge to all qualified *Fitness and Wellness* adopters:

- **CengageNOW™ Instant Access Code.** ISBN-10: 0-495-39420-3. Get instant access to CengageNOW™! This exciting online resource is a powerful new learning companion that helps students gauge their unique study needs—and provides them with a Personalized Change Plan that enhances their problem-solving skills and conceptual understanding. A click of the mouse allows students to enter and explore the system whenever they choose, with no instructor setup necessary. The Personalized Change Plan section guides students through a behavior change process tailored specifically to their needs and personal motivation. An excellent tool to give as a project, this plan is easy to assign, track, and grade, even for large sections.
- **CengageNOW™ Printed Access Code.** ISBN-10: 0-495-39419-X. CengageNOW™ is a powerful new online learning companion that helps students gauge their unique study needs—and provides them with a Personalized Change Plan that enhances their problem-solving skills and conceptual understanding. A click of the mouse allows students to enter and explore the system whenever they choose, with

no instructor setup necessary. The Personalized Change Plan section guides students through a behavior change process tailored specifically to their needs and personal motivation. An excellent tool to give as a project, this plan is easy to assign, track, and grade, even for large sections.

- **Instructor's Manual with Test Bank.** ISBN-10: 0-495-38845-9. This comprehensive resource provides learning objectives, detailed chapter outlines, a list of chapter-specific labs, a list of websites, classroom activities, and teaching strategies. The test bank provides true/false, multiple-choice, critical-thinking, short answer, and essay questions.
- **PowerLecture CD-ROM.** ISBN-10: 0-495-38847-5. Designed to make lecture preparation easier, this CD-ROM includes more than 200 customizable PowerPoint® presentation slides with images from the text, new ABC video clips, and electronic versions of the Instructor's Manual and Test Bank. Also included is the ExamView® Computerized Test Bank, an easy-to-use assessment and tutorial system that allows you to create, deliver, and customize tests (both print and online) in minutes.
- **Transparency Acetates.** ISBN-10: 0-495-38853-X. More than 100 transparency acetates are available, including text art and supplementary outlines.
- **Telecourse Guide for Dallas TeleLearning "Becoming Physically Fit."** ISBN-10: 0-495-38844-0. "Becoming Physically Fit" is a new telecourse produced by the Dallas TeleLearning of the LeCroy Center for Educational Telecommunications. This course is designed to move students toward improving their personal physical fitness and obtain an overall healthier lifestyle at a pace specific to each individual. Students are asked to make behavioral as well as physical changes to their lifestyle. The successful implementation of these changes serves to motivate students to maintain personal fitness, proper nutrition, and lifelong healthy lifestyle choices. For more information on the course, visit http://telelearning.dcccd.edu.
- **Behavior Change Workbook.** ISBN-10: 0-495-01145-2, ISBN-13: 978-0-495-01145-3. The Behavior Change Workbook includes a brief discussion of the current theories behind making positive lifestyle changes, along with exercises to help students make those changes in their everyday lives.

- **Careers in Health, Physical Education, and Sport, 2e.** ISBN-10: 0-495-38839-4. This unique booklet takes students through the complicated process of picking the type of career they want to pursue; explains how to prepare for the transition into the working world; and provides insight into different types of career paths, education requirements, and reasonable salary expectations. A designated chapter discusses some of the legal issues that surround the workplace, including discrimination and harassment. This supplement is complete with personal development activities designed to encourage students to focus on and develop better insight into their future.
- **Walk4Life® Pedometer.** ISBN-10: 0-495-01315-3, ISBN-13: 978-0-495-01315-0. Provided through an alliance with Walk4Life®, the Walk4Life® Elite Model pedometer tracks steps, elapsed time, and distance. Including a calorie counter and a clock, it is an excellent class activity and tool to encourage students to track their steps and walk toward better fitness awareness.
- **Diet Analysis™+ 8.0 Win/Mac Online Access Card.** ISBN-10: 0-534-63981-X. The market-leading diet assessment program used by colleges and universities, Diet Analysis™+ allows students to easily create personalized profiles based on their height, weight, age, sex, and activity level. Its dynamic interface makes it easy for users to track vitamins, minerals, calories, fiber, and fats in foods, as well as to determine whether their nutrient needs are being met. Students can use this information to adjust their diet, gain a better understanding of how nutrition relates to their personal health goals, and complete nutrition analysis assignments. Thoroughly revised and updated with the latest USDA standards, the software is available online or on a Win/Mac-compatible CD-ROM. Both versions provide practical and instructive features with a comprehensive database, making it a favorite among professors and students alike. Diet Analysis™+ 8.0 is appropriate for all nutrition and health courses in which the professor wants to incorporate nutritional assessment.
- **Diet Analysis™+ 8.0.1 Win/Mac CD-ROM.** ISBN-10: 0-495-55715-3. The market-leading diet assessment program used by colleges and universities, Diet Analysis™+ allows students to easily create personalized profiles based on their height, weight, age, sex, and activity level. Its dynamic interface makes it easy for users to track

vitamins, minerals, calories, fiber, and fats in foods, as well as to determine whether their nutrient needs are being met. Students can use this information to adjust their diet, gain a better understanding of how nutrition relates to their personal health goals, and complete nutrition analysis assignments. Thoroughly revised and updated with the latest USDA standards, the software is available online or on a Win/Mac-compatible CD-ROM. Both versions provide practical and instructive features with a comprehensive database, making it a favorite among professors and students alike. Diet Analysis™+ 8.0 is appropriate for all nutrition and health courses in which the professor wants to incorporate nutritional assessment.

- **Readings for a Healthy Living.** ISBN-10: 0-759-35944-X. This reader features 12 articles written by author Dianne Hales and published in *Parade* magazine. Readings include "Take Your Meds—The Right Way," "You Can Think Yourself Thin," "Getting Yourself Back on Track," "Too Tough to Seek Help," and "The Best Medical Help Online."
- **TestWell Online Assessment Access Card.** ISBN-10: 0-495-01264-5. This web-based assessment tool allows students to answer 100 questions specific to their health status in relation to the six dimensions of wellness. Students are provided a 10-step Behavior Change Guide for long-term positive behavior modifications. It can be used as a pre- or post-test to assess students' health status, and it can provide a venue for learning about the different dimensions of wellness. It executes immediate feedback based on students' responses and can contribute to classroom participation and overall learning assessment. Test-Well offers a fun and easy web-based activity for student enrichment.
- **Health and Wellness Resource Center.** http://academic.cenage.com/health This comprehensive website provides easy-to-find answers to health questions and access to full text articles from hundreds of journals, pamphlets, and reference materials.

Acknowledgments

We would like to thank the reviewers for their valuable comments and contributions to the eighth edition. We also wish to thank Jonathan and Cherie Hoeger, Jessica Bringhurst, Austin Legg, David Gonzalez, Amber Neroes, Brent and Amber Fawson, Kristin Aldrich, Josh Bean, Dr. Lynda Ransdell, Michelle StanWiens, and Christian Atance, all of whom contributed to the new photography in this edition.

A thank-you note from Patty to the course instructor at the end of the semester read:

Thank you for making me a new person. I truly appreciate the time you spent with me. Without your kindness and motivation, I would never have made it. It's great to be fit and trim. I've never had this feeling before, and I wish everyone could feel like this once in their life.

Thank you, Your trim Patty!

Patty had never been taught the principles governing a sound weight loss program. She needed this knowledge, and like most Americans who have never experienced the process of becoming physically fit, she needed to be in a structured exercise setting to truly feel the joy of fitness.

Of even greater significance, Patty maintained her aerobic and strength-training programs. A year after ending her calorie-restricted diet, her weight actually increased by 10 pounds—but her body fat decreased from 22.5 percent to 21.2 percent. As discussed in Chapter 6, the weight increase is related mostly to changes in lean tissue lost during the weight-reduction phase. Despite only a slight drop in weight during the second year following the calorie-restricted diet, Patty's two-year follow-up revealed a further decrease in body fat, to 19.5 percent. Patty understands the new quality of life reaped through a sound fitness program.

Lifestyle, Health, and Quality of Life

Research findings have shown that physical inactivity and negative lifestyle habits pose a serious threat to health. Movement and physical activity are basic functions for which the human organism was created. Advances in modern technology, however, have all but eliminated the need for physical activity in daily life. Physical activity no longer is a natural part of our existence. This epidemic of physical inactivity is the second greatest threat to U.S. public health and has been termed **Sedentary Death Syndrome, or SeDS.** (The number-one threat is tobacco use—the largest cause of preventable deaths.)

Today we live in an automated society. Most of the activities that used to require strenuous physical exertion can be accomplished by machines with the simple pull of a handle or push of a button. If people go to a store that is only a couple of blocks away,

most drive their automobiles and then spend a couple of minutes driving around the parking lot to find a spot 50 yards closer to the store's entrance. The groceries do not even have to be carried out anymore. A store employee willingly takes them out in a cart and places them in the vehicle. During a visit to a multilevel shopping mall, nearly everyone chooses to ride the escalators instead of taking the stairs.

Automobiles, elevators, escalators, telephones, intercoms, remote controls, electric garage door openers—all are modern-day commodities that minimize the amount of movement and effort required of the human body.

One of the most significant detrimental effects of modern-day technology has been an increase in **chronic diseases** related to a lack of physical activity. These include hypertension (high blood pressure), heart disease, chronic low back pain, and obesity, among others. They sometimes are referred to as **hypokinetic diseases.** ("Hypo" means low or little, and "kinetic" implies motion.) Lack of adequate physical activity is a fact of modern life that most people can avoid no longer. If we want to enjoy contemporary commodities and still expect to live life to its fullest, a personalized lifetime exercise program must become a part of our daily lives.

With the developments in technology, three additional factors have changed our lives significantly and have had a negative effect on human health: nutrition, stress, and environment. Fatty foods, sweets, alcohol, tobacco, excessive stress, and environmental

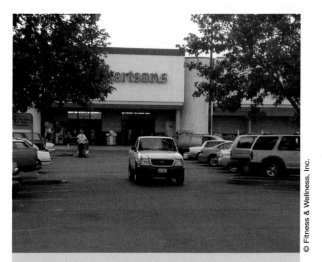

The epitome of physical inactivity is to drive around a parking lot for several minutes in search of a parking spot 10 to 20 yards closer to the store's entrance.

© Fitness & Wellness, Inc.

Introduction to Physical Fitness and Wellness

© Fitness & Wellness, Inc.

There is no drug in current or prospective use that holds as much promise for sustained health as a lifetime program of physical exercise.[1]

OBJECTIVES

- Understand the importance of sound physical fitness and wellness
- Define physical fitness and list components of health-related and skill-related fitness
- Learn the benefits of a comprehensive fitness and wellness program
- Learn motivational and behavior modification techniques to enhance compliance with a healthy lifestyle program
- Determine whether medical clearance is required for safe participation in exercise

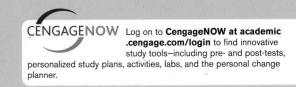

Most people go to school to help them make a better living. A fitness and wellness course will teach you how to live better—how to truly live your life to its fullest potential. Real success is about more than money: Making a good living will not help you unless you live a wellness lifestyle that will allow you to enjoy what you have. Your lifestyle is the most important factor affecting your personal well-being, but most people don't know how to make the right choices to live their best life.

During the last three decades, the benefits of physical activity have been substantiated by scientific evidence linking increased physical activity and positive lifestyle habits to better health and improved quality of life. Even though a few individuals live long because of favorable genetic factors, for most people the quality of life during middle age and the "golden years" is more often related to wise choices initiated during youth and continued throughout life.

Based on the abundance of scientific research on physical activity and exercise, a clear distinction has been established between the two. **Physical activity** is defined as bodily movement produced by skeletal muscles that requires the expenditure of energy and produces progressive health benefits. Examples of physical activity are walking to and from work and the store, taking the stairs instead of elevators and escalators, gardening, doing household chores, dancing, and washing the car by hand.

Physical inactivity, by contrast, implies a level of activity that is lower than that required to maintain good health.

Exercise is considered a type of physical activity that requires planned, structured, and repetitive bodily movement to improve or maintain one or more components of physical fitness. Walking, jogging, cycling, aerobics, swimming, strength training, and stretching—as a regular weekly program—are all examples of exercise.

Unfortunately, the current way of life in most developed nations does not provide the human body with sufficient physical exercise to maintain adequate health. Furthermore, many lifestyle patterns are such a serious threat to health that they actually speed up deterioration of the human body. In a few short years, lack of wellness leads to loss of vitality and gusto for life, as well as premature morbidity and mortality.

The typical North American is not a good role model in terms of physical fitness. According to the Centers for Disease Control and Prevention (CDC), the majority of U.S. adults are not sufficiently physically active to promote good health. The data indicate that only 46 percent of adults meet the minimal recommendation of 30 minutes of moderate physical activity at least 5 days per week, 25 percent report no leisure physical activity at all, and 16 percent are completely inactive (that is, spending less than 10 minutes per week in moderate- or vigorous-intensity physical

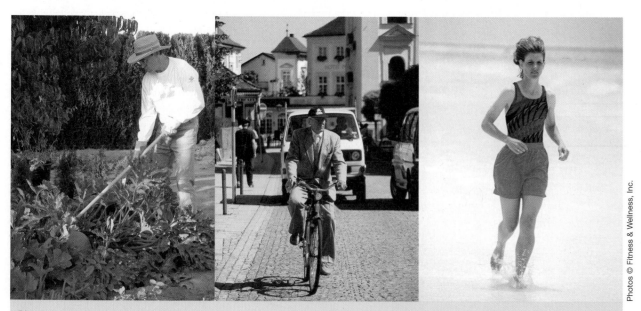

Physical activity and exercise lead to less disease, a longer life, and enhanced quality of life.

Photos © Fitness & Wellness, Inc.

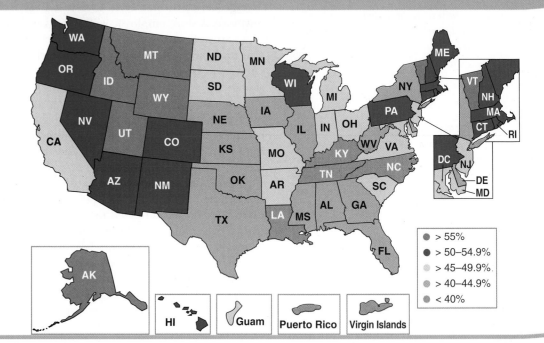

FIGURE 1.1

U.S. prevalence of recommended physical activity.*

- ● > 55%
- ● > 50–54.9%
- ● > 45–49.9%
- ● > 40–44.9%
- ● < 40%

*Moderate-intensity physical activity at least 5 days a week for 30 minutes a day or vigorous-intensity physical activity 3 days a week for 20 minutes a day.
SOURCE: Centers for Disease Control and Prevention, Atlanta, 2005.

activity). The prevalence of physical activity by state in the United States is displayed in Figure 1.1.

Even though most people in the United States believe that a positive lifestyle has a great impact on health and longevity, most do not know how to implement a fitness and wellness program that will yield the desired results. Patty Neavill is an example of someone who frequently tried to change her life but was unable to do so because she did not know how to implement a sound exercise and weight control program. At age 24, Patty, a college sophomore, was discouraged by her weight, level of fitness, self-image, and quality of life in general.

She had struggled with weight most of her life. Like thousands of other people, she had made many unsuccessful attempts to lose weight. Patty put aside her fears and decided to enroll in a fitness course. As part of the course requirement, she took a battery of fitness tests at the beginning of the semester. Patty's cardiorespiratory fitness and strength ratings were poor, her flexibility classification was average, she weighed more than 200 pounds, and she was 41 percent body fat.

Following the initial fitness assessment, Patty met with her course instructor, who prescribed an exercise and nutrition program such as the one presented in this book. Patty fully committed to carry out the prescription. She walked or jogged five times a week, worked out with weights twice a week, and played volleyball or basketball two to four times each week. Her daily caloric intake was set in the range of 1,500 to 1,700 calories. She took care to meet the minimum required amounts from the basic food groups each day, which contributed about 1,200 calories to her diet. The remainder of the calories came primarily from complex carbohydrates. At the end of the 16-week semester, Patty's cardiorespiratory fitness, strength, and flexibility ratings had all improved to the "good" category, she had lost 50 pounds, and her percent body fat had dropped to 22.5!

KEY TERMS

Physical activity Bodily movement produced by skeletal muscles that requires energy expenditure and produces progressive health benefits.

Exercise A type of physical activity that requires planned, structured, and repetitive bodily movement done to improve or maintain one or more components of physical fitness.

hazards (such as wastes, noise, and air pollution) have detrimental effects on people's health.

The leading causes of death in the United States today (see Figure 1.2) are lifestyle related. About 59 percent of all deaths in the United States are caused by cardiovascular disease and cancer.[2] Almost 80 percent of these deaths could be prevented by adhering to a healthy lifestyle. The third leading cause of death—chronic lower respiratory (lung) disease—is related largely to tobacco use. Accidents are the fourth leading cause of death. Even though not all accidents are preventable, many are. Fatal accidents often are related to abusing drugs and not wearing seat belts.

According to Dr. David Satcher, former U.S. Surgeon General, more than 50 percent of the people who die in the United States each year die because of what they do. Estimates indicate that more than half of disease is lifestyle related, a fifth is attributed to environmental factors, and a tenth is influenced by the health care the individual receives. Only 16 percent is related to genetic factors. Thus, the individual controls as much as 84 percent of disease susceptibility and quality of life. The data also indicate that 83 percent of deaths that occur before age 65 are preventable. In essence, most people in the United States are threatened by the very lives they lead today.[3]

Based on 2007 government data, the average **life expectancy** in the United States is now 75.2 years for men and 80.4 years for women. Unlike previous life expectancy calculations, the World Health Organization (WHO) has calculated **healthy life expectancy (HLE)** estimates for 191 nations. The United States ranks 24th in this report, with an HLE of 70 years. Japan is first, with an HLE of 74.5 years (see Figure 1.3).

The ranking for the United States is a major surprise for a developed country with one of the best medical care systems in the world. The rating indicates that Americans die earlier and spend more time disabled than people in most other advanced countries. The WHO points to several factors that may account for this unexpected finding:

1. The extremely poor health of some groups, such as Native Americans, rural African Americans, and the inner-city poor. Their health status is more characteristic of poor, developing nations than a rich, industrialized country.
2. The HIV epidemic, which causes more deaths and disability than in other developed nations
3. The high use of tobacco products
4. A high incidence of coronary heart disease
5. Fairly high levels of violence, notably homicides, compared with other developed countries

Although life expectancy in the United States has gradually increased by 30 years over the last century, scientists from the National Institute of Aging believe that in the coming decades the average lifespan may decrease by as much as 5 years. This decrease in life expectancy will be related primarily to the growing epidemic of obesity. According to CDC estimates, more than 23 percent of the adult popu-

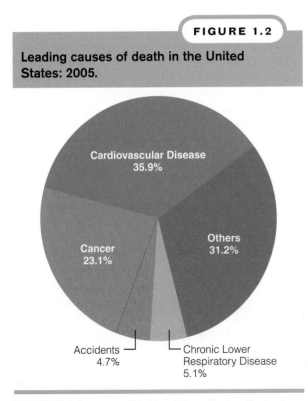

FIGURE 1.2

Leading causes of death in the United States: 2005.

Cardiovascular Disease
35.9%

Cancer
23.1%

Others
31.2%

Accidents
4.7%

Chronic Lower
Respiratory Disease
5.1%

SOURCE: U.S. Department of Health and Human Services, Centers for Disease Control and Prevention, *National Vital Statistics Report; Deaths: Final Data for 2004*, 55:19 (August 21, 2007).

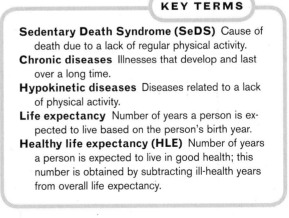

KEY TERMS

Sedentary Death Syndrome (SeDS) Cause of death due to a lack of regular physical activity.

Chronic diseases Illnesses that develop and last over a long time.

Hypokinetic diseases Diseases related to a lack of physical activity.

Life expectancy Number of years a person is expected to live based on the person's birth year.

Healthy life expectancy (HLE) Number of years a person is expected to live in good health; this number is obtained by subtracting ill-health years from overall life expectancy.

FIGURE 1.3

Healthy life expectancy for selected countries.

Country	Years
Ireland	69.6
USA	70.0
Germany	70.4
United Kingdom	71.7
Austria	71.6
Belgium	71.6
Greece	72.5
Netherlands	72.0
Norway	71.7
Spain	72.8
Italy	72.7
Canada	72.0
Switzerland	72.5
France	73.1
Sweden	73.0
Japan	74.5

Years (scale 60 65 70 75 80)

■ Healthy life expectancy

SOURCE: WHO, http://www.who.int/inf-pr-2000/en/pr2000-life.html. Retrieved Nov. 24, 2007.

lation in the United States is obese. Additional information on the obesity epidemic and its detrimental health consequences is given in Chapter 6.

2007 ACSM/AHA Physical Activity and Public Health Recommendations

In August of 2007, the American College of Sports Medicine (ACSM) and the American Heart Association (AHA) released joint physical activity recommendations for healthy adults.[4] These recommendations were issued to update and clarify previous recommendations, including the 1996 landmark report by the U.S. Surgeon General on physical activity and health.[5]

The updated recommendations indicate that to promote and maintain good health, all healthy adults between 18 and 65 years of age need:

1. **Moderate-intensity aerobic physical activity** for a minimum of 30 minutes five days a week or **vigorous-intensity aerobic physical activity** for a minimum of 20 minutes three days a week. A combination of moderate- and vigorous-intensity activities can be used to meet the aerobic activity recommendation. That is, a person could participate in moderate-intensity activity twice a week for 30 minutes and high-intensity activity for 20 minutes on another two days.
2. Activities that maintain or increase muscular strength and muscular endurance a minimum of two days per week on nonconsecutive days

The ACSM/AHA report further states that a greater amount of physical activity, to exceed the minimum recommendations in items 1 and 2 above, will provide even greater benefits and is recommended for individuals who wish to further improve personal fitness, reduce the risk for chronic disease and disabilities, prevent premature mortality, or prevent unhealthy weight gain.

The update also states that only about half of the U.S. adult population meet the above recommendations. About 53 percent of college graduates adhere to the recommendations, followed by individuals with some college education and high school graduates, and the least likely to meet the recommendations are those with less than a high school diploma (37.8 percent).

Importance of Increased Physical Activity

The U.S. Surgeon General has stated that poor health as a result of lacking physical activity is a serious public health problem that must be met head-on at once. Regular moderate physical activity provides substantial benefits in health and well-being for the vast majority of people who are not physically active. For those who are already moderately active, even greater health benefits can be achieved by increasing the level of physical activity.

Among the benefits of regular physical activity and exercise are significantly reduced risks for developing or dying from heart disease, stroke, type 2 diabetes, colon and breast cancers, high blood pressure, and osteoporotic fractures.[6] Regular physical activity also is important for the health of muscles, bones, and joints, and it seems to reduce symptoms of depression and anxiety, improve mood, and enhance one's ability to perform daily tasks throughout life. It also can help control health care costs and maintain a high quality of life into old age.

Moderate physical activity has been defined as any activity that requires an energy expenditure of 150 calories per day, or 1,000 calories per week. The general health recommendation is that people strive to accumulate at least 30 minutes of physical activity a minimum of five days per week. Whereas 30 minutes of continuous activity is preferred, on days when time is limited, three activity sessions of at least 10 minutes each provide about half the aerobic benefits. Examples of moderate physical activity are walking, cycling, playing basketball or volleyball, swimming, doing water aerobics, dancing fast, pushing a stroller, raking leaves, shoveling snow, washing or waxing a car, washing windows or floors, and even gardening.

Because of the ever-growing epidemic of obesity in the United States, a 2002 guideline by American and Canadian scientists from the Institute of Medicine of the National Academy of Sciences increased the recommendation to 60 minutes of moderate-intensity physical activity every day.[7] This recommendation was based on evidence indicating that people who maintain healthy weight typically accumulate one hour of daily physical activity.

Subsequently, the 2005 Dietary Guidelines for Americans released by the U.S. Department of Health and Human Services and the Department of Agriculture recommend that up to 60 minutes of moderate- to vigorous-intensity physical activity per day may be necessary to prevent weight gain, and between 60 and 90 minutes of moderate-intensity physical activity daily is recommended to sustain weight loss for previously overweight people.[8]

In sum, although health benefits are derived from 30 minutes per day, people with a tendency to gain weight need to be physically active daily for an hour to an hour and a half to prevent weight gain. And 60 to 90 minutes of activity per day provides additional health benefits, including a lower risk for cardiovascular disease and diabetes.

CRITICAL THINKING

Do you consciously incorporate physical activity into your daily lifestyle? • Can you provide examples? • Do you think you get sufficient daily physical activity to maintain good health?

Wellness

After the initial fitness boom swept across the United States in the 1970s, it became clear that improving physical fitness alone was not always enough to lower the risk for disease and ensure better health. For example, individuals who run 3 miles a day, lift weights regularly, participate in stretching exercises, and watch their body weight can be classified as having good or excellent fitness. If these same people, however, have high blood pressure, smoke, are under constant stress, consume too much alcohol, and eat too many fatty foods, they are exposing themselves to **risk factors** for disease of which they may not be aware.

Good health no longer is viewed as simply the absence of disease. The notion of good health has evolved notably in the last few years and continues to change as scientists learn more about lifestyle factors that bring on illness and affect wellness. Once the idea took hold that fitness by itself would not necessarily decrease the risk for disease and ensure better health, the wellness concept developed in the 1980s.

Wellness is an all-inclusive umbrella covering a variety of health-related factors. A wellness lifestyle requires the implementation of positive programs to change behavior and thereby improve health and quality of life, prolong life, and achieve total well-being. To enjoy a wellness lifestyle, a person has to practice behaviors that will lead to positive outcomes in seven dimensions of wellness: physical, emotional, intellectual, social, environmental, spiritual, and occupational (see Figure 1.4). These dimensions are interrelated; one frequently affects the others. For example, a person who is "emotionally down" often has no desire to exercise, study, go to work, socialize with friends, or attend church.

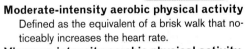

KEY TERMS

Moderate-intensity aerobic physical activity Defined as the equivalent of a brisk walk that noticeably increases the heart rate.

Vigorous-intensity aerobic physical activity Defined as an activity similar to jogging that causes rapid breathing and a substantial increase in heart rate.

Risk factors Characteristics that predict the chances for developing a certain disease.

Wellness The constant and deliberate effort to stay healthy and achieve the highest potential for well-being.

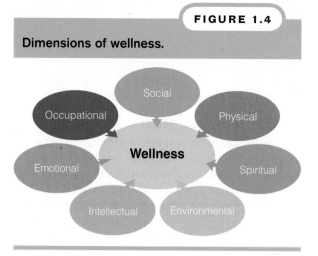

FIGURE 1.4

Dimensions of wellness.

The concept behind the seven dimensions of wellness shows that high-level wellness clearly goes beyond optimum fitness and the absence of disease. Wellness incorporates fitness, proper nutrition, stress management, disease prevention, social support, self-worth, nurturance (a sense of being needed), spirituality, personal safety, substance control and not smoking, regular physical examinations, health education, and environmental support.

For a wellness way of life, individuals must be physically fit and manifest no signs of disease, and they also must avoid all risk factors for disease (such as physical inactivity, hypertension, abnormal cholesterol levels, cigarette smoking, excessive stress, faulty nutrition, or careless sex). Even though an individual tested in a fitness center might demonstrate adequate or even excellent fitness, indulgence in unhealthy lifestyle behaviors will increase the risk for chronic diseases and decrease the person's well-being. Additional information on wellness and how to implement a wellness program is given in Chapter 8.

Unhealthy behaviors contribute to the staggering U.S. health care costs. Risk factors for disease carry a heavy price tag. Health care costs in the United States rose from $12 billion in 1950 to $2 trillion in 2005, or about 16 percent of the gross domestic product (GDP). In 1980, health care costs represented 8.8 percent of the GDP, and they are projected to reach about 20 percent by the year 2015. Based on estimates, 1 percent of Americans account for 30 percent of these costs. Half of the people use up about 97 percent of the health care dollars. In terms of yearly health care costs per person, the United States spends more than any other industrialized nation. In 2004, U.S. health care costs per capita were about $6,280; they are expected to reach almost $9,000 in 2010. Yet, overall, the U.S. health care system ranks only 37th in the world.

One of the reasons for the low overall ranking is the overemphasis on state-of-the-art cures instead of prevention programs. The United States is the best place in the world to treat people once they are sick, but the system does a poor job of keeping people healthy in the first place.

Physical Fitness

Individuals are physically fit when they can meet both the ordinary and the unusual demands of daily life safely and effectively without being overly fatigued and still have energy left for leisure and recreational activities. **Physical fitness** can be classified as health related, skill related, and physiological.

Health-Related Fitness

Health-related fitness has four components: cardiorespiratory endurance, muscular strength and endurance, muscular flexibility, and body composition (see Figure 1.5), defined respectively as:

1. *Cardiorespiratory endurance:* the ability of the heart, lungs, and blood vessels to supply oxygen to the cells to meet the demands of prolonged physical activity (also referred to as aerobic exercise)
2. *Muscular strength and endurance:* the ability of the muscles to generate force
3. *Muscular flexibility:* the achievable range of motion at a joint or group of joints without causing injury

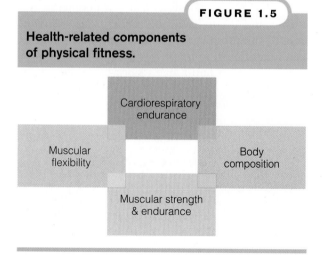

FIGURE 1.5

Health-related components of physical fitness.

4. *Body composition:* the amount of lean body mass and adipose tissue (fat mass) in the human body

Skill-Related Fitness

Fitness in motor skills is essential in activities such as basketball, racquetball, golf, hiking, soccer, and water skiing. Good skill-related fitness also enhances overall quality of life by helping people cope more effectively in emergency situations (see Chapter 4). The components of **skill-related fitness** are agility, balance, coordination, power, reaction time, and speed (see Figure 1.6):

1. *Agility:* the ability to change body position and direction quickly and efficiently. Agility is important in sports such as basketball, soccer, and racquetball, in which the participant must change direction rapidly and at the same time maintain proper body control.
2. *Balance:* the ability to maintain the body in equilibrium. Balance is vital in activities such as gymnastics, diving, ice skating, skiing, and even football and wrestling, in which the athlete attempts to upset the opponent's equilibrium.
3. *Coordination:* integration of the nervous system and the muscular system to produce correct, graceful, and harmonious body movements. This component is important in a wide variety of motor activities, such as golf, baseball, karate, soccer, and racquetball, in which hand-eye or foot-eye movements, or both, must be integrated.
4. *Power:* the ability to produce maximum force in the shortest time. The two components of power are muscle speed and force (strength). An effective combination of these two components allows a person to produce explosive movements such as are required in jumping; putting the shot; and spiking, throwing, and hitting a ball.

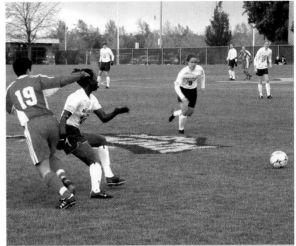

Good skill-related fitness enhances success in sports performance.

© Fitness & Wellness, Inc.

5. *Reaction time:* the time required to initiate a response to a given stimulus. Good reaction time is important for starts in track and swimming; for quick reactions when playing tennis at the net; and in sports such as ping-pong, boxing, and karate.
6. *Speed:* the ability to propel the body or a part of the body rapidly from one point to another. Examples of activities that require good speed for success are soccer, basketball, stealing a base in baseball, and sprints in track.

Physiological Fitness

Physiological fitness is a new term used primarily in the field of medicine in reference to biological systems that are affected by physical activity and the role the latter plays in the prevention of illness, in-

FIGURE 1.6

Motor skill–related components of physical fitness.

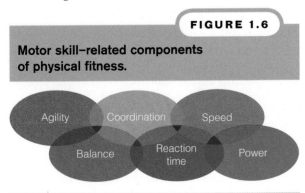

KEY TERMS

Physical fitness The general capacity to adapt and respond favorably to physical effort.

Health-related fitness A physical state encompassing cardiorespiratory endurance, muscular strength and endurance, muscular flexibility, and body composition.

Skill-related fitness Components of fitness important for successful motor performance in athletic events and in lifetime sports and activities.

Physiological fitness Biological systems that are affected by physical activity; also the role of activity in disease prevention.

cluding cardiovascular disease, diabetes, obesity, and osteoporosis.

In terms of preventive medicine, the main emphasis of fitness programs should be on the health-related components. As these components improve, so does physiological fitness. Skill-related fitness is crucial for success in sports and athletics, and it also contributes to wellness. Improving skill-related fitness affords an individual more enjoyment and success in lifetime sports, and regular participation in skill-related fitness activities also helps develop health-related fitness. Further, total fitness is achieved by taking part in specific programs to improve health-related and skill-related components alike.

Benefits of Fitness and Wellness

The benefits to be enjoyed from participating in a regular fitness and wellness program are many. In addition to a longer life (see the next three Figures), the greatest benefit of all is that physically fit people who lead a positive lifestyle have a healthier and better quality of life. These people live life to its fullest and have fewer health problems than inactive individuals who also indulge in negative lifestyle habits.

Compiling an all-inclusive list of the benefits to be reaped through participation in a fitness and wellness program is a challenge, but the following list summarizes many of them:

- Improves and strengthens the cardiorespiratory system
- Promotes better muscle tone, muscular strength, and endurance
- Improves muscular flexibility
- Enhances athletic performance
- Helps maintain recommended body weight
- Helps preserve lean body mass
- Increases resting metabolic rate
- Improves the body's ability to use fat during physical activity
- Improves posture and physical appearance
- Improves functioning of the immune system
- Lowers the risk for chronic diseases and illness (such as cardiovascular diseases and cancer)
- Decreases the mortality rate from chronic diseases
- Thins the blood so it doesn't clot as readily (thereby decreasing the risk for coronary heart disease and strokes)
- Helps the body manage cholesterol more effectively

- Prevents or delays the development of high blood pressure and lowers blood pressure in people with hypertension
- Helps prevent and control diabetes
- Helps achieve peak bone mass in young adults and maintain bone mass later in life, thereby decreasing the risk for osteoporosis
- Helps people sleep better
- Helps prevent chronic back pain
- Relieves tension and helps in coping with life stresses
- Raises levels of energy and job productivity
- Extends longevity and slows the aging process
- Promotes psychological well-being through better morale, self-image, and self-esteem
- Reduces feelings of depression and anxiety
- Motivates a person toward positive lifestyle changes (improving nutrition, quitting smoking, controlling alcohol and drug use)
- Speeds recovery time following physical exertion
- Speeds recovery following injury or disease
- Regulates and improves overall body functions
- Helps maintain independent living, especially in older adults
- Enhances quality of life: People feel better and live a healthier and happier life.

In addition to the benefits listed, **epidemiological** research studies linking physical activity habits and mortality rates have shown lower premature mortality rates in physically active people. Pioneer work in this area demonstrated that as the amount of weekly physical activity increased, the risk for cardiovascular death decreased.[9] In this study, conducted among 16,936 Harvard alumni, the greatest decrease in cardiovascular deaths was observed in those who burned more than 2,000 calories per week through physical activity.

Another major study subsequently upheld the findings of the Harvard alumni study.[10] Based on data from 13,344 individuals who were followed over an average of eight years, the results confirmed that the level of cardiorespiratory fitness is related to mortality from all causes. These findings showed a graded and consistent inverse relationship between physical fitness and mortality, regardless of age and other risk factors.

In essence, the higher the level of cardiorespiratory fitness, the longer the life (see Figure 1.7). The death rate from all causes for the low-fitness men was 3.4 times higher than for the high-fitness men. For the low-fitness women, the death rate was 4.6 times higher than for the high-fitness women. The

FIGURE 1.7

Death rates by physical fitness levels.

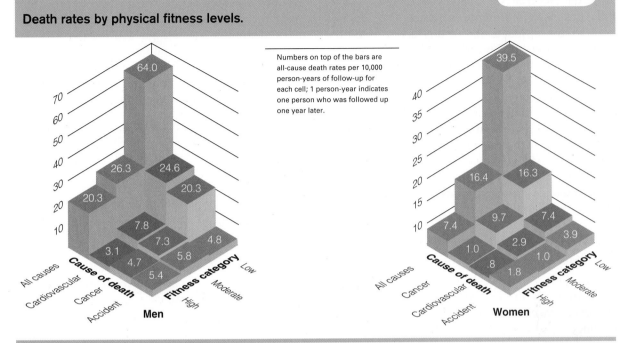

Numbers on top of the bars are all-cause death rates per 10,000 person-years of follow-up for each cell; 1 person-year indicates one person who was followed up one year later.

SOURCE: S. N. Blair et al., "Physical Fitness and All-Cause Mortality: A Prospective Study of Healthy Men and Women," *Journal of the American Medical Association* 262 (1989): 2395–2401.

study also reported a greatly reduced rate of premature deaths, even at moderate fitness levels, which most adults can achieve easily. People gain further protection when they combine higher fitness levels with reduction in other risk factors such as hypertension, elevated cholesterol, cigarette smoking, and excessive body fat.

Additional research that looked at changes in fitness and mortality found a substantial (44 percent) reduction in mortality risk when the study participants abandoned a sedentary lifestyle and became moderately fit.[11] The lowest death rate was found in people who were fit and remained fit, and the highest rate was found in men who remained unfit (see Figure 1.8).

Further research in this area substantiated the previous findings and also indicated that primarily vigorous activities are associated with greater longevity.[12] Vigorous activity was defined as activity that requires a *metabolic equivalent* (**MET**) level equal to

FIGURE 1.8

Effects of fitness changes on mortality rates.

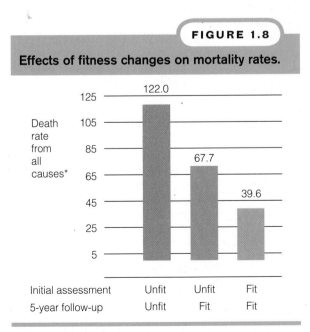

| Initial assessment | Unfit | Unfit | Fit |
| 5-year follow-up | Unfit | Fit | Fit |

SOURCE: S. N. Blair et al., "Changes in Physical Fitness and All-Cause Mortality: A Prospective Study of Healthy and Unhealthy Men," *JAMA* 273 (1995): 1193–1198.

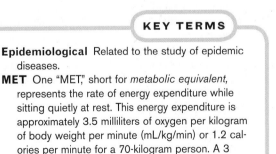

KEY TERMS

Epidemiological Related to the study of epidemic diseases.

MET One "MET," short for *metabolic equivalent*, represents the rate of energy expenditure while sitting quietly at rest. This energy expenditure is approximately 3.5 milliliters of oxygen per kilogram of body weight per minute (mL/kg/min) or 1.2 calories per minute for a 70-kilogram person. A 3 MET activity requires three times the energy expenditure of sitting quietly at rest.

or greater than 6 (see Chapter 4, Table 4.1, page 112). This level represents exercising at an energy level six times that of the resting energy requirement. Examples of vigorous activities used in the previous study include brisk walking; jogging; swimming laps; playing squash, racquetball, or tennis; and shoveling snow. Results also indicated that vigorous exercise is as important as maintaining recommended weight and not smoking.

The results of these studies indicate clearly that fitness improves wellness, quality of life, and longevity. If people are able, they should do vigorous exercise, because it is associated most closely with longer life.

National Health Objectives for the Year 2010

Every 10 years, the U.S. Department of Health and Human Services releases a list of objectives for preventing disease and promoting health. From its onset in 1980, this 10-year plan has helped instill a new sense of purpose and focus for public health and preventive medicine. These national health objec-

tives are intended as realistic goals to improve the health of all Americans in the first decade of the new millennium. Two unique goals of the 2010 objectives are that they emphasize increased quality and years of healthy life and that they seek to eliminate health disparities among all groups of people. The objectives address three important points:[13]

1. *Personal responsibility.* Individuals need to become ever more health-conscious. Responsible and informed behaviors are the key to good health.
2. *Health benefits for all people.* Lower socioeconomic conditions and poor health often are interrelated. Extending the benefits of good health to all people is crucial to the health of the nation.
3. *Health promotion and disease prevention.* A shift from treatment to preventive techniques will drastically cut health care costs and help all Americans achieve a better quality of life.

Development of these health objectives involves more than 10,000 people representing 300 national organizations, including the Institute of Medicine

---

FIGURE 1.9

Selected national health objectives for the year 2010.

1. Increase quality and years of healthy life.
2. Eliminate health disparities.
3. Improve the health, fitness, and quality of life of all Americans through the adoption and maintenance of regular, daily physical activity.
4. Promote health and reduce chronic disease risk, disease progression, debilitation, and premature death associated with dietary factors and nutritional status among all people in the United States.
5. Reduce disease, disability, and death related to tobacco use and exposure to secondhand smoke.
6. Increase the quality, availability, and effectiveness of educational and community-based programs designed to prevent disease and improve the health and quality of life of the American people.

7. Promote health for all people through a healthy environment.
8. Reduce the incidence and severity of injuries from unintentional causes, as well as violence and abuse.
9. Promote worker health and safety through prevention.
10. Improve access to comprehensive, high-quality health care.
11. Ensure that every pregnancy in the United States is intended.
12. Improve maternal and pregnancy outcomes and reduce rates of disability in infants.
13. Improve the quality of health-related decisions through effective communication.
14. Decrease the incidence of functional limitations due to arthritis, osteoporosis, and chronic back conditions.
15. Decrease cancer incidence, morbidity, and mortality.

16. Promote health and prevent secondary conditions among persons with disabilities.
17. Enhance the cardiovascular health and quality of life of all Americans through prevention and control of risk factors, and promotion of healthy lifestyle behaviors.
18. Prevent HIV transmission and associated morbidity and mortality.
19. Improve the mental health of all Americans.
20. Raise the public's awareness of the signs and symptoms of lung disease.
21. Increase awareness of healthy sexual relationships and prevent all forms of sexually transmitted diseases.
22. Reduce the incidence of substance abuse by all people, especially children.

SOURCE: U.S. Department of Health and Human Services.

of the National Academy of Sciences, all state health departments, and the federal Office of Disease Prevention and Health Promotion. A summary of key 2010 objectives is provided in Figure 1.9. Living according to the fitness and wellness principles provided in this book will enhance the quality of your life and allow you to be an active participant in achieving the Healthy People 2010 Objectives.

The Path to Fitness and Wellness

Current scientific data and the fitness movement that began more than three decades ago in the United States have led many people to see the benefits of participating in fitness programs that will improve and maintain health. Because fitness and wellness needs vary from one person to another, exercise and wellness prescriptions must be personalized for best results. This book provides the necessary guidelines for developing a lifetime program to improve fitness and promote preventive health care and personal wellness. As you study the book and complete the assignments in each chapter, you will learn to:

- Determine whether medical clearance is required for you to participate safely in exercise
- Assess your overall level of physical fitness, including cardiorespiratory endurance, muscular strength and endurance, muscular flexibility, and body composition
- Prescribe personal programs for total fitness development
- Learn behavior modification techniques that will allow you to change unhealthy lifestyle patterns
- Develop sound diet and weight-control programs
- Implement a healthy lifestyle program that includes prevention of cardiovascular diseases and cancer, management of stress, and cessation of smoking, if applicable
- Discern myths from facts pertaining to exercise and health-related concepts

Behavior Modification

Scientific evidence of the benefits derived from living a healthy lifestyle continues to mount each day. Although the data are impressive, most people still

---

BEHAVIOR MODIFICATION PLANNING

Healthy Lifestyle Habits

Research indicates that adherence to the following 12 lifestyle habits will significantly improve health and extend life:

1. Participate in a lifetime physical activity program.
2. Do not smoke cigarettes.
3. Eat right.
4. Avoid snacking.
5. Maintain recommended body weight through adequate nutrition and exercise.
6. Sleep 7 to 8 hours each night.
7. Lower your stress levels.
8. Drink alcohol moderately or not at all.
9. Surround yourself with healthy friendships.
10. Seek to live and work in a healthy environment.
11. Increase education.
12. Take personal safety measures to lessen the risk for avoidable accidents.

Try It

Look at the list above and indicate which habits are already part of your lifestyle. What changes could you make to incorporate additional healthy habits into your daily life?

---

don't adhere to a healthy lifestyle. To understand why this is so, one has to examine what motivates people and what actions are required to make permanent changes in behavior, called **behavior modification.**

Let's look at an all too common occurrence on college campuses. Most students understand that they should be exercising. They contemplate enrolling in a fitness course. The motivating factor might be enhanced physical appearance, health benefits, or simply fulfillment of a college requirement. They sign up for the course, participate for a few months, finish the course—and stop exercising! Various excuses are offered: too busy, no one to exercise with, already have the grade, inconvenient open-gym hours, job conflicts. A few months later, they realize once again that exercise is vital and repeat the cycle (see Figure 1.10).

The information in this book will be of little value to you if you are unable to abandon negative

---

KEY TERMS

Behavior modification The process used to permanently change negative behaviors in favor of positive behaviors that will lead to better health and well-being.

FIGURE 1.10

Exercise–exercise dropout cycle.

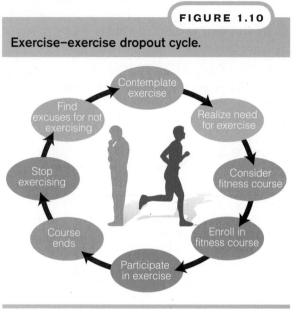

habits and adopt and maintain new, healthy behaviors. Before looking at the physical fitness and wellness guidelines, you will need to take a critical look at your behaviors and lifestyle—and most likely make some permanent changes to promote your overall health and wellness.

Changing Behavior

The very first step in addressing behavioral change is to recognize that indeed a problem exists. Five general categories of behaviors are addressed in the process of willful change:

1. Stopping a negative behavior
2. Preventing relapse of a negative behavior
3. Developing a positive behavior
4. Strengthening a positive behavior
5. Maintaining a positive behavior

Changing chronic, unhealthy behaviors to stable, healthy behaviors is often challenging. Change usually does not happen all at once but, rather, is a lengthy process with several stages.

The simplest model of change is the two-stage model of unhealthy behavior and healthy behavior. This model states that either you do it or you don't. Most people who use this model attempt self-change but end up asking themselves why they're unsuccessful: They just can't do it (for example, start and adhere to exercise or quit smoking). Their intention to change may be good, but to accomplish it they need knowledge about how

to achieve change. The following discussion may help.

To aid in this process, psychologists James Prochaska, John Norcross, and Carlo DiClemente developed a behavioral change model.[14] The model's five stages are important for understanding the process of willful change. The stages of change describe underlying processes that people go through to change most problem behaviors and adopt healthy ones. Most frequently, the model is used to change health-related behaviors such as physical inactivity, smoking, poor nutrition, inadequate weight control, stressfulness, and alcohol abuse. The five stages of change are precontemplation, contemplation, preparation, action, and maintenance. A sixth stage of change, termination/adoption, was subsequently added.

After years of study, researchers have found that applying specific behavior-change techniques during each stage of the model increases the rate of success for change. Understanding each stage of this model will help you determine where you are in relation to your personal healthy lifestyle behaviors. It also will help you identify techniques to make successful changes.

Precontemplation

People in the **precontemplation stage** are not considering or do not want to change a specific behavior. They typically deny having a problem and presently do not intend to change. These people are usually unaware or underaware of the problem. Other people around them, however, including family, friends, health care practitioners, and coworkers, identify the problem quite clearly.

Precontemplators do not care about the problem behavior and might even avoid information and materials that address the issue. They avoid free screenings and workshops that could help identify and change the problem, even if they receive financial incentives for attending. Frequently these people actively resist change and seem resigned to accept the unhealthy behavior as their "fate."

Precontemplators are the most difficult people to reach for behavioral change. They often think that change isn't even a possibility. Educating them about the problem behavior is critical to helping them start contemplating the process of change. It is said that knowledge is power, and the challenge is to find ways to help them realize that they will be ultimately responsible for the consequences of their behavior. Sometimes they initiate change only when under pressure from others.

Contemplation

In the **contemplation stage,** people acknowledge that they have a problem and begin to think seriously about overcoming it. Although they are not quite ready for change yet, they are weighing the pros and cons. People may remain in this stage for years, but in their minds they are planning to take some action within the next six months or so. Education and peer support are valuable during this stage.

Preparation

In the **preparation stage,** people are seriously considering and planning to change a behavior within the next month. They are taking initial steps for change and may even try it for a short while, such as stopping smoking for a day or exercising a few times during this month. In this stage, people define a general goal for behavior change (say, to quit smoking by the last day of the month) and write specific objectives to accomplish this goal (see the discussion on SMART goals, pages 19–20). Continued peer and environmental support are recommended during the preparation stage.

Action

The **action stage** requires the most commitment of time and energy by the individual. Here people are actively doing things to change or modify the problem behavior or to adopt a new healthy behavior. The action stage requires that the person follow the specific guidelines set forth for that behavior. An example is a person who has actually stopped smoking completely, is exercising aerobically three times per week according to exercise prescription guidelines (see Chapter 3), or is maintaining a healthy diet.

Relapse, in which the individual regresses to a previous stage, is common during the action stage. Once people maintain the action stage for six consecutive months, they move into the maintenance stage.

Maintenance

During the **maintenance stage,** the person continues to adhere to the behavior change for up to five years. The maintenance stage requires continually adhering to the specific guidelines that govern the target behavior (for example, complete smoking cessation, aerobic exercise three times per week, or proper stress management techniques). At this time, a person works to reinforce the gains made through the various stages of change and strives to prevent lapses and relapses.

Termination/Adoption

Once a person has maintained a behavior more than five years, he or she enters the **termination/ adoption stage** without fear of relapse. In the case of negative behaviors that have been terminated, this stage of change is referred to as termination. If the person has adopted a positive behavior for more than five years, this stage is designated the adoption stage. Many experts believe that after this period of time, any former addictions, problems, or lack of compliance with healthy behaviors no longer present an obstacle in the quest for wellness. The change has become a part of one's lifestyle. This phase is the ultimate goal for everyone who seeks a healthier lifestyle.

Use the form provided in Figure 1.11 to determine where you stand in respect to behaviors that you want to change or new ones that you wish to adopt. As you fill out this form, you will realize that you are at different stages for different behaviors. For instance, you may be in the termination stage for aerobic exercise and smoking, in the action stage for strength training, but only in the contemplation stage for a healthy diet. Realizing where you are with respect to different behaviors will help you design a better action plan for a healthy lifestyle.

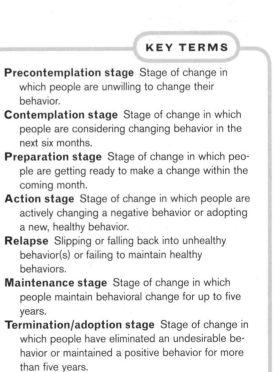

KEY TERMS

Precontemplation stage Stage of change in which people are unwilling to change their behavior.

Contemplation stage Stage of change in which people are considering changing behavior in the next six months.

Preparation stage Stage of change in which people are getting ready to make a change within the coming month.

Action stage Stage of change in which people are actively changing a negative behavior or adopting a new, healthy behavior.

Relapse Slipping or falling back into unhealthy behavior(s) or failing to maintain healthy behaviors.

Maintenance stage Stage of change in which people maintain behavioral change for up to five years.

Termination/adoption stage Stage of change in which people have eliminated an undesirable behavior or maintained a positive behavior for more than five years.

FIGURE 1.11

Identifying your current stage of change.

Please indicate which response most accurately describes your current _____
behavior (in the blank space identify the behavior: smoking, physical activity, stress, nutrition, weight control, etc.).
Next, select the statement below (select only one) that best represents your current behavior pattern. To select the
most appropriate statement, fill in the blank for one of the first three statements if your current behavior is a problem
behavior. (For example, you might say, "I currently smoke, and I do *not* intend to change in the foreseeable future,"
or "I currently *do not* exercise, but I am contemplating changing in the next 6 months.") If you have already started to
make changes, fill in the blank in one of the last three statements. (In this case, you might say: "I currently *eat a low-fat
diet* but I have done so only within the last 6 months," or "I currently *practice adequate stress management techniques*, and
I have done so for more than 6 months.") As you can see, you may use this form to identify your stage of change for
any type of health-related behavior.

1. I currently _____, and I do not intend to change in the foreseeable future.

2. I currently _____, but I am contemplating changing in the next 6 months.

3. I currently _____ regularly but intend to change in the next month.

4. I currently _____, but I have done so only within the last 6 months.

5. I currently _____, and I have done so for more than 6 months.

6. I currently _____, and I have done so for more than 5 years.

STAGES OF CHANGE

1 = Precontemplation	4 = Action
2 = Contemplation	5 = Maintenance
3 = Preparation	6 = Termination/Adoption

Using the form provided in Activity 1.1 at the end of the chapter, select two or three behaviors that you have targeted for the next three months. Developing new behavioral patterns takes time, and trying to work on too many components at once most likely will lower your chances for success. Start with components in which you think you will have a high chance for success.

CRITICAL THINKING

What factors do you think keep you from participating in a regular exercise program? • How about factors that keep you from managing your daily caloric intake?

Motivation and Locus of Control

Motivation often explains why some people succeed and others do not. Although motivation comes from within, external factors are what trigger the inner desire to accomplish a given task. These external factors, then, control behavior.

Understanding **locus of control** is helpful to the study of motivation. People who believe that they have control over events in their lives are said to have an *internal* locus of control. By contrast, people who believe that what happens to them is the result of chance or environmental factors and is unrelated to their behavior have an *external* locus of control. The latter group often have difficulty getting out of the precontemplation or contemplation stages.

People with an internal locus of control are apt to be healthier and have an easier time initiating and adhering to a wellness program than those who perceive that they have little control and think of themselves as powerless and vulnerable. The latter people also are at greater risk for illness. When illness does strike, restoring a sense of control is vital to regaining health.

Few people have either a completely external or a completely internal locus of control. They fall somewhere along a continuum. The more external the locus, the greater is the challenge in changing and adhering to exercise and other healthy lifestyle

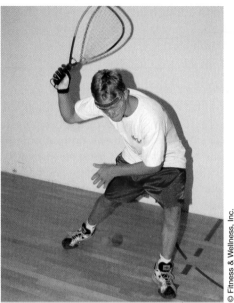

Many people refrain from physical activity because they lack the necessary skills to enjoy and reap the benefits of regular participation.

© Fitness & Wellness, Inc.

behaviors. Fortunately, a person can develop a more internal locus of control. Understanding that most events in life are not determined genetically or environmentally helps people pursue goals and gain control over their lives. Three impediments, however, can keep people from entering the preparation or action stages: problems of competence, of confidence, and of motivation.

1. *Problems of competence.* Lacking the skills to perform a given task leads to less competence. If your friends play basketball regularly but you don't know how to play, you might not be inclined to participate. The solution to this problem of competence is to master the skills you need for participation. Most people are not born with all-inclusive natural abilities, including those for playing sports. A college professor continuously watched a group of students play an entertaining game of basketball every Friday at noon. Having no basketball skills, he was reluctant to play (contemplation stage). Eventually, however, the desire to join in the fun was strong enough that he enrolled in a beginning course at the college so he would learn to play the game (preparation stage). To his surprise, most of the students were impressed that he was willing to do this. Now, with greater compe-

tence, he became able to join in on Friday's pick-up games (action stage).

Another alternative is to select an activity in which you are skilled. It may not be basketball, but it well could be aerobics. And don't be afraid to try new activities. Similarly, if your body weight is a problem, you could learn to cook low-calorie meals. Try different recipes until you find foods you like. Patty's story at the beginning of this chapter exemplifies a lack of competence. Patty was motivated and knew she could do it, but she lacked the skills to reach her goal. All along, Patty was fluctuating between the contemplation and action stages. Once she mastered the skills, she was able to achieve and maintain her goal.

2. *Problems of confidence.* Problems with confidence arise when you have the skills but don't believe you can get it done. Fear and feelings of inadequacy often interfere with the ability to perform the task. Don't talk yourself out of something until you have given it a fair try. If the skills are there, the sky is the limit. Initially, try to visualize yourself doing the task and getting it done. Repeat this several times, then actually give it a try. You will surprise yourself.

Sometimes, lack of confidence sets in when the task seems to be insurmountable. In these situations, dividing a goal into smaller, realistic objectives helps to accomplish the task. You may know how to swim, but the goal of swimming a continuous mile could take you several weeks to accomplish. Set up your training program so that you swim a little farther each day, until you are able to swim the entire mile. If you don't meet your objective on a given day, try it again, reevaluate, cut back a little, and, most important, don't give up.

3. *Problems of motivation.* With problems of motivation, both the competence and the confidence are there, but individuals are unwilling to change because the reasons for change are not important to them. For example, a person begins contemplating a smoking cessation program when the reasons for quitting outweigh

---

KEY TERMS

Motivation The desire and will to do something.
Locus of control The extent to which a person believes that he or she can influence the external environment.

the reasons for smoking. Lack of knowledge and lack of goals are the primary causes of unwillingness to change (precontemplators). Knowledge often determines goals, and goals determine motivation. How badly you want something dictates how hard you'll work at it. Many people are unaware of the magnitude of the benefits of a wellness program. When it comes to a healthy lifestyle, however, there may not be a second chance. A stroke, a heart attack, or cancer can have irreparable or fatal consequences. Greater understanding of what leads to disease may be all that is needed to initiate change.

Also, feeling physically fit is difficult to explain unless you have experienced it yourself. The benefits that Patty expressed with gratitude to her instructor—fitness, self-esteem, confidence, health, and quality of life—cannot be conveyed to someone who is constrained by sedentary living. In a way, wellness is like reaching the top of a mountain. The quiet, the clean air, the lush vegetation, the flowing water in the river, the wildlife, and the majestic valley below are difficult to explain to someone who has spent a lifetime within city limits.

Behavior Modification Principles

Over the course of many years, we all develop habits that we would like to change at some point. The adage "Old habits die hard" comes to mind. Acquiring positive behaviors that will lead to better health and well-being requires continual effort. When wellness is concerned, the sooner we implement a healthy lifestyle program, the greater are the health benefits and quality of life that lie ahead. Adopting the following behavior modification principles can help change behavior.

Self-Analysis

The first step in modifying behavior is a decisive desire to do so. If you have no interest in changing a behavior, you won't do it (precontemplator). A person who has no intention of quitting smoking will not quit, regardless of what anyone says or how strong the evidence is against it. As part of your self-analysis, you may want to prepare a list of reasons for continuing or discontinuing the behavior. When

the reasons for changing outweigh the reasons for not changing, you are ready for the next step (contemplation stage).

Behavior Analysis

Now you have to determine the frequency, circumstances, and consequences of the behavior to be altered or implemented. If the desired outcome is to consume less fat, you first must find out what foods in your diet are high in fat, when you eat them, and when you don't eat them (preparation stage). Knowing when you don't eat fatty foods points to circumstances under which you exert control of your diet and will help as you set goals.

Goal Setting

A **goal** motivates change in behavior. The stronger the goal, or desire, the more motivated you will be either to change unwanted behaviors or to implement new healthy behaviors. The final topic of this chapter, SMART goals, will help you write goals and prepare an action plan to achieve them. This will aid with behavior modification.

Social Support

Surrounding yourself with people who will work toward a common goal with you or will encourage you along the way will be helpful. Attempting to quit smoking, for instance, is easier when the person is around others who are trying to quit as well. The person also may get help from friends who have quit already. Peer support is a strong incentive for behavior change. During this process, people who will not be supportive should be avoided. Friends who have no desire to quit smoking may tempt the person to smoke and encourage relapse. People who achieved the same goal earlier might not be supportive either. For instance, someone might say, "I can do six consecutive miles." The response should be, "I'm proud that I can jog three consecutive miles."

Monitoring

During the action and maintenance stages, continuous behavior monitoring increases awareness of the desired outcome. Sometimes this principle in itself is sufficient to cause change. For example, keeping track of daily food intake reveals sources of calories and fat in the diet. This can help a person cut down gradually or completely eliminate some high-fat foods before consuming them. If the goal is to increase daily intake of fruits and vegetables, keeping track of the number of servings eaten each day raises awareness and may help increase their intake.

A Positive Outlook

Having a positive outlook means taking an optimistic approach from the beginning and believing in yourself. Following the guidelines in this chapter will help you pace yourself so you can work toward change. Also, you may become motivated by looking at the outcomes—how much healthier you will be, how much better you will look, or how much farther you can jog.

Reinforcement

People tend to repeat behaviors that are rewarded and disregard those that are not rewarded or are punished. If you have successfully cut down your fat intake during the week, reward yourself by going to a show or buying a new pair of shoes. Do not reinforce yourself with destructive behaviors such as eating a high-fat dinner. If you fail to change a desired behavior (or to implement a new one), you

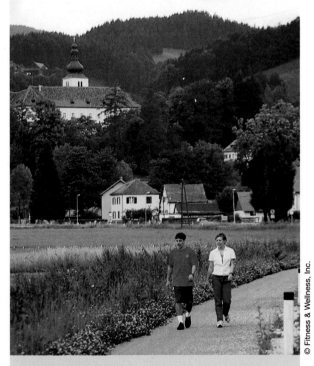

Social support enhances regular participation and the process of behavior modification.

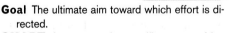

© Fitness & Wellness, Inc.

may want to put off buying those new shoes. When a positive behavior becomes habitual, give yourself an even better reward. Treat yourself to a weekend away from home, buy a new bike, or get that tennis racket you always wanted.

SMART Goals

Only a well-conceived action plan will help you attain goals. Determining what you want to accomplish is the starting point, but to reach your goal you need to write **SMART** goals. The SMART acronym means that goals are *s*pecific, *m*easurable, *a*cceptable, *r*ealistic, and *t*imely.

1. *Specific.* When writing goals, state exactly and in a positive manner what you would like to accomplish. For example, if you are overweight at 150 pounds and at 27 percent body fat, simply stating, "I will lose weight" is not a specific goal. Instead, rewrite your goal to state, "I will reduce my body fat to 20 percent body fat (137 pounds) in 12 weeks."

   Be sure to write down your goals. An unwritten goal is simply a wish. A written goal, in essence, becomes a contract with yourself. Show this goal to a friend or an instructor and have him or her witness the contract you made with yourself by signing alongside your signature.

   Once you have identified and written down a specific goal, write the specific **objectives** required to reach that goal. These objectives are the necessary steps along the way. For example, a goal might be to achieve recommended body weight. Several specific objectives could be to:

   a. Lose an average of 1 pound (or 1 fat percentage point) per week
   b. Monitor body weight before breakfast every morning
   c. Assess body composition every three weeks
   d. Limit fat intake to less than 25 percent of total daily caloric intake

> ### KEY TERMS
>
> **Goal** The ultimate aim toward which effort is directed.
> **SMART** An acronym for *s*pecific, *m*easurable, *a*cceptable, *r*ealistic, and *t*imely.
> **Objectives** Steps required to reach a goal.

e. Eliminate all pastries from the diet during this time

f. Walk/jog in the proper target zone for 60 minutes, six times per week

2. *Measurable.* Whenever possible, goals and objectives should be measurable. For example, "I will lose weight" is not measurable, but "I will reduce body fat to 20 percent" is measurable. Also note that all of the sample specific objectives (a.) through (f.) in item 1 above are measurable. For instance, you can figure out easily whether you are losing a pound or a percentage point per week; you can conduct a nutrient analysis to assess your average fat intake; or you can monitor your weekly exercise sessions to make sure you are meeting this specific objective.

3. *Acceptable.* Goals that you set for yourself are more motivational than goals that someone else sets for you. These goals will motivate and challenge you and should be consistent with other goals you have. As you set an acceptable goal, ask yourself: Do I have the time, commitment, and necessary skills to accomplish it? If not, you need to restate your goal so that it is acceptable to you.

In instances where successful completion of a goal involves others, such as an athletic team or an organization, an acceptable goal must be compatible with those of the other people involved. If a team's practice schedule is Monday through Friday from 4:00 to 6:00 p.m., it is unacceptable for you to train only three times per week or at a different time of the day.

Acceptable goals are embraced with positive thoughts. Visualize and believe in your success. As difficult as some tasks may seem, where there's a will, there's a way. A plan of action, prepared according to the guidelines in this chapter, will help you achieve your goals.

4. *Realistic.* Goals should be within reach. If you currently weigh 190 pounds and your target weight (at 20 percent body fat) is 140 pounds, setting a goal to lose 50 pounds in a month would be unsound, if not impossible. Such a goal does not allow for the implementation of adequate behavior modification techniques or ensure weight maintenance at the target weight. Unattainable goals only set you up for failure, discouragement, and loss of interest. On the other hand, do not write goals that are too easy to achieve and do not challenge you. If a goal is too easy, you may lose interest and stop working toward it.

At times, problems arise even with realistic goals. Try to anticipate potential difficulties as much as possible, and plan for ways to deal with them. If your goal is to jog for 30 minutes on six consecutive days, what are the alternatives if the weather turns bad? Possible solutions are to jog in the rain; find an indoor track; jog at a different time of day, when the weather is better; or participate in a different aerobic activity, such as stationary cycling, swimming, or step aerobics.

Monitoring your progress as you move toward a goal also reinforces behavior. Keep an exercise log, or do a body composition assessment periodically, which enables you to determine your progress at any given time.

5. *Timely.* A goal should always have a specific date set for completion. The above example to reach 20 percent body fat in 12 weeks demonstrates timeliness. The chosen date should be realistic but not too distant in the future. Allow yourself enough time to achieve the goal, but not too much time, as this could affect your performance. With a deadline, a task is much easier to work toward.

Goal Evaluation

In addition to the SMART guidelines provided above, you should conduct periodic evaluations of your goals. Reevaluations are vital for success. You may find that after you have fully committed and put all your effort into a goal, that goal may be unreachable. If so, reassess the goal.

Recognize that you will face obstacles and that you will not always meet your goals. Use your setbacks to learn from them. Rewrite your goal and create a plan that will help you get around self-defeating behaviors in the future. Once you achieve a goal, set a new one to improve upon it or maintain what you have achieved. Goals keep you motivated.

In addition to previously discussed guidelines, throughout this book you will find information on behavioral change. For example, Chapter 3 includes the Exercise Readiness Questionnaire, tips to start and adhere to an exercise program, and how to set your fitness goals; Chapter 4 offers tips to enhance your aerobic workout; Chapter 6 gives suggestions on how to adhere to a lifetime weight management program; Chapter 7 sets forth stress management techniques; and Chapter 8 outlines a six-step smoking cessation plan.

A Word of Caution Before You Start Exercise

Even though exercise testing and participation is relatively safe for most apparently healthy men and women under ages 45 and 55, respectively, a small but real risk exists for exercise-induced abnormalities in people with a history of cardiovascular problems and those who are at higher risk for disease.[15] These people should be screened before initiating or increasing the intensity of an exercise program.

Before you start an exercise program or participate in any exercise testing, you should fill out the Clearance for Exercise Participation questionnaire provided in Activity 1.2. A "yes" answer to any of these questions may signal the need for a physician's approval before you participate. If you don't have any "yes" responses, you may proceed to Chapter 2 to assess your current level of fitness.

---

www WEB INTERACTIVE

LifeScan will help you learn more about the health risks you might be taking each day. Take the health questionnaire to determine your personal lifestyle risks. Your score pertains to general results, nutrition results, and height/weight results. Your ranking among the top ten causes of death is provided, as well as suggestions on how to improve. **http://wellness.uwsp.edu/other/lifescan/**

ASSESS YOUR BEHAVIOR

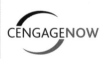

*Log on to **academic.cengage.com/login** and take a wellness inventory to assess the behaviors that might benefit most from healthy change.*

1. Are you aware of lifestyle factors that may negatively impact your health?

2. Do you accumulate at least 30 minutes of moderate-intensity physical activity five days per week?

3. Do you make a constant and deliberate effort to stay healthy and achieve the highest potential for well-being?

ASSESS YOUR KNOWLEDGE

CENGAGENOW *Log on to **academic.cengage.com/login** to assess your understanding of this chapter's topics by taking the chapter pre-test and exploring the modules recommended in your Personalized Study Plan.*

1. Bodily movement produced by skeletal muscles is called
   a. physical activity.
   b. kinesiology.
   c. exercise.
   d. aerobic exercise.
   e. muscle strength.

2. Most people in the United States
   a. get adequate physical activity on a regular basis.
   b. meet health-related fitness standards.
   c. regularly participate in skill-related activities.
   d. Choices a, b, and c are correct.
   e. None of the above choices is correct.

3. The leading cause of death in the United States is
   a. cancer.
   b. accident.
   c. chronic lower respiratory disease.
   d. disease of the cardiovascular system.
   e. drug-related illness.

CONTINUED

4. The constant and deliberate effort to stay healthy and achieve the highest potential for well-being is defined as
   a. health.
   b. physical fitness.
   c. wellness.
   d. health-related fitness.
   e. metabolic fitness.

5. Which of the following is *not* a component of health-related fitness?
   a. Cardiorespiratory endurance
   b. Body composition
   c. Agility
   d. Muscular strength and endurance
   e. Muscular flexibility

6. Research on the effects of fitness on mortality indicates that the largest drop in premature mortality is seen between the
   a. average and excellent fitness groups.
   b. least fit and moderately fit groups.
   c. good and high fitness groups.
   d. moderately fit and good fitness groups.
   e. The drop is similar between all fitness groups.

7. What is the greatest benefit of being physically fit?
   a. Absence of disease
   b. Higher quality of life
   c. Improved sports performance
   d. Better personal appearance
   e. Maintenance of ideal body weight

8. Which of the following is a stage in the behavioral modification model?
   a. Recognition
   b. Motivation
   c. Relapse
   d. Preparation
   e. Goal setting

9. A precontemplator is a person who
   a. has no desire to change a behavior.
   b. is looking to make a change in the next six months.
   c. is preparing for change in the next 30 days.
   d. willingly adopts healthy behaviors.
   e. is talking to a therapist to overcome a problem behavior.

10. A SMART goal is effective when it is
    a. realistic.
    b. measurable.
    c. specific.
    d. acceptable.
    e. All are correct choices.

Correct answers can be found at the back of the book.

Clearance for Exercise Participation

Name _____   Date _____

Course _____   Section _____

I. Health History

Even though participation in exercise is relatively safe for most apparently healthy individuals, the reaction of the cardiovascular system to increased levels of physical activity cannot always be totally predicted. Consequently, there is a small but real risk of certain changes occurring during exercise partici- pation. These changes include abnormal blood pressure, irregular heart rhythm, fainting, and in rare instances a heart attack or cardiac arrest. Therefore, you must provide honest answers to this questionnaire.

Have you ever had or do you now have any of the following conditions?

☐ Yes ☐ No   1. Cardiovascular disease (any type of heart or blood vessel disease, including strokes)

☐ Yes ☐ No   2. Elevated blood lipids (cholesterol and triglycerides)

☐ Yes ☐ No   3. Chest pain at rest or during exertion

☐ Yes ☐ No   4. Shortness of breath or other respiratory problems

☐ Yes ☐ No   5. Uneven, irregular, or skipped heartbeats (including a racing or fluttering heart)

☐ Yes ☐ No   6. Elevated blood pressure

☐ Yes ☐ No   7. Often feel faint or have spells of severe dizziness

☐ Yes ☐ No   8. Obesity (BMI of 30 or above)

☐ Yes ☐ No   9. Diabetes

☐ Yes ☐ No   10. Any joint, bone, or muscle problems (e.g., arthritis, low back pain, rheumatism)

☐ Yes ☐ No   11. An eating disorder (anorexia nervosa, bulimia, binge-eating)

☐ Yes ☐ No   12. Any other concern regarding your ability to participate safely in an exercise program? If so, explain:

Indicate if any of the following two conditions apply:

☐ Yes ☐ No   13. Do you smoke cigarettes?

☐ Yes ☐ No   14. Men—Are you age 45 or older?

☐ Yes ☐ No   15. Women—Are you age 55 or older?

Exercise may not be recommended under some of the conditions listed above; others may simply indicate special consideration. If any of the conditions apply, you should consult your physician before participating in an exercise program. You also should promptly report to your instructor any exercise-related abnormalities you experienced during the course of the semester.

Student's Signature: _____   Date: _____

II. Do you feel that it is safe for you to proceed with an exercise program? Explain any concerns or limitations that you may have regarding your safe participation in a comprehensive exercise program to improve cardiorespiratory endurance, muscular strength and endurance, and muscular flexibility.

_____

_____

_____

_____

_____

_____

_____

_____

_____

_____

III. In a few words, describe your previous experiences with sports participation, whether you have taken part in a structured exercise program, and express your own feelings about exercise participation.

_____

_____

_____

_____

_____

_____

_____

_____

_____

_____

Assessment of Physical Fitness

© Fitness & Wellness, Inc.

OBJECTIVES

- Identify the health-related components of physical fitness
- Be able to assess cardiorespiratory fitness
- Understand the difference between muscular strength and muscular endurance
- Learn to assess muscular-strength fitness
- Be able to assess muscular flexibility

- Understand the components of body composition
- Be able to assess body composition
- Learn to determine recommended body weight
- Learn to assess disease risk based on body mass index (BMI) and waist circumference

CENGAGENOW Log on to **CengageNOW at academic .cengage.com/login** to find innovative study tools—including pre- and post-tests, personalized study plans, activities, labs, and the personal change planner.

The health-related components of physical fitness—cardiorespiratory endurance, muscular strength and endurance, muscular flexibility, and body composition—are the topics of this chapter, along with basic techniques frequently used to assess these components. Through these assessment techniques you will be able to determine your level of physical fitness regularly as you engage in an exercise program. Fitness testing in a comprehensive program is important to:

1. Educate yourself regarding the various fitness components
2. Assess your fitness level for each health-related fitness component and compare the results with health fitness and physical fitness standards
3. Identify areas of weakness for training emphasis
4. Motivate you to participate in exercise
5. Use as a starting point for your personalized exercise prescriptions
6. Evaluate the progress and effectiveness of your program
7. Make adjustments in your exercise prescription, if necessary
8. Reward yourself for complying with your exercise program (a change to a higher fitness level is a reward in and of itself)

You are encouraged to conduct at least pre– and post–exercise program fitness tests. A personal fitness profile is provided in Activity 2.1, page 57, for you to record the results of each fitness test in this chapter (pre-test). At the end of the term, you can use the back of Activity 2.1, page 58, to record the results of your post-test. You also may choose to use the computer software available with this textbook.

In Chapter 3 you will learn to write personal fitness goals for this course (see Activity 3.4, pages 95–98). You should base these goals on the actual results of your initial fitness assessments. As you proceed with your exercise program, you should allow a minimum of eight weeks before doing your post-fitness assessments.

As discussed in Chapter 1, exercise testing or exercise participation is not advised for individuals with certain medical or physical conditions. Therefore, before starting an exercise program or participating in any exercise testing, you should fill out the Clearance for Exercise Participation questionnaire given in Chapter 1, Activity 1.2, page 25. A "yes" answer to any of the questions suggests that you consult a physician before initiating, continuing, or increasing your level of physical activity.

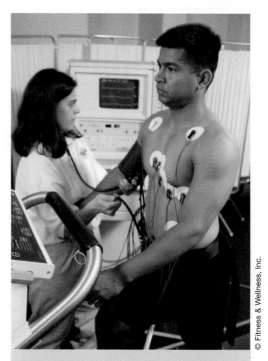

© Fitness & Wellness, Inc.

An exercise tolerance test with 12-lead electrocardiographic monitoring (stress ECG) may be required of some individuals prior to participation in exercise.

Responders Versus Nonresponders

Individuals who follow similar training programs show a wide variation in physiological responses. Heredity plays a crucial role in how each person responds to and improves after beginning an exercise program. Several studies have documented that following exercise training, most individuals, called **responders,** readily show improvements, but a few, **nonresponders,** exhibit small or no improvements at all. This concept is referred to as the **principle of individuality.**

After several months of aerobic training, increases in **maximal oxygen uptake (VO_{2max})** are between 15 and 20 percent, on the average, although individual responses can range from 0 (in a few selected cases) to more than 50 percent improvement, even when all participants follow exactly the same training program. Nonfitness and low-fitness participants, however, should not label themselves as nonresponders based on the previous discussion. Nonresponders constitute less than 5 percent of exercise participants. Although additional research is necessary, lack of improve-

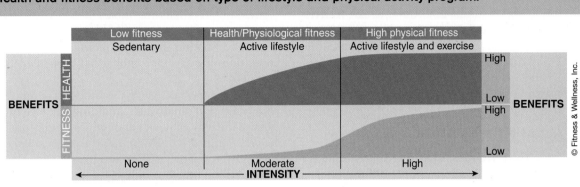

© Fitness & Wellness, Inc.

FIGURE 2.1

Health and fitness benefits based on type of lifestyle and physical activity program.

ment in cardiorespiratory endurance among nonresponders might be related to low levels of leg strength. A lower-body strength-training program has been shown to help these individuals improve VO_{2max} through aerobic exercise.[1]

Following assessment of cardiorespiratory fitness, if your fitness level is less than adequate, do not let that discourage you, but make it a priority to be physically active every day. In addition to regular exercise, lifestyle behaviors such as walking, taking stairs, cycling to work, parking farther from the office, doing household tasks, gardening, and doing yardwork provide substantial benefits. In this regard, monitoring of daily physical activity and exercise habits should be used in conjunction with fitness testing to evaluate compliance among nonresponders. After all, it is through increased daily activity that we reap the health benefits that improve quality of life.

Fitness Assessment Battery

No single test can provide a complete measure of physical fitness. Because health-related fitness has four components, a battery of tests is necessary to determine an individual's overall level of fitness. In the next few pages are descriptions of several tests used to assess the health-related fitness components. When interpreting the results of fitness tests, two standards can be applied: health fitness and physical fitness.

Health Fitness Standard

As illustrated in Figure 2.1, although improvements in fitness (VO_{2max}—see discussion of cardiorespiratory endurance on the next page) with a moderate

aerobic activity program are not as notable, significant health benefits are reaped with such a program. Health benefits include a reduction in blood lipids and blood pressure, weight loss, stress release, and lower risks for type 2 diabetes, cardiovascular disease, certain cancers, and premature mortality.

More specifically, improvements in the **metabolic profile** (better insulin sensitivity, glucose tolerance, and cholesterol levels) can be notable in spite of little or no improvement in aerobic capacity or weight loss. These improvements in the metabolic profile through an active lifestyle and moderate physical activity are referred to as **metabolic fitness.**

KEY TERMS

Responders Individuals who exhibit improvements in fitness as a result of exercise training.

Nonresponders Individuals who exhibit small or no improvements in fitness as compared with others who undergo the same training program.

Principle of individuality Training concept stating that genetics plays a major role in individual responses to exercise training and that these differences must be considered when designing exercise programs for different people.

Maximal oxygen uptake (VO_{2max}) Maximum amount of oxygen the human body is able to utilize per minute of physical activity.

Metabolic profile Result of the assessment of diabetes and cardiovascular disease risk through plasma insulin, glucose, lipid, and lipoprotein levels.

Metabolic fitness Denotes improvements in the metabolic profile through a moderate-intensity exercise program in spite of little or no improvement in health-related fitness.

The health fitness or criterion-referenced standards used in this book are based on epidemiological data linking minimum fitness values to disease prevention and better health. Attaining the **health fitness standards** requires only moderate amounts of physical activity. For example, a 2-mile walk in less than 30 minutes, five to six times per week, seems to be sufficient to achieve the health fitness standard for cardiorespiratory endurance.

Physical Fitness Standard

The **physical fitness standard** is set higher than the health fitness standard and requires a more vigorous exercise program. Whenever possible, participating in a vigorous exercise program is preferable because it provides even greater health and fitness benefits.[2] Such a program is recommended for individuals who wish to further improve personal fitness, reduce the risk for chronic disease and disabilities, and prevent premature mortality or unhealthy weight gain.

By participating in vigorous exercise, physically fit people of all ages have the freedom to enjoy most of life's daily and recreational activities to their fullest potential. The current health fitness standards are not enough to achieve this goal.

Sound physical fitness gives the individual a level of independence throughout life that many people no longer enjoy. Most older people should be able to carry out activities similar to those they conducted in their youth, though not with the same intensity. Although a person does not have to be an elite athlete, activities such as changing a tire, chopping wood, climbing several flights of stairs, playing a game of basketball, mountain biking, playing soccer with grandchildren, walking several miles around a lake, and hiking through a national park require more than the "average fitness" level of the American people.

If the main objective of the fitness program is to lower the risk for disease, attaining the health fitness standards may be enough to ensure better health. But if the individual wants to participate in moderate to vigorous fitness activities, achieving a high physical fitness standard is recommended. For the purposes of this book, both health fitness and physical fitness standards are given for each fitness test. You will have to decide your personal objectives for the fitness program.

Cardiorespiratory Endurance

Cardiorespiratory endurance is the single most important component of health-related physical fitness. The exception occurs among older adults, for whom muscular strength is particularly important. As a person breathes, part of the oxygen in the air is taken up in the lungs and transported in the blood to the heart. The heart then pumps the oxygenated blood through the circulatory system to all organs and tissues of the body. At the cellular level, oxygen is used to convert food substrates, primarily carbo-

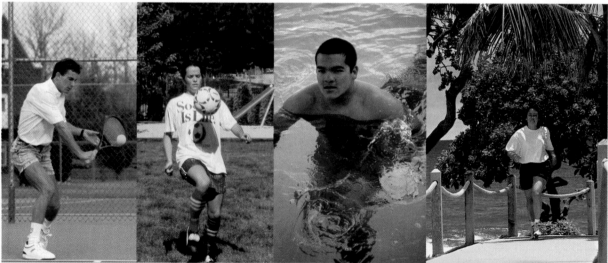

Aerobic activities promote cardiorespiratory development and help decrease the risk for chronic diseases.

Photos © Fitness & Wellness, Inc.

hydrates and fats, into the energy necessary to conduct body functions, maintain a constant internal equilibrium, and perform physical tasks.

Some examples of activities that promote **cardiorespiratory endurance,** or aerobic fitness, are brisk walking, jogging, cycling, rowing, swimming, cross-country skiing, aerobics, soccer, basketball, and racquetball. Guidelines to develop a lifetime cardiorespiratory endurance exercise program are given in Chapter 3, and an introduction and description of benefits of leading aerobic activities are given in Chapter 4.

A sound cardiorespiratory endurance program contributes greatly to good health. The typical American is not exactly a good role model in terms of cardiorespiratory fitness. A poorly conditioned heart that has to pump more often just to keep a person alive is subject to more wear and tear than is a well-conditioned heart. In situations that place strenuous demands on the heart, such as doing yardwork, lifting heavy objects or weights, or running to catch a bus, the unconditioned heart may not be able to sustain the strain.

Everyone who initiates a cardiorespiratory exercise program can expect a number of benefits from training. Among these are decreases in resting heart rate, blood pressure, blood lipids (cholesterol and triglycerides), recovery time following exercise, and risk for hypokinetic diseases (those associated with physical inactivity and sedentary living). Simultaneously, cardiac muscle strength and oxygen-carrying capacity increase.

Cardiorespiratory endurance is determined by VO_{2max}, the maximum amount of oxygen the human body is able to utilize per minute of physical activity. This value can be expressed in liters per minute (L/min) or milliliters per kilogram (2.2 pounds) of body weight per minute (mL/kg/min). The relative value in mL/kg/min is used most often because it considers total body mass (weight) in kilograms. When comparing two individuals with the same absolute value, the one with the lesser body mass will have a higher relative value, indicating that more oxygen is available to each kilogram (2.2 pounds) of

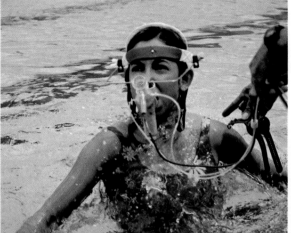

© Fitness & Wellness, Inc.

Maximal oxygen uptake (VO_{2max}) can be determined through direct gas analysis, as shown during a water aerobics exercise test.

body weight. Because all tissues and organs of the body need oxygen to function, higher oxygen consumption indicates a more efficient cardiorespiratory system.

Physical exertion requires more energy to perform the activity. As a result, the heart, lungs, and blood vessels have to deliver more oxygen to the cells to supply the required energy. During prolonged exercise, an individual with a high level of cardiorespiratory endurance is able to deliver the required amount of oxygen to the tissues with relative ease. The cardiorespiratory system of a person with a low level of endurance has to work much harder, as the heart has to pump more often to supply the same amount of oxygen to the tissues, and consequently fatigues faster. Hence, a higher capac-

---

CRITICAL THINKING

While your absolute maximal oxygen uptake remains unchanged, your relative maximal oxygen uptake can increase without engaging in an aerobic exercise program. • How can you accomplish this, and would you benefit from doing so?

KEY TERMS

Health fitness standard The lowest fitness requirements for maintaining good health, decreasing the risk for chronic diseases, and lowering the incidence of musculoskeletal injuries.

Physical fitness standard Required criteria to achieve a high level of physical fitness; ability to do moderate to vigorous physical activity without undue fatigue.

Cardiorespiratory endurance Ability of the lungs, heart, and blood vessels to deliver adequate amounts of oxygen to the cells to meet the demands of prolonged physical activity.

ity to deliver and utilize oxygen (oxygen uptake) indicates a more efficient cardiorespiratory system.

Oxygen uptake, expressed in L/min, is valuable in determining the caloric expenditure of physical activity. The human body burns about 5 calories for each liter of oxygen consumed, and oxygen uptake ranges from about .3 to .5 L/min during resting conditions to about 3 L/min during maximal exercise for moderately fit individuals and over 5 L/min in highly conditioned athletes. During aerobic exercise, the average person trains at between 50 and 75 percent of VO_{2max}. Thus, we burn between 1.5 to 2.5 calories/min at rest to a range of 7 to 12 calories/min during vigorous-intensity aerobic exercise.

Let's use a practical illustration. A person with a VO_{2max} of 3.5 L/min who trains at 60 percent of maximum uses 2.1 (3.5 × .60) liters of oxygen per minute of physical activity. This indicates that 10.5 calories are burned during each minute of exercise (2.1 × 5). If the activity is carried out for 30 minutes, 315 calories (10.5 × .30) have been burned. Because a pound of body fat represents 3,500 calories, the previous example indicates that this individual would have to exercise for a total of 333 minutes (3,500 ÷ 10.5) to burn the equivalent of a pound of body fat. At 30 minutes per exercise session, approximately 11 sessions would be required to expend the 3,500 calories.

Assessing Cardiorespiratory Endurance

Even though most cardiorespiratory endurance tests probably are safe to administer to apparently healthy individuals (those with no major heart disease risk factors or symptoms), the American College of Sports Medicine recommends that a physician be present for all maximal exercise tests on apparently healthy men over age 45 and women over age 55.[3]

A maximal test is any test that requires the participant's all-out or nearly all-out effort, such as the 1.5-Mile Run Test or a maximal exercise treadmill test (stress electrocardiogram). For submaximal exercise tests (such as a walking test), a physician should be present when testing higher-risk and symptomatic individuals and people with medical conditions, regardless of age.

1.5-Mile Run Test

The test used most often to determine cardiorespiratory endurance is the 1.5-Mile Run Test. The fitness category is determined according to the time a person takes to run or walk a 1.5-mile course. The

only equipment necessary to conduct this test is a stopwatch and a track or a premeasured 1.5-mile course.

Although the 1.5-Mile Run Test is quite simple to administer, a note of caution is in order: As the objective is to cover the distance in the shortest time, it is considered a maximal exercise test. The 1.5-Mile Run Test should be limited to conditioned individuals who have been cleared for exercise. It is not recommended for unconditioned beginners, symptomatic individuals, those with known cardiovascular disease or risk factors for heart disease, or men over age 45 and women over age 55. Unconditioned beginners are encouraged to have at least six weeks of aerobic training before they take the test.

TABLE 2.1

Estimated Maximal Oxygen Uptake (in mL/kg/min) for 1.5-Mile Run Test

Time	VO_{2max}	Time	VO_{2max}	Time	VO_{2max}
6:10	80.0	10:30	48.6	14:50	34.0
6:20	79.0	10:40	48.0	15:00	33.6
6:30	77.9	10:50	47.4	15:10	33.1
6:40	76.7	11:00	46.6	15:20	32.7
6:50	75.5	11:10	45.8	15:30	32.2
7:00	74.0	11:20	45.1	15:40	31.8
7:10	72.6	11:30	44.4	15:50	31.4
7:20	71.3	11:40	43.7	16:00	30.9
7:30	69.9	11:50	43.2	16:10	30.5
7:40	68.3	12:00	42.0	16:20	30.2
7:50	66.8	12:10	41.7	16:30	29.8
8:00	65.2	12:20	41.0	16:40	29.5
8:10	63.9	12:30	40.4	16:50	29.1
8:20	62.5	12:40	39.8	17:00	28.9
8:30	61.2	12:50	39.2	17:10	28.5
8:40	60.2	13:00	38.6	17:20	28.3
8:50	59.1	13:10	38.1	17:30	28.0
9:00	58.1	13:20	37.8	17:40	27.7
9:10	56.9	13:30	37.2	17:50	27.4
9:20	55.9	13:40	36.8	18:00	27.1
9:30	54.7	13:50	36.3	18:10	26.8
9:40	53.5	14:00	35.9	18:20	26.6
9:50	52.3	14:10	35.5	18:30	26.3
10:00	51.1	14:20	35.1	18:40	26.0
10:10	50.4	14:30	34.7	18:50	25.7
10:20	49.5	14:40	34.3	19:00	25.4

Adapted from "A Means of Assessing Maximal Oxygen Intake," by K. H. Cooper, *Journal of the American Medical Association*, 203 (1968), 201–204; *Health and Fitness Through Physical Activity*, by M. L. Pollock (New York: John Wiley and Sons, 1978); and *Training for Sport Activity*, by J. H. Wilmore (Boston: Allyn & Bacon, 1982).

Prior to taking the 1.5-Mile Run Test, you should do a few warm-up exercises—some stretching, walking, and slow jogging. Next, time yourself during the 1.5-mile run to see how fast you cover the distance. If you notice any unusual symptoms during the test, do not continue. Stop immediately and see your physician, or retake the test after another six weeks of aerobic training. At the end of the test, cool down by walking or jogging slowly for another three to five minutes. Referring to your performance time, look up your estimated VO_{2max} in Table 2.1 and the corresponding fitness category in Table 2.2.

For example, a 20-year-old female runs the 1.5-mile course in 12 minutes and 40 seconds. Table 2.1 shows a VO_{2max} of 39.8 mL/kg/min for a time of 12:40. According to Table 2.2, this VO_{2max} places her in the "good" cardiorespiratory fitness category.

1.0-Mile Walk Test*

The 1.0-Mile Walk Test calls for a 440-yard track (four laps to a mile) or a premeasured 1.0-mile course. Body weight in pounds must be determined prior to the walk. A stopwatch is required to measure total walking time and exercise heart rate.

You can proceed to walk the 1-mile course at a brisk pace, so that the exercise heart rate at the end

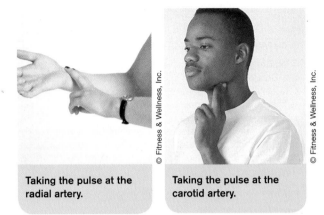

Taking the pulse at the radial artery.

Taking the pulse at the carotid artery.

© Fitness & Wellness, Inc.

of the test is above 120 beats per minute (bpm). At the end of the 1.0-mile walk, check your walking time and immediately count your pulse for 10 seconds. You can take your pulse on the wrist by placing two fingers over the radial artery (inside of the wrist on the side of the thumb) or over the carotid artery in the neck just below the jaw next to the voice box.

Next, multiply the 10-second pulse count by 6 to obtain the exercise heart rate in bpm. Now convert the walking time from minutes and seconds to minute units. Each minute has 60 seconds, so the seconds are divided by 60 to obtain the fraction of a minute. For instance, a walking time of 12 minutes and 15 seconds equals 12 + (15 ÷ 60), or 12.25 minutes. To obtain the estimated VO_{2max} in mL/kg/min

---

*Source: "Validation of the Rockport Fitness Walking Test in College Males and Females," by F. A. Dolgener, L. D. Hensley, J. J. Marsh, and J. K. Fjelstul, *Research Quarterly for Exercise and Sport* 65 (1994): 152–158.

TABLE 2.2

Cardiorespiratory Fitness Categories According to Maximal Oxygen Uptake (in mL/kg/min)

				Fitness Category		
Gender	Age	Poor	Fair	Average	Good	Excellent
Men	≤29	≤24.9	25–33.9	34–43.9	44–52.9	≥53
	30–39	≤22.9	23–30.9	31–41.9	42–49.9	≥50
	40–49	≤19.9	20–26.9	27–38.9	39–44.9	≥45
	50–59	≤17.9	18–24.9	25–37.9	38–42.9	≥43
	60–69	≤15.9	16–22.9	23–35.9	36–40.9	≥41
Women	≤29	≤23.9	24–30.9	31–38.9	39–48.9	≥49
	30–39	≤19.9	20–27.9	28–36.9	37–44.9	≥45
	40–49	≤16.9	17–24.9	25–34.9	35–41.9	≥42
	50–59	≤14.9	15–21.9	22–33.9	34–39.9	≥40
	60–69	≤12.9	13–20.9	21–32.9	33–36.9	≥37

High physical fitness standard

Health fitness or criterion-referenced standard

Tips to Increase Daily Physical Activity

Adults need recess, too! There are 1,440 minutes in every day. Schedule a minimum of 30 of these minutes for physical activity. With a little creativity and planning, even the person with the busiest schedule can make room for physical activity. For many folks, before or after work or meals is often an available time to cycle, walk, or play. Think about your weekly or daily schedule and look for or make opportunities to be more active. Every little bit helps. Consider the following suggestions:

- Walk, cycle, jog, skate, etc., to school, work, the store, or place of worship.
- Use a pedometer to count your daily steps.
- Walk while doing errands.
- Get on or off the bus several blocks away.
- Park the car farther away from your destination.
- At work, walk to nearby offices instead of sending e-mails or using the phone.
- Walk or stretch a few minutes every hour that you are at your desk.
- Take fitness breaks—walking or doing desk exercises—instead of taking cigarette breaks or coffee breaks.
- Incorporate activity into your lunch break (walk to the restaurant).
- Take the stairs instead of the elevator or escalator.
- Play with children, grandchildren, or pets. Everybody wins. If you find it too difficult to be active after work, try it before work.

- Do household tasks.
- Work in the yard or garden.
- Avoid labor-saving devices. Turn off the self-propelled option on your lawnmower or vacuum cleaner.
- Use leg power. Take small trips on foot to get your body moving.
- Exercise while watching TV (for example, use hand weights, stationary bicycle/treadmill/stairclimber, or stretch).
- Spend more time playing sports than sitting in front of the TV or the computer.
- Dance to music.
- Keep a pair of comfortable walking or running shoes in your car and office. You'll be ready for activity wherever you go!
- Make a Saturday morning walk a group habit.
- Learn a new sport or join a sports team.
- Avoid carts when golfing.
- When out of town, stay in hotels with fitness centers.

SOURCE: Adapted from Centers for Disease Control and Prevention, Atlanta, 2005.

Try It

Keep a three-day log of all your activities. List the activities performed, time of day, and how long you were engaged in these activities. You may be surprised by your findings.

---

for the 1.0-Mile Walk Test, plug your values into the following equation:

$$VO_{2max} = 88.768 - (0.0957 \times W) + (8.892 \times G) - (1.4537 \times T) - (0.1194 \times HR),$$

where:

W = weight in pounds
G = gender (use 0 for women and 1 for men)
T = total time for the mile walk in minutes
HR = exercise heart rate in bpm at the end of the mile walk

For example, a woman who weighs 140 pounds completed the mile walk in 14 minutes and 39 seconds, with an exercise heart rate of 148 bpm. The estimated VO_{2max} is:

W = 140 lbs
G = 0 (female gender = 0)
T = 14:39 = 14 + (39 ÷ 60) = 14.65 min
HR = 148 bpm
VO_{2max} = 88.768 – (0.0957 × 140) + (8.892 × 0)
        – (1.4537 × 14.65) – (0.1194 × 148)
VO_{2max} = 36.4 mL/kg/min.

As with the 1.5-Mile Run Test, the fitness categories based on VO_{2max} are found in Table 2.2. Record your cardiorespiratory fitness test results on your fitness profile in Activity 2.1, Pre-Test, page 57.

Muscular Strength and Endurance

Adequate levels of strength enhance a person's health and well-being throughout life. The need for good **muscular fitness** is not confined to highly trained athletes, fitness enthusiasts, and individuals who have jobs that require heavy muscular work. In fact, a well-planned strength-training program leads to increased muscle strength and endurance, muscle tone, tendon and ligament strength, and bone density—all of which help to improve and maintain everyday functional physical capacity.

Strength is crucial for top performance in daily activities such as sitting, walking, running, lifting and carrying objects, doing housework, and even enjoying recreational activities. Strength is also valuable in improving personal appearance and self-image, developing sports skills, promoting stability of joints, and meeting certain emergencies in life in which strength is necessary to cope effectively.

Muscular strength also seems to be the most important health-related component of physical fitness in the older-adult population. Whereas proper cardiorespiratory endurance helps maintain a healthy heart, good strength levels do more to promote independent living than any other fitness component. More than anything else, older adults want to enjoy good health and function independently. Many, however, are confined to nursing homes because they lack sufficient strength to move about. They usually cannot walk very far, and some have to be helped in and out of beds, chairs, and tubs.

A strength-training program can have a tremendous impact on quality of life. Research has shown leg strength improvements as high as 200 percent in previously inactive adults over age 90.[4] As strength improves, so does the ability to move about, the capacity for independent living, and life enjoyment during the "golden years." More specifically, good strength enhances quality of life in that it:

- Increases lean (muscle) tissue
- Stresses the bones, preserves bone density, and decreases the risk for osteoporosis
- Helps increase and maintain **resting metabolism**
- Encourages weight loss and maintenance
- Improves balance and restores mobility
- Makes lifting and reaching easier
- Decreases the risk for injuries and falls
- Reduces chronic low back pain and alleviates arthritic pain
- Lowers cholesterol, high blood pressure, and the risk for developing diabetes
- Promotes psychological well-being

Furthermore, with time, regular strength training decreases the heart-rate and blood-pressure responses to lifting a heavy resistance (a weight). This adaptation reduces the demands on the cardiovascular system when one performs activities such as carrying a child, the groceries, or a suitcase.

Muscular Strength and Muscular Endurance

Although **muscular strength** and **muscular endurance** are interrelated, the two have a basic difference. Muscular strength is the ability to exert maximum force against resistance. Muscular endurance (also called localized muscular endurance) is the ability of the muscle to exert submaximal force repeatedly over a period of time. Muscular endurance depends to a large extent on muscular strength and to a lesser extent on cardiorespiratory endurance. Weak muscles cannot repeat an action several times or sustain it for long. Keeping these concepts in mind, strength tests and training programs have been designed to measure and develop absolute muscular strength, muscular endurance, or a combination of the two.

Determining Strength

Muscular strength usually is determined by using the **one repetition maximum (1 RM)** technique. Although this assessment gives a good measure of absolute strength, it does require a considerable amount of time to administer. Muscular endurance commonly is established by the number of repetitions an individual can perform against a submaximal resistance or by the length of time a person can sustain a given contraction.

Muscular Endurance Test

We live in a world in which muscular strength and endurance are both required, and muscular endurance depends to a large extent on muscular strength. Accordingly, a muscular endurance test has been selected to determine the level of strength. Three exercises that help assess endurance of the upper-body, lower-body, and midbody muscle groups have been selected for your muscular endurance test. To perform the test, you will need a stopwatch, a metronome, a bench or gymnasium bleacher 16¼" high, and a partner.

KEY TERMS

Muscular fitness   A term that is used to define good levels of both muscular strength and muscular endurance.

Resting metabolism   The energy requirement to maintain the body's vital processes in the resting state.

Muscular strength   Ability to exert maximum force against resistance.

Muscular endurance   Ability of a muscle to exert submaximal force repeatedly over a period of time.

One repetition maximum (1 RM)   The maximal amount of resistance a person is able to lift in a single effort.

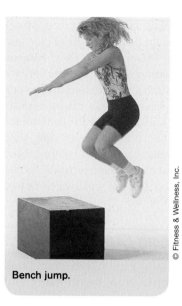

Bench jump.

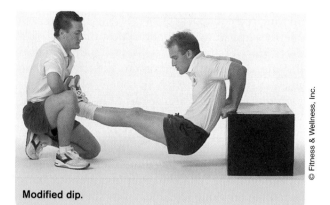

Modified dip.

The exercises conducted for this test are the Bench Jump, Modified Dip (men) or Modified Push-Up (women), and Bent-Leg Curl-Up. Individuals who are susceptible to low back injury may do the Abdominal Crunch instead of the Bent-Leg Curl-Up Test. All tests should be conducted with the aid of a partner. The correct procedures for performing these exercises follow.

Bench Jump

For the Bench Jump, use a bench or gymnasium bleacher 16¼″ high, and attempt to jump up and down on the bench as many times as you can in 1 minute. If you cannot jump the full minute, step up and down. A repetition is counted each time both feet return to the floor.

Modified Dip

The Modified Dip is an upper-body exercise that is done by men only. Using a bench or gymnasium bleacher, place your hands on the bench with the fingers pointing forward. Have a partner hold your feet in front of you. Bend your hips at approximately 90 degrees. (You also may use three sturdy chairs; put your hands on two chairs placed by the sides of your body and your feet on the third chair in front of you.)

Next, lower your body by flexing your elbows until you reach a 90-degree angle at this joint, and then return to the starting position. The repetition does not count if you fail to reach 90 degrees. Perform the repetitions to a two-step cadence (down-up) regulated with a metronome set at 56 beats per

minute. Perform as many continuous repetitions as possible. If you fail to follow the metronome cadence, you no longer can count the repetitions.

Modified Push-Up

Women perform the Modified Push-Up instead of the Modified Dip. Lie down on the floor (face down), bend your knees (feet up in the air), and place your hands on the floor by your shoulders with the fingers pointing forward. Your lower body will be supported at the knees (rather than the feet) throughout the test. Your chest must touch the floor on each repetition.

Perform the repetitions to a two-step cadence (up-down) regulated with a metronome set at 56 beats per minute. Do as many continuous repetitions as possible. If you fail to follow the metronome cadence, you cannot count any more repetitions.

Bent-Leg Curl-Up

For the Bent-Leg Curl-Up, lie down on the floor, face up, and bend both legs at the knees at approximately 100 degrees. Your feet should be on the

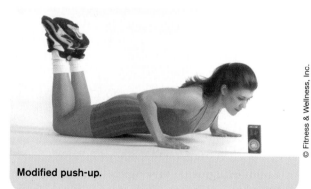

Modified push-up.

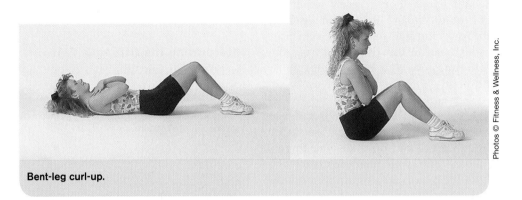

Bent-leg curl-up.

floor, and you must hold them in place yourself throughout the test. Cross your arms in front of your chest, each hand on the opposite shoulder.

Now raise your head off the floor, placing your chin 1″ to 2″ from your chest. This is the starting and finishing position for each curl-up. The back of the head may not come in contact with the floor; the hands cannot be removed from the shoulders; and neither the feet nor the hips can be raised off the floor at any time during the test. The test is terminated if any of these four conditions occur. When you curl up, your upper body must come to an upright position before going back down. The repetitions are performed to a two-step cadence (up-down) regulated with the metronome set at 40 beats per minute.

For this exercise you should allow a brief practice period of 5 to 10 seconds to familiarize yourself with the cadence (the up movement is initiated with the first beat, then you must wait for the next beat to initiate the down movement; one repetition is accomplished every two beats of the metronome). Count as many repetitions as you are able to perform following the proper cadence. The test is terminated if you fail to maintain the appropriate cadence or if you accomplish 100 repetitions. Have your partner check the angle at the knees throughout the test to make sure that you maintain the 100-degree angle as closely as possible.

Abdominal Crunch

The Abdominal Crunch is recommended only for individuals who are unable to perform the Bent-Leg Curl-Up because of susceptibility to low back injury. Exercise form must be monitored carefully during the test because many participants have difficulty maintaining proper form for this test. People often slide their bodies, bend their elbows, or shrug their shoulders during the test. These actions make the

test easier and misrepresent performance. Further, lack of spinal flexibility does not allow some individuals to move the required (3½″) range of motion. Others are unable to keep their heels on the floor during the test. Some research has questioned the validity of this test as an effective measure of abdominal strength or abdominal endurance.[5,6] With these caveats in mind, the procedure is as follows.

Tape a 3½″ × 30″ strip of cardboard onto the floor. Lie on the floor in a supine position (face up) with your knees bent at approximately 100 degrees and your legs slightly apart. Your feet should be on the floor, and you must hold them in place yourself throughout the test. Straighten your arms, and place them on the floor alongside your trunk with your palms down and fingers fully extended. The

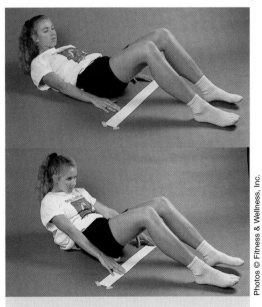

Abdominal crunch.

fingertips of both hands should barely touch the closest edge of the cardboard. Bring your head off the floor until your chin is 1″ to 2″ away from your chest. Keep your head in this position during the entire test. (Do not move your head by flexing or extending the neck.) You now are ready to begin the test.

Perform the repetitions to a two-step cadence (up-down) regulated with a metronome set at 60 beats per minute. As you curl up, slide your fingers over the cardboard until your fingertips reach the far end (3½″) of the board, then return to the starting position.

Allow a brief practice period of about 10 seconds to familiarize yourself with the cadence. Initiate the up movement with the first beat and the down movement with the next beat. Accomplish one repetition every two beats of the metronome. Count as many repetitions as you are able to perform while following the proper cadence. You may not count a repetition if your fingertips fail to reach the distant end of the cardboard.

Terminate the test if you: (a) fail to maintain the appropriate cadence, (b) bend your elbows, (c) shrug your shoulders, (d) slide your body, (e) fail to keep your heels on the floor, (f) do not keep your chin close to your chest, (g) accomplish 100 repetitions, or (h) can no longer perform the test. Have your partner check the angle at the knees throughout the test to make sure you maintain the 100-degree angle as closely as possible. For this test you also may use a Crunch-Ster Curl-Up Tester, available from Novel Products.*

Interpreting the Strength Test

According to the number of repetitions you performed on each test item, look up the percentile

*Novel Products, Inc., Figure Finder Collection, PO Box 408, Rockton, IL 61072-0408; 1-800-323-5143.

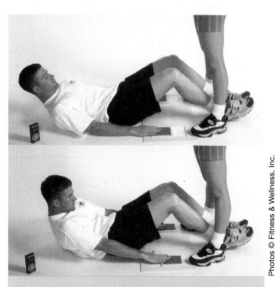

Abdominal crunch test using a Crunch-Ster Curl-Up Tester.

Photos © Fitness & Wellness, Inc.

TABLE 2.3

Muscular Endurance Scoring Table

Percentile Rank	MEN Bench Jumps	Modified Dips	Bent-Leg Curl-Ups	Abdominal Crunches
99	66	54	100	100
95	63	50	81	100
90	62	38	65	100
80	58	32	51	66
70	57	30	44	45
60	56	27	31	38
50	54	26	28	33
40	51	23	25	29
30	48	20	22	26
20	47	17	17	22
10	40	11	10	18
5	34	7	3	16

Percentile Rank	WOMEN Bench Jumps	Modified Push-ups	Bent-Leg Curl-Ups	Abdominal Crunches
99	58	95	100	100
95	54	70	100	100
90	52	50	97	69
80	48	41	77	49
70	44	38	57	37
60	42	33	45	34
50	39	30	37	31
40	38	28	28	27
30	36	25	22	24
20	32	21	17	21
10	28	18	9	15
5	26	15	4	0

■ High physical fitness standard   ■ Health fitness standard

TABLE 2.4

Fitness Categories Based on Percentile Ranks

Percentile Rank	Fitness Category	Points
≥90	Excellent	5
70–80	Good	4
50–60	Average	3
30–40	Fair	2
≤20	Poor	1

TABLE 2.5

Muscular Strength/Endurance Fitness Categories by Total Points

Total Points	Strength Endurance Category
≥13	Excellent
10–12	Good
7–9	Average
4–6	Fair
≤3	Poor

rank for each exercise in the far left column of Table 2.3. Based on your percentile ranks, you can determine your muscular endurance fitness category for each exercise using the guidelines provided in Table 2.4. Look up the number of points assigned for each fitness category in Table 2.4. Now total the points and determine your overall strength endurance fitness category according to the ratings provided in Table 2.5.

Record the results of your strength tests in Activity 2.1, Pre-Test, page 57.

Muscular Flexibility

Flexibility refers to the achievable range of motion at a joint or group of joints without causing injury. Most people who exercise don't take the time to stretch. And many of those who do stretch don't stretch properly. When joints are not regularly moved through their full range of motion, muscles and ligaments shorten in time, and flexibility decreases.

Developing and maintaining some level of flexibility are important factors in all health enhancement programs, and even more so as we age. Good flexibility promotes healthy muscles and joints.

Sports medicine specialists believe that many muscular/skeletal problems and injuries, especially in adults, are related to a lack of flexibility. At times in daily life we have to make rapid or strenuous movements we are not accustomed to making. A tight muscle that is abruptly forced beyond its normal range of motion often leads to injuries.

Improving elasticity of muscles and connective tissue around joints enables an individual to have greater freedom of movement and the ability to participate in many types of sports and recreational activities. Adequate flexibility also makes activities of daily living such as turning, lifting, and bending easier to perform. A person must take care, however, not to overstretch joints. Too much flexibility leads to unstable and loose joints, which may actually increase injury rate.

A decline in flexibility can cause poor posture and subsequent aches and pains that lead to limited movement of joints. Inordinate tightness is uncomfortable and debilitating. Approximately 80 percent of all low back problems in the United States stem from improper alignment of the vertebral column and pelvic girdle, a direct result of inflexible and weak muscles. This backache syndrome costs U.S. industry billions of dollars each year in lost productivity, health services, and worker compensation.

Muscular flexibility is highly specific and varies from one joint to the other (hip, trunk, shoulder), as well as from one individual to the next. Muscular flexibility relates primarily to genetic factors and the index of physical activity. Beyond that, factors such as joint structure, ligaments, tendons, muscles, skin, tissue injury, adipose (fat) tissue, body temperature, age, and gender influence the range of motion about a joint.

On the average, women are more flexible than men and seem to retain this advantage throughout life. Aging decreases the extensibility of soft tissue, decreasing flexibility in both genders. The most significant contributors to loss of flexibility, however, are sedentary living and lack of physical activity.

Most experts agree that participating in a regular flexibility program is beneficial because it:

- Helps to maintain good joint mobility
- Increases resistance to muscle injury and soreness

KEY TERMS

Flexibility The achievable range of motion at a joint or group of joints without causing injury.

- Prevents low back and other spinal column problems
- Improves and maintains good postural alignment
- Enhances proper and graceful body movement
- Improves personal appearance and self-image
- Facilitates the development of motor skills throughout life

Flexibility exercises also have been prescribed successfully to treat **dysmenorrhea**[7] (painful menstruation), general neuromuscular tension (stress), and knots (trigger points) in muscles and fascia. Regular **stretching** helps decrease the aches and pains caused by psychological stress and contributes to a decrease in anxiety, blood pressure, and breathing rate.[8]

Further, mild stretching exercises, in conjunction with calisthenics, are helpful in warm-up routines to prepare the body for more vigorous aerobic or strength-training exercises and as cool-down routines following exercise to help the person return to a normal resting state. Fatigued muscles tend to contract to a shorter than average resting length, and stretching exercises help fatigued muscles reestablish their normal resting length.

Similar to muscular strength, good range of motion is critical in older life. Because of decreased flexibility, older adults lose mobility and are unable to perform simple daily tasks such as bending forward and turning. Many older adults do not turn their heads or rotate their trunks to look over their shoulder but, rather, step around 90 degrees to 180 degrees to see behind them.

Physical activity and exercise also can be hampered severely by restricted range of motion. Because of the pain involved during activity, older people who have tight hip flexors (muscles) cannot jog or walk very far. A vicious circle ensues, because the condition usually worsens with further inactivity. A simple stretching program can alleviate or prevent this problem and help people return to an exercise program.

Assessing Flexibility

Two flexibility tests are used to produce a flexibility profile: the Modified Sit-and-Reach Test and the Total Body Rotation Test.

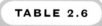

TABLE 2.6

Modified Sit-and-Reach Scoring Table

	MEN						WOMEN				
Percentile Rank	Age Category <18	19–35	36–49	>50	Fitness Category	Percentile Rank	Age Category <18	19–35	36–49	>50	Fitness Category
99	20.8	20.1	18.9	16.2		99	22.6	21.0	19.8	17.2	
95	19.6	18.9	18.2	15.8	Excellent	95	19.5	19.3	19.2	15.7	Excellent
90	18.2	17.2	16.1	15.0		90	18.7	17.9	17.4	15.0	
80	17.8	17.0	14.6	13.3	Good	80	17.8	16.7	16.2	14.2	Good
70	16.0	15.8	13.9	12.3		70	16.5	16.2	15.2	13.6	
60	15.2	15.0	13.4	11.5	Average	60	16.0	15.8	14.5	12.3	Average
50	14.5	14.4	12.6	10.2		50	15.2	14.8	13.5	11.1	
40	14.0	13.5	11.6	9.7	Fair	40	14.5	14.5	12.8	10.1	Fair
30	13.4	13.0	10.8	9.3		30	13.7	13.7	12.2	9.2	
20	11.8	11.6	9.9	8.8		20	12.6	12.6	11.0	8.3	
10	9.5	9.2	8.3	7.8	Poor	10	11.4	10.1	9.7	7.5	Poor
5	8.4	7.9	7.0	7.2		5	9.4	8.1	8.5	3.7	
1	7.2	7.0	5.1	4.0		1	6.5	2.6	2.0	1.5	

High physical fitness standard

Health fitness standard

From *Lifetime Physical Fitness & Wellness: A Personalized Program*, by W. W. K. Hoeger (Belmont, CA: Wadsworth Cengage Learning, 2009).

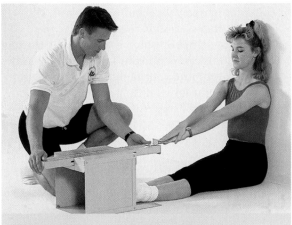

Starting position for Modified Sit-and-Reach Test.

© Fitness & Wellness, Inc.

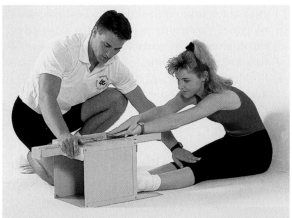

Modified Sit-and-Reach Test.

© Fitness & Wellness, Inc.

Modified Sit-and-Reach Test

To perform the Modified Sit-and-Reach Test, you will need the Acuflex I* sit-and-reach flexibility tester, or you may simply place a yardstick on top of a box approximately 12″ high.

To administer this test:

1. Warm up properly before the first trial.
2. Remove your shoes. Sit on the floor with your hips, back, and head against a wall, legs fully extended, and the bottom of your feet against the Acuflex I or the sit-and-reach box.
3. Place your hands one on top of the other and reach forward as far as possible without letting your hips, back, or head come off the wall.
4. Another person then should slide the reach indicator on the Acuflex I (or yardstick) along the top of the box until the end of the indicator touches the tips of your fingers. The indicator then must be held firmly in place throughout the rest of the test.
5. Your head and back now can come off the wall, and you may reach forward gradually three times, the third time stretching forward as far as possible on the indicator (or yardstick), holding the final position at least 2 seconds. Be sure to keep the back of your knees against the floor throughout the test.
6. Record to the nearest half inch the final number of inches you reached.
7. You are allowed two trials, and an average of the two scores is used as the final test score.

*The Acuflex I and II flexibility testers for the Modified Sit-and-Reach and the Total Body Rotation Tests can be obtained from Novel Products, Inc., Figure Finder Collection, PO Box 408, Rockton, IL 61072-0408; 1-800-323-5143.

The percentile ranks and fitness categories for this test are given in Tables 2.6 and 2.4, respectively.

Total Body Rotation Test

An Acuflex II total body rotation flexibility tester or a measuring scale with a sliding panel is needed to administer the Total Body Rotation Test. The Acuflex II or scale is placed on the wall at shoulder height and should be adjustable to accommodate individual differences in height. If an Acuflex II is not available, you can build your own scale. Glue or tape a measuring tape above the sliding panel and another below it, centered at the 15″ mark. Each tape should be at least 30″ long. Draw a line on the floor, centered at the 15″ mark. Use the following procedure:

1. Warm up properly before beginning this test.
2. To start, stand sideways, an arm's length away from the wall, with your feet straight ahead, slightly separated, and your toes right up to the corresponding line drawn on the floor. Hold out the arm opposite the wall horizontally from the body and make a fist. The Acuflex II, measuring scale, or tapes should be at shoulder height at this time.
3. Now rotate the body, the extended arm going backward (always maintaining a horizontal plane) and making contact with the panel,

KEY TERMS

Dysmenorrhea Painful menstruation.
Stretching Moving the joints beyond the accustomed range of motion.

gradually sliding it forward as far as possible. If no panel is available, slide your fist alongside the tapes as far as possible. Hold the final position at least 2 seconds.

4. Position the hand with the little-finger side forward during the entire sliding movement. Proper hand position is crucial. Some people attempt to open the hand or push with extended fingers or slide the panel with the knuckles—none of which is acceptable. During the test you can bend your knees slightly, but you cannot move your feet; they always must point straight forward. You must keep your body as straight (vertical) as possible.

TABLE 2.7

Total Body Rotation Scoring Table

| | Percentile Rank | Left Rotation | | | | Right Rotation | | | | Fitness Category |
| | | Age Category | | | | Age Category | | | | |
		<18	19–35	36–49	>50	<18	19–35	36–49	>50	
Men	99	29.1	28.0	26.6	21.0	28.2	27.8	25.2	22.2	
	95	26.6	24.8	24.5	20.0	25.5	25.6	23.8	20.7	Excellent
	90	25.0	23.6	23.0	17.7	24.3	24.1	22.5	19.3	
	80	22.0	22.0	21.2	15.5	22.7	22.3	21.0	16.3	Good
	70	20.9	20.3	20.4	14.7	21.3	20.7	18.7	15.7	
	60	19.9	19.3	18.7	13.9	19.8	19.0	17.3	14.7	Average
	50	18.6	18.0	16.7	12.7	19.0	17.2	16.3	12.3	
	40	17.0	16.8	15.3	11.7	17.3	16.3	14.7	11.5	Fair
	30	14.9	15.0	14.8	10.3	15.1	15.0	13.3	10.7	
	20	13.8	13.3	13.7	9.5	12.9	13.3	11.2	8.7	
	10	10.8	10.5	10.8	4.3	10.8	11.3	8.0	2.7	Poor
	05	8.5	8.9	8.8	0.3	8.1	8.3	5.5	0.3	
	01	3.4	1.7	5.1	0.0	6.6	2.9	2.0	0.0	
Women	99	29.3	28.6	27.1	23.0	29.6	29.4	27.1	21.7	
	95	26.8	24.8	25.3	21.4	27.6	25.3	25.9	19.7	Excellent
	90	25.5	23.0	23.4	20.5	25.8	23.0	21.3	19.0	
	80	23.8	21.5	20.2	19.1	23.7	20.8	19.6	17.9	Good
	70	21.8	20.5	18.6	17.3	22.0	19.3	17.3	16.8	
	60	20.5	19.3	17.7	16.0	20.8	18.0	16.5	15.6	Average
	50	19.5	18.0	16.4	14.8	19.5	17.3	14.6	14.0	
	40	18.5	17.2	14.8	13.7	18.3	16.0	13.1	12.8	Fair
	30	17.1	15.7	13.6	10.0	16.3	15.2	11.7	8.5	
	20	16.0	15.2	11.6	6.3	14.5	14.0	9.8	3.9	
	10	12.8	13.6	8.5	3.0	12.4	11.1	6.1	2.2	Poor
	5	11.1	7.3	6.8	0.7	10.2	8.8	4.0	1.1	
	1	8.9	5.3	4.3	0.0	8.9	3.2	2.8	0.0	

High physical fitness standard

Health fitness standard

From *Lifetime Physical Fitness & Wellness: A Personalized Program,* by W. W. K. Hoeger (Belmont, CA: Wadsworth, Cengage Learning, 2009).

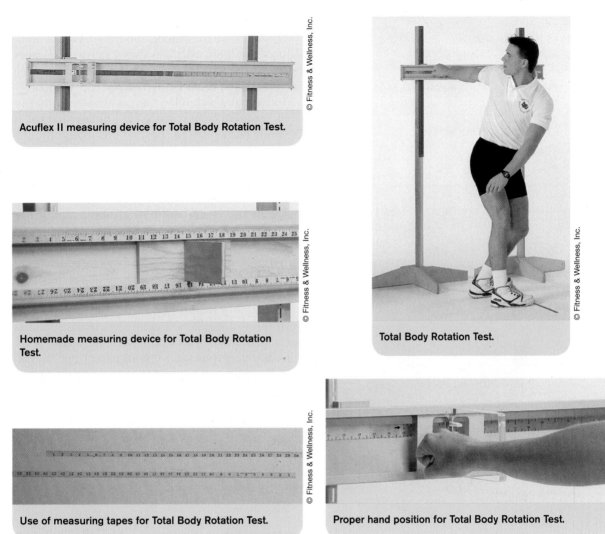

Acuflex II measuring device for Total Body Rotation Test.

Homemade measuring device for Total Body Rotation Test.

Total Body Rotation Test.

Use of measuring tapes for Total Body Rotation Test.

Proper hand position for Total Body Rotation Test.

5. Conduct the test on either the right or the left side of the body. Two trials are allowed on the selected side. The farthest point reached, measured to the nearest half inch and held for at least 2 seconds, is recorded. The average of the two trials is the final test score.

6. Refer to Tables 2.7 and 2.4 to determine the respective percentile rank and fitness category for this test.

Interpreting Flexibility Tests

The fitness category for each flexibility test is obtained based on your percentile rank for each test, using the guidelines provided in Table 2.4. You also should look up the number of points assigned for each fitness category in this table. Your overall flexibility fitness category is obtained by totaling these points and using

the ratings provided in Table 2.8. Record your flexibility test results in Activity 2.1, Pre-Test, page 57.

Body Composition

Currently, starting at age 25, the average man and woman in the United States gains 1 to 2 pounds of body weight per year. Thus, by age 65, the average American will have gained in excess of 40 pounds of weight. Because of the typical reduction in physical activity in our society, however, each year the average person also loses a half pound of lean tissue. Therefore, this span of 40 years has resulted in an actual fat gain of at least 60 pounds, accompanied by a 20-pound loss of lean body mass[9] (see Figure 2.2). These changes cannot be detected unless body composition is assessed periodically.

TABLE 2.8

Muscular Flexibility Fitness Categories by Total Points

Total Points	Flexibility Category
≥9	Excellent
7–8	Good
5–6	Average
3–4	Fair
≤2	Poor

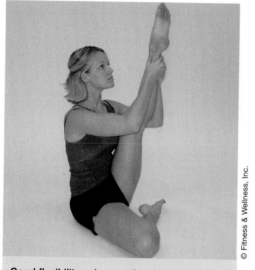

© Fitness & Wellness, Inc.

Good flexibility enhances the development of sports-related skills.

Body composition refers to the fat and nonfat components of the human body. The fat component of the body usually is called fat mass or **percent body fat.** The nonfat component of the body is termed **lean body mass.**

Total fat in the human body is classified into two types: essential fat and storage fat. **Essential fat** is the body fat needed for normal physiological functions. Essential fat constitutes about 3 percent of the total weight in men and 12 percent in women (see Figure 2.3). The percentage is higher in women because it includes gender-specific fat, such as that found in the breast tissue, the uterus, and other gender-related fat deposits. Without it, human health deteriorates. **Storage fat,** the body fat stored in adipose tissue, is found mostly beneath the skin (subcutaneous fat) and around major organs in the body.

Obesity is a health hazard of epidemic proportions in most developed countries. By itself, it has been associated with several serious health problems and accounts for 15 to 20 percent of the annual mortality rate in the United States (see Figure 2.4). It is one of the six major risk factors for coronary heart disease. It also is a risk factor for other diseases of the cardiovascular system, including hypertension, congestive heart failure, elevated blood lipids, atherosclerosis, strokes, thromboembolitic disease, varicose veins, and intermittent claudication.

FIGURE 2.2

Typical body composition changes for adults in the United States.

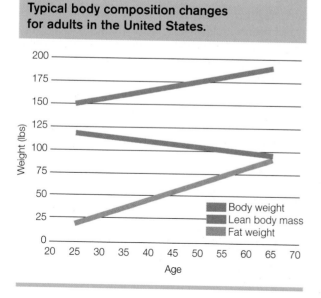

FIGURE 2.3

Typical body composition of an adult man and woman.

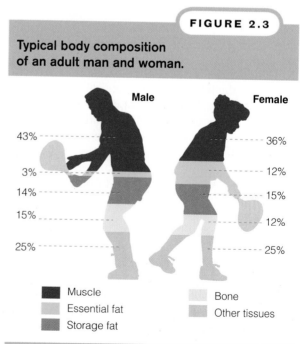

FIGURE 2.4

Percentage of adult population that is overweight and obese in the United States.

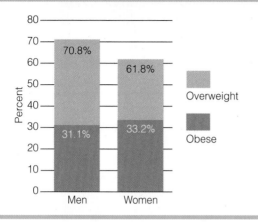

SOURCE: "Prevalence of Overweight and Obesity in the US," by C. L. Ogden et al., *JAMA* 295 (2006): 1549–1555.

Underweight people, too, have health problems and a higher mortality rate. Although the social pressure to be thin has waned slightly in recent years, pressure to attain model-like thinness is still with us and contributes to the gradual increase in incidence of eating disorders (such as anorexia nervosa and bulimia nervosa, discussed in Chapter 5). Extreme weight loss can spawn medical conditions such as heart damage, gastrointestinal problems, shrinkage of internal organs, immune system abnormalities, disorders of the reproductive system, loss of muscle tissue, damage to the nervous system, and even death.

For many years, people relied on height/weight charts to determine **recommended body weight,** but we now know that these tables are highly inaccurate for many people. The standard height/weight tables, first published in 1912, were based on average weights (including shoes and clothing) for men and women who obtained life insurance policies between 1888 and 1905. The recommended weight on height/weight tables is obtained according to gender, height, and frame size. As no scientific guidelines are given to determine frame size, most people choose their frame size based on the column where the weight comes closest to their own!

The proper way to determine recommended weight is to find out what percent of total body weight is fat and what amount is lean tissue (body composition). Once the fat percentage is known, recommended weight can be calculated from recommended body fat.

Obesity is related to an excess of body fat. If body weight is the only criterion, an individual easily can be considered overweight according to height/weight charts, yet not be genuinely obese. Typical examples are football players, body builders, weight lifters, and other athletes with large muscle size. Some athletes who appear to be 20 or 30 pounds overweight really have little body fat.

At the other end of the spectrum, some people who weigh very little and are viewed by many as "skinny" or underweight actually can be classified as obese because of their high body fat content. People who weigh as little as 120 pounds but are more than 30 percent fat (about a third of their total body weight) are not rare. These people often are sedentary or are dieting constantly. Physical inactivity and constant negative caloric balance both lead to a loss in lean body mass (see Chapter 6). Body weight alone clearly does not always tell the true story.

Assessing Body Composition

Body composition can be assessed through several procedures. The most common techniques are skinfold thickness, girth measurements, bioelectrical impedance, hydrostatic (underwater) weighing, and to a lesser extent, air displacement and dual energy X-ray absorptiometry (DEXA). These procedures all yield estimates of body fat; thus, each technique may yield slightly different values. Therefore, when assessing body composition, the same technique should be used for pre- and post-test comparisons.

DEXA is most frequently used in research and by medical facilities. A radiographic technique, it uses very low dose beams of X-ray energy (hundreds of times lower than a typical body X-ray) to measure total body fat mass, fat distribution pattern (see "Waist Circumference" on page 52), and bone density. Many exercise scientists consider DEXA to be the standard technique to assess body composition.

KEY TERMS

Body composition The fat and nonfat components of the human body.

Percent body fat (fat mass) Fat component of the body.

Lean body mass Nonfat component of the body.

Essential fat Body fat needed for normal physiological functions.

Storage fat Body fat stored in adipose tissue.

Recommended body weight The weight at which there appears to be no harm to human health.

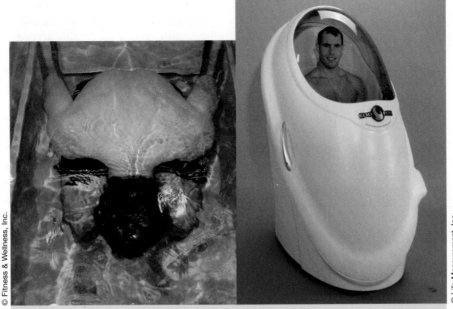

Hydrostatic weighing (left) and air displacement (right) techniques used for assessing body composition.

Hydrostatic, or underwater, weighing is commonly used in exercise physiology and fitness laboratories. In essence, a person's "regular" weight is compared with a weight taken underwater. Because fat is more buoyant than lean tissue, comparing the two weights can determine a person's percent of fat.

Air displacement, a relatively new technique, uses computerized pressure sensors to determine the amount of air displaced by a person sitting inside an airtight chamber. Body volume is calculated by subtracting the air volume with the person inside the chamber from the volume of the empty chamber. Additional research is needed, however, to determine the accuracy of this technique, especially among different age groups, ethnic backgrounds, and athletic populations.

Bioelectrical impedance is much simpler to administer, but its accuracy is highly questionable. In this technique, sensors are applied to the skin, and a weak (totally painless) electrical current is run through the body to estimate body fat, lean body mass, and body water. The technique is based on the principle that fat tissue is a less efficient conductor of electrical current than lean tissue is. The easier the conductance, the leaner the individual. Body weight scales with sensors on the surface are also available to perform this procedure, but again, the accuracy of this technique is highly questionable.

The most common and practical technique available to assess body composition uses skinfold thickness. Two additional techniques, not used to assess body composition but to determine excessive body weight (discussed later in this chapter), are body mass index and waist circumference.

Skinfold Thickness

Assessment of body composition is done most frequently using skinfold thickness. This technique is based on the principle that approximately half of the body's fatty tissue is directly beneath the skin. Valid and reliable estimates of this tissue give a good indication of percent body fat.

The skinfold thickness test is performed with the aid of pressure calipers. To reflect the total percentage of fat, three sites are measured:

- For women: triceps, suprailium, and thigh
- For men: chest, abdomen, and thigh

All measurements are taken on the right side of the body with the person standing. The correct anatomical landmarks for skinfolds are as follows and are also shown in Figure 2.5:

- Chest: a diagonal fold halfway between the shoulder crease and the nipple

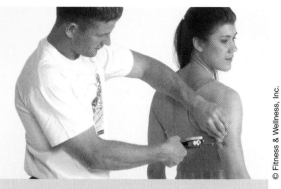

Skinfold thickness technique used for assessing body composition.

© Fitness & Wellness, Inc.

- Abdomen: a vertical fold about 1″ to the right of the umbilicus
- Triceps: a vertical fold on the back of the upper arm, halfway between the shoulder and the arm
- Thigh: a vertical fold on the front of the thigh, midway between the knee and the hip

- Suprailium: a diagonal fold above the crest of the ilium (on the side of the hip)

Each site is measured by grasping a double thickness of skin firmly with the thumb and forefinger, pulling the fold slightly away from the muscle tissue. Hold the calipers perpendicular to the fold, and take the measurements ½″ below the finger hold. Measure each site three times, and read the values to the nearest .1 to .5 mm. Record the average of the two closest readings as the final value. Take the readings without delay to avoid excessive compression of the skinfold. Releasing and refolding the skinfold is required between readings. Be sure to wear shorts and a loose-fitting T-shirt (no leotards), and do not use lotion on your skin the day when skinfolds are to be taken.

After determining the average value for each site, percent fat can be obtained by adding together all three skinfold measurements and looking up the respective values in Table 2.9 for women, Table 2.10 for men under age 40, and Table 2.11 for men over

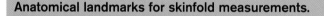

FIGURE 2.5

Anatomical landmarks for skinfold measurements.

SKINFOLD MEASUREMENT

1. Select the proper anatomical sites. For men, use chest, abdomen, and thigh skinfolds. For women, use triceps, suprailium, and thigh skinfolds. Take all measurements on the right side of the body with the person standing.

2. Measure each site by grasping a double thickness of skin firmly with the thumb and forefinger, pulling the fold slightly away from the muscular tissue. Hold caliper perpendicular to the fold, and take the measurement one-half inch below the finger hold. Measure each site three times and read the values to the nearest .1 to .5 mm. Record the average of the two closest readings as the final value. Take the readings without delay to avoid excessive compression of the skinfold. Release and refold the skinfold between readings.

3. When doing pre- and post-assessments, conduct the measurement at the same time of day. The best time is early in the morning to avoid water hydration changes resulting from activity or exercise.

4. Obtain percent fat by adding the three skinfold measurements and looking up the respective values.

For example, if the skinfold measurements for an 18-year-old female are: (a) triceps = 16, (b) suprailium = 4, and (c) thigh = 30 (total = 50), the percent body fat is 20.6%.

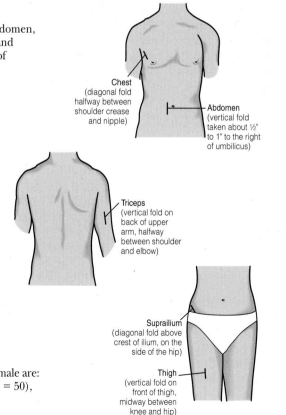

Chest
(diagonal fold halfway between shoulder crease and nipple)

Abdomen
(vertical fold taken about ½″ to 1″ to the right of umbilicus)

Triceps
(vertical fold on back of upper arm, halfway between shoulder and elbow)

Suprailium
(diagonal fold above crest of ilium, on the side of the hip)

Thigh
(vertical fold on front of thigh, midway between knee and hip)

Percent Fat Estimates for Women, Calculated from Triceps, Suprailium, and Thigh Skinfold Thickness

Sum of 3 Skinfolds	Under 22	23 to 27	28 to 32	33 to 37	38 to 42	43 to 47	48 to 52	53 to 57	Over 58
23–25	9.7	9.9	10.2	10.4	10.7	10.9	11.2	11.4	11.7
26–28	11.0	11.2	11.5	11.7	12.0	12.3	12.5	12.7	13.0
29–31	12.3	12.5	12.8	13.0	13.3	13.5	13.8	14.0	14.3
32–34	13.6	13.8	14.0	14.3	14.5	14.8	15.0	15.3	15.5
35–37	14.8	15.0	15.3	15.5	15.8	16.0	16.3	16.5	16.8
38–40	16.0	16.3	16.5	16.7	17.0	17.2	17.5	17.7	18.0
41–43	17.2	17.4	17.7	17.9	18.2	18.4	18.7	18.9	19.2
44–46	18.3	18.6	18.8	19.1	19.3	19.6	19.8	20.1	20.3
47–49	19.5	19.7	20.0	20.2	20.5	20.7	21.0	21.2	21.5
50–52	20.6	20.8	21.1	21.3	21.6	21.8	22.1	22.3	22.6
53–55	21.7	21.9	22.1	22.4	22.6	22.9	23.1	23.4	23.6
56–58	22.7	23.0	23.2	23.4	23.7	23.9	24.2	24.4	24.7
59–61	23.7	24.0	24.2	24.5	24.7	25.0	25.2	25.5	25.7
62–64	24.7	25.0	25.2	25.5	25.7	26.0	26.2	26.4	26.7
65–67	25.7	25.9	26.2	26.4	26.7	26.9	27.2	27.4	27.7
68–70	26.6	26.9	27.1	27.4	27.6	27.9	28.1	28.4	28.6
71–73	27.5	27.8	28.0	28.3	28.5	28.8	29.0	29.3	29.5
74–76	28.4	28.7	28.9	29.2	29.4	29.7	29.9	30.2	30.4
77–79	29.3	29.5	29.8	30.0	30.3	30.5	30.8	31.0	31.3
80–82	30.1	30.4	30.6	30.9	31.1	31.4	31.6	31.9	32.1
83–85	30.9	31.2	31.4	31.7	31.9	32.2	32.4	32.7	32.9
86–88	31.7	32.0	32.2	32.5	32.7	32.9	33.2	33.4	33.7
89–91	32.5	32.7	33.0	33.2	33.5	33.7	33.9	34.2	34.4
92–94	33.2	33.4	33.7	33.9	34.2	34.4	34.7	34.9	35.2
95–97	33.9	34.1	34.4	34.6	34.9	35.1	35.4	35.6	35.9
98–100	34.6	34.8	35.1	35.3	35.5	35.8	36.0	36.3	36.5
101–103	35.2	35.4	35.7	35.9	36.2	36.4	36.7	36.9	37.2
104–106	35.8	36.1	36.3	36.6	36.8	37.1	37.3	37.5	37.8
107–109	36.4	36.7	36.9	37.1	37.4	37.6	37.9	38.1	38.4
110–112	37.0	37.2	37.5	37.7	38.0	38.2	38.5	38.7	38.9
113–115	37.5	37.8	38.0	38.2	38.5	38.7	39.0	39.2	39.5
116–118	38.0	38.3	38.5	38.8	39.0	39.3	39.5	39.7	40.0
119–121	38.5	38.7	39.0	39.2	39.5	39.7	40.0	40.2	40.5
122–124	39.0	39.2	39.4	39.7	39.9	40.2	40.4	40.7	40.9
125–127	39.4	39.6	39.9	40.1	40.4	40.6	40.9	41.1	41.4
128–130	39.8	40.0	40.3	40.5	40.8	41.0	41.3	41.5	41.8

Body density is calculated based on the generalized equation for predicting body density of women developed by A. S. Jackson, M. L. Pollock, and A. Ward, reported in *Medicine and Science in Sports and Exercise,* 12 (1980), 175–182. Percent body fat is determined from the calculated body density using the Siri formula.

40. You can record your results in Activity 2.1, Pre-Test, page 57. Then compute your recommended body weight using the range given in Table 2.12 and the computation form in Activity 2.2, page 59.

The recommended percent body fat values given in Table 2.12 include essential fat and storage fat, discussed previously. For example, the recommended body fat range for women under age 30 is 17 to 25 percent. This indicates that only 5 to 13 percent of the total recommended fat is storage fat, and the other 12 percent is essential fat. The recommended range has been selected based on research indicating that some storage fat is required for optimal health and greater longevity.

The recommended body fat range selected in this book incorporates the recommendations of most

TABLE 2.10

Percent Fat Estimates for Men Under Age 40 Calculated from Chest, Abdomen, and Thigh Skinfold Thickness

Sum of 3 Skinfolds	Age							
	Under 19	20 to 22	23 to 25	26 to 28	29 to 31	32 to 34	35 to 37	38 to 40
8–10	.9	1.3	1.6	2.0	2.3	2.7	3.0	3.3
11–13	1.9	2.3	2.6	3.0	3.3	3.7	4.0	4.3
14–16	2.9	3.3	3.6	3.9	4.3	4.6	5.0	5.3
17–19	3.9	4.2	4.6	4.9	5.3	5.6	6.0	6.3
20–22	4.8	5.2	5.5	5.9	6.2	6.6	6.9	7.3
23–25	5.8	6.2	6.5	6.8	7.2	7.5	7.9	8.2
26–28	6.8	7.1	7.5	7.8	8.1	8.5	8.8	9.2
29–31	7.7	8.0	8.4	8.7	9.1	9.4	9.8	10.1
32–34	8.6	9.0	9.3	9.7	10.0	10.4	10.7	11.1
35–37	9.5	9.9	10.2	10.6	10.9	11.3	11.6	12.0
38–40	10.5	10.8	11.2	11.5	11.8	12.2	12.5	12.9
41–43	11.4	11.7	12.1	12.4	12.7	13.1	13.4	13.8
44–46	12.2	12.6	12.9	13.3	13.6	14.0	14.3	14.7
47–49	13.1	13.5	13.8	14.2	14.5	14.9	15.2	15.5
50–52	14.0	14.3	14.7	15.0	15.4	15.7	16.1	16.4
53–55	14.8	15.2	15.5	15.9	16.2	16.6	16.9	17.3
56–58	15.7	16.0	16.4	16.7	17.1	17.4	17.8	18.1
59–61	16.5	16.9	17.2	17.6	17.9	18.3	18.6	19.0
62–64	17.4	17.7	18.1	18.4	18.8	19.1	19.4	19.8
65–67	18.2	18.5	18.9	19.2	19.6	19.9	20.3	20.6
68–70	19.0	19.3	19.7	20.0	20.4	20.7	21.1	21.4
71–73	19.8	20.1	20.5	20.8	21.2	21.5	21.9	22.2
74–76	20.6	20.9	21.3	21.6	22.0	22.2	22.7	23.0
77–79	21.4	21.7	22.1	22.4	22.8	23.1	23.4	23.8
80–82	22.1	22.5	22.8	23.2	23.5	23.9	24.2	24.6
83–85	22.9	23.2	23.6	23.9	24.3	24.6	25.0	25.3
86–88	23.6	24.0	24.3	24.7	25.0	25.4	25.7	26.1
89–91	24.4	24.7	25.1	25.4	25.8	26.1	26.5	26.8
92–94	25.1	25.5	25.8	26.2	26.5	26.9	27.2	27.5
95–97	25.8	26.2	26.5	26.9	27.2	27.6	27.9	28.3
98–100	26.6	26.9	27.3	27.6	27.9	28.3	28.6	29.0
101–103	27.3	27.6	28.0	28.3	28.6	29.0	29.3	29.7
104–106	27.9	28.3	28.6	29.0	29.3	29.7	30.0	30.4
107–109	28.6	29.0	29.3	29.7	30.0	30.4	30.7	31.1
110–112	29.3	29.6	30.0	30.3	30.7	31.0	31.4	31.7
113–115	30.0	30.3	30.7	31.0	31.3	31.7	32.0	32.4
116–118	30.6	31.0	31.3	31.6	32.0	32.3	32.7	33.0
119–121	31.3	31.6	32.0	32.3	32.6	33.0	33.3	33.7
122–124	31.9	32.2	32.6	32.9	33.3	33.6	34.0	34.3
125–127	32.5	32.9	33.2	33.5	33.9	34.2	34.6	34.9
128–130	33.1	33.5	33.8	34.2	34.5	34.9	35.2	35.5

Body density is calculated based on the generalized equation for predicting body density of men developed by A. S. Jackson and M. L. Pollock, British *Journal of Nutrition,* 40 (1978), 497–504. Percent body fat is determined from the calculated body density using the Siri formula.

TABLE 2.11

Percent Fat Estimates for Men Over Age 40 Calculated from Chest, Abdomen, and Thigh Skinfold Thickness

Sum of 3 Skinfolds	Age							
	41 to 43	44 to 46	47 to 49	50 to 52	53 to 55	56 to 58	59 to 61	Over 62
8–10	3.7	4.0	4.4	4.7	5.1	5.4	5.8	6.1
11–13	4.7	5.0	5.4	5.7	6.1	6.4	6.8	7.1
14–16	5.7	6.0	6.4	6.7	7.1	7.4	7.8	8.1
17–19	6.7	7.0	7.4	7.7	8.1	8.4	8.7	9.1
20–22	7.6	8.0	8.3	8.7	9.0	9.4	9.7	10.1
23–25	8.6	8.9	9.3	9.6	10.0	10.3	10.7	11.0
26–28	9.5	9.9	10.2	10.6	10.9	11.3	11.6	12.0
29–31	10.5	10.8	11.2	11.5	11.9	12.2	12.6	12.9
32–34	11.4	11.8	12.1	12.4	12.8	13.1	13.5	13.8
35–37	12.3	12.7	13.0	13.4	13.7	14.1	14.4	14.8
38–40	13.2	13.6	13.9	14.3	14.6	15.0	15.3	15.7
41–43	14.1	14.5	14.8	15.2	15.5	15.9	16.2	16.6
44–46	15.0	15.4	15.7	16.1	16.4	16.8	17.1	17.5
47–49	15.9	16.2	16.6	16.9	17.3	17.6	18.0	18.3
50–52	16.8	17.1	17.5	17.8	18.2	18.5	18.8	19.2
53–55	17.6	18.0	18.3	18.7	19.0	19.4	19.7	20.1
56–58	18.5	18.8	19.2	19.5	19.9	20.2	20.6	20.9
59–61	19.3	19.7	20.0	20.4	20.7	21.0	21.4	21.7
62–64	20.1	20.5	20.8	21.2	21.5	21.9	22.2	22.6
65–67	21.0	21.3	21.7	22.0	22.4	22.7	23.0	23.4
68–70	21.8	22.1	22.5	22.8	23.2	23.5	23.9	24.2
71–73	22.6	22.9	23.3	23.6	24.0	24.3	24.7	25.0
74–76	23.4	23.7	24.1	24.4	24.8	25.1	25.4	25.8
77–79	24.1	24.5	24.8	25.2	25.5	25.9	26.2	26.6
80–82	24.9	25.3	25.6	26.0	26.3	26.6	27.0	27.3
83–85	25.7	26.0	26.4	26.7	27.1	27.4	27.8	28.1
86–88	26.4	26.8	27.1	27.5	27.8	28.2	28.5	28.9
89–91	27.2	27.5	27.9	28.2	28.6	28.9	29.2	29.6
92–94	27.9	28.2	28.6	28.9	29.3	29.6	30.0	30.3
95–97	28.6	29.0	29.3	29.7	30.0	30.4	30.7	31.1
98–100	29.3	29.7	30.0	30.4	30.7	31.1	31.4	31.8
101–103	30.0	30.4	30.7	31.1	31.4	31.8	32.1	32.5
104–106	30.7	31.1	31.4	31.8	32.1	32.5	32.8	33.2
107–109	31.4	31.8	32.1	32.4	32.8	33.1	33.5	33.8
110–112	32.1	32.4	32.8	33.1	33.5	33.8	34.2	34.5
113–115	32.7	33.1	33.4	33.8	34.1	34.5	34.8	35.2
116–118	33.4	33.7	34.1	34.4	34.8	35.1	35.5	35.8
119–121	34.0	34.4	34.7	35.1	35.4	35.8	36.1	36.5
122–124	34.7	35.0	35.4	35.7	36.1	36.4	36.7	37.1
125–127	35.3	35.6	36.0	36.3	36.7	37.0	37.4	37.7
128–130	35.9	36.2	36.6	36.9	37.3	37.6	38.0	38.5

Body density is calculated based on the generalized equation for predicting body density of men developed by A. S. Jackson and M. L. Pollock, *British Journal of Nutrition,* 40 (1978), 497–504. Percent body fat is determined from the calculated body density using the Siri formula.

TABLE 2.12

Recommended Body Composition According to Percent Body Fat

Age	Males	Females
≤29	12–20%	17–25%
30–49	13–21%	18–26%
≥50	14–22%	19–27%

High physical fitness standard

Health fitness or criterion referenced standard

health and fitness experts throughout the United States. If you desire to have just one target weight, you may select your body weight according to your personal preference, as long as it falls within the recommended range. The lower end of the range constitutes the high physical fitness standard; the high end represents the health fitness standard.

Body Mass Index

Another technique scientists use to determine thinness and excessive fatness relies on **body mass index (BMI).** This incorporates height and weight to estimate critical fat values at which the risk for disease increases. BMI is calculated by dividing the weight in kilograms by the square of the height in meters, or multiplying your weight in pounds by 705 and dividing this figure by the square of the height in inches. For example, the BMI for an individual who weighs 172 pounds (78 kg) and is 67″ (1.7 meters) tall would be 27 [78 ÷ (1.7)²] or [172 × 705 ÷ (67)²].

Because of its simplicity and measurement consistency across populations, BMI is used almost exclusively to determine health risks and mortality rates associated with excessive body weight. You can compute and record your own BMI and recommended body weight according to BMI guidelines using the form provided in Activity 2.2 (pages 59–60). You can also obtain your BMI for selected weights and heights by looking it up in Table 2.13.

KEY TERMS

Body mass index (BMI) Incorporates height and weight to estimate critical fat values at which risk for disease increases.

TABLE 2.13

Body Mass Index

Determine your BMI by looking up the number where your weight and height intersect on the table. According to your results, look up your disease risk in Table 2.14.

Height	110	115	120	125	130	135	140	145	150	155	160	165	170	175	180	185	190	195	200	205	210	215	220	225	230	235	240	245	250
5′0″	21	22	23	24	25	26	27	28	29	30	31	32	33	34	35	36	37	38	39	40	41	42	43	44	45	46	47	48	49
5′1″	21	22	23	24	25	26	26	27	28	29	30	31	32	33	34	35	36	37	38	39	40	41	42	43	43	44	45	46	47
5′2″	20	21	22	23	24	25	26	27	27	28	29	30	31	32	33	34	35	36	37	37	38	39	40	41	42	43	44	45	46
5′3″	19	20	21	22	23	24	25	26	27	27	28	29	30	31	32	33	34	35	35	36	37	38	39	40	41	42	43	43	44
5′4″	19	20	21	21	22	23	24	25	26	27	27	28	29	30	31	32	33	33	34	35	36	37	38	39	39	40	41	42	43
5′5″	18	19	20	21	22	22	23	24	25	26	27	27	28	29	30	31	32	32	33	34	35	36	37	37	38	39	40	41	42
5′6″	18	19	19	20	21	22	23	23	24	25	26	27	27	28	29	30	31	31	32	33	34	35	36	36	37	38	39	40	40
5′7″	17	18	19	20	20	21	22	23	23	24	25	26	27	27	28	29	30	31	31	32	33	34	34	35	36	37	38	38	39
5′8″	17	17	18	19	20	21	21	22	23	24	24	25	26	27	27	28	29	30	30	31	32	33	33	34	35	36	36	37	38
5′9″	16	17	18	18	19	20	21	21	22	23	24	24	25	26	27	27	28	29	30	30	31	32	32	33	34	35	35	36	37
5′10″	16	17	17	18	19	19	20	21	22	22	23	24	24	25	26	27	27	28	29	29	30	31	32	32	33	34	34	35	36
5′11″	15	16	17	17	18	19	20	20	21	22	22	23	24	24	25	26	26	27	28	29	29	30	31	31	32	33	33	34	35
6′0″	15	16	16	17	18	18	19	20	20	21	22	22	23	24	24	25	26	26	27	28	28	29	30	31	31	32	33	33	34
6′1″	15	15	16	16	17	18	18	19	20	20	21	22	22	23	24	24	25	26	26	27	28	28	20	30	30	31	32	32	33
6′2″	14	15	15	16	17	17	18	19	19	20	21	21	22	22	23	24	24	25	26	26	27	28	28	29	30	30	31	31	32
6′3″	14	14	15	16	16	17	17	18	19	19	20	21	21	22	22	23	24	24	25	26	26	27	27	28	29	29	30	31	31
6′4″	13	14	15	15	16	16	17	18	18	19	19	20	21	21	22	23	23	24	24	25	26	26	27	27	28	29	29	30	30

TABLE 2.14

Disease Risk According to Body Mass Index (BMI)

BMI	Disease Risk	Category
<18.5	Increased	Underweight
18.5–21.99	Low	Acceptable
22.0–24.99	Very low	Acceptable
25.0–29.99	Increased	Overweight
30.0–34.99	High	Obesity I
35.0–39.99	Very high	Obesity II
>40.0	Extremely high	Obesity III

TABLE 2.15

Disease Risk According to Waist Circumference (WC)

Men	Women	Disease Risk
<35.5	<32.5	Low
35.5–40.0	32.5–35.0	Moderate
>40.0	>35.0	High

According to the BMI, the lowest risk for chronic disease is in the 22 to 25 range (see Table 2.14). Individuals are classified as overweight between 25 and 30. BMIs above 30 are defined as obesity and below 18.5 as underweight. Compared with individuals with a BMI between 22 and 25, people with a BMI between 25 and 30 (overweight) exhibit mortality rates up to 25 percent higher; rates for those with a BMI above 30 (obese) are 50 to 100 percent higher.[10]

BMI is a useful tool to screen the general population, but, similar to height/weight charts, it fails to differentiate fat from lean body mass or where most of the fat is located. Using BMI, strength-trained individuals and athletes with a large amount of muscle mass (such as body builders and football players) can easily fall in the moderate or even high-risk categories. Therefore, body composition and waist circumference (see below) are better procedures to determine health risk and recommended body weight.

Waist Circumference

Scientific evidence suggests that the way people store fat affects their risk for disease. The total amount of body fat by itself is not the best predictor of increased risk for disease, but rather the location of the fat. **Android obesity** is seen in individuals who tend to store fat in the trunk or abdominal area (which pro-

duces the "apple" shape). **Gynoid obesity** is seen in people who store fat primarily around the hips and thighs (which creates the "pear" shape).

Obese individuals with abdominal fat are clearly at higher risk for heart disease, hypertension, type 2 diabetes ("non-insulin-dependent" diabetes), and stroke than are obese people with similar amounts of body fat stored primarily in the hips and thighs. Evidence also indicates that among individuals with a lot of abdominal fat, those whose fat deposits are located around internal organs (intra-abdominal or abdominal visceral fat) have an even greater risk for disease than those with fat mainly just beneath the skin (subcutaneous fat).

Complex scanning techniques to identify individuals at risk because of high intra-abdominal fatness are costly, so a simple **waist circumference (WC)** measure, designed by the National Heart, Lung, and Blood Institute, is used to assess this risk. A waist circumference of more than 40 inches in men and 35 inches in women indicates a higher risk for cardiovascular disease, hypertension, and type 2 diabetes (see Table 2.15). Thus, weight loss is encouraged when individuals exceed these measurements.

WC may even be a better predictor of disease risk than BMI. Thus, BMI in conjunction with WC provides the best combination to identify individuals at higher risk due to excessive body fat. Table 2.16 provides guidelines to identify people at risk according to BMI and WC.

KEY TERMS

Android obesity Obesity pattern seen in individuals who tend to store fat in the trunk or abdominal area.

Gynoid obesity Obesity pattern seen in people who store fat primarily around the hips and thighs.

Waist circumference (WC) A waist girth measurement to assess potential risk for disease based on intra-abdominal fat content.

CRITICAL THINKING

How do you feel about your current body weight? • What influence does society have on the way you perceive yourself in terms of your weight? • Do the results from your body composition measurements make you feel any different about the way you see your current body weight and image?

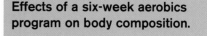

TABLE 2.16

Disease Risk According to Body Mass Index (BMI) and Waist Circumference (WC)

Classification	BMI (kg/m²)	Disease Risk Relative to Normal Weight and WC	
		Men ≤40" (102 cm) Women ≤35" (88 cm)	Men >40" (102 cm) Women >35" (88 cm)
Underweight	<18.5	Increased	Low
Normal	18.5–24.9	Very low	Increased
Overweight	25.0–29.9	Increased	High
Obesity Class I	30.0–34.9	High	Very high
Obesity Class II	35.0–39.9	Very high	Very high
Obesity Class III	≥40.0	Extremely high	Extremely high

Adapted from: Expert Panel, "Executive Summary of the Clinical Guidelines on the Identification, Evaluation, and Treatment of Overweight and Obesity in Adults," *Archives of Internal Medicine* 158 (1998) 1855–1867.

FIGURE 2.6

Effects of a six-week aerobics program on body composition.

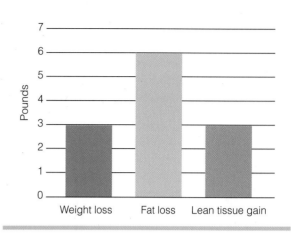

SOURCE: "Fitness Benefits of Aerobic Dance," by W. W. K. Hoeger. Data collected at the University of Texas of The Permian Basin, 1985.

Effects of Exercise and Diet on Body Composition

If you engage in a diet and exercise program, you should repeat body composition measurements about once a month to monitor changes in lean and fat tissue. This is important because lean body mass is affected by weight-reduction programs as well as physical activity. A negative caloric balance does lead to a decrease in lean body mass. These effects will be explained in detail in Chapter 6. As lean body mass changes, so will your recommended body weight.

Changes in body composition resulting from a weight-control/exercise program are illustrated by a coed aerobics course taught during a six-week summer term. Students participated in aerobic dance routines four times a week, 60 minutes each time. On the first and the last days of class, several physiological parameters, including body composition, were assessed. Students also were given information on diet and nutrition and followed their own weight-control program. At the end of the six weeks, the average weight loss for the entire class was 3 pounds. When body composition was assessed, however, class members were surprised to find that the average fat loss was actually 6 pounds, accompanied by a 3-pound increase in lean body mass (see Figure 2.6).

When dieting, have your body composition reassessed periodically because of the effects of negative caloric balance on lean body mass. As discussed in Chapter 6, dieting does decrease lean body mass. This loss of lean body mass can be offset or eliminated by combining a sensible diet with exercise.

www WEB INTERACTIVE

Calculate your body mass index (BMI) using your height and weight. BMI is a ratio of weight to height, a mathematical formula that correlates with body fat. BMI is a better predictor of disease risk than is body weight alone. This site also features tools to calculate your ideal weight and your target heart rate.
http://www.halls.md/body-mass-index/bmi.htm

*Log on to **academic.cengage.com/login** and take a wellness inventory to assess the behaviors that might benefit most from healthy change.*

1. Do you consciously attempt to incorporate as much physical activity as possible in your activities of daily living (walk, take stairs, cycle, participate in sports and recreational activities)?

2. Are your strength levels sufficient for you to perform tasks of daily living (climbing stairs, carrying a backpack, opening jars, doing housework, mowing the yard) without requiring additional assistance or feeling unusually fatigued?

3. Do you know what your percent body fat is according to a reliable body composition assessment technique administered by a qualified technician?

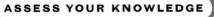

*Log on to **academic.cengage.com/login** to assess your understanding of this chapter's topics by taking the chapter pre-test and exploring the modules recommended in your Personalized Study Plan.*

1. The metabolic profile is used in reference to
a. insulin sensitivity.
b. glucose tolerance.
c. cholesterol levels.
d. cardiovascular disease.
e. All of the above are correct choices.

2. Cardiorespiratory endurance is determined by the
a. amount of oxygen the body is able to utilize per minute of physical activity.
b. length of time it takes the heart rate to return to 120 bpm following the 1.5-Mile Run Test.
c. difference between the maximal heart rate and the resting heart rate.
d. product of the heart rate and blood pressure at rest versus exercise.
e. time it takes a person to reach a heart rate between 120 and 170 bpm during the 1.0-Mile Walk Test.

3. An "excellent" cardiorespiratory fitness rating in mL/kg/min for young male adults is about
a. 10.
b. 20.
c. 30.
d. 40.
e. 50.

4. Which of the following parameters is used to estimate maximal oxygen uptake according to the 1.0-Mile Walk Test?
a. Body weight
b. Gender
c. Total 1.0-mile walk time
d. Exercise heart rate
e. All of the above are used to estimate VO_{2max}.

5. The ability of a muscle to exert submaximal force repeatedly over time is known as
a. muscular strength.
b. plyometric training.
c. muscular endurance.
d. isokinetic training.
e. isometric training.

6. A 70th percentile rank places an individual in the _____ fitness category.
a. excellent
b. good
c. average
d. fair
e. poor

7. Muscular flexibility is defined as the
a. capacity of joints and muscles to work in a synchronized manner.
b. achievable range of motion at a joint or group of joints without causing injury.
c. capability of muscles to stretch beyond their normal resting length without injury to the muscles.
d. capacity of muscles to return to their proper length following the application of a stretching force.
e. limitations placed on muscles as the joints move through their normal planes.

8. During the starting position of the Modified Sit-and-Reach Test
a. the hips, back, and head are placed against a wall.
b. you measure the distance from the hips to the feet.
c. you make a fist with the hands.
d. you stretch forward as far as possible over the reach indicator.
e. All of the above are correct choices.

CONTINUED

9. Essential fat in women is
   a. 3 percent.
   b. 5 percent.
   c. 10 percent.
   d. 12 percent.
   e. 17 percent.

10. Which of the following is *not* a technique used in the assessment of body fat?
   a. Hydrostatic weighing
   b. Skinfold thickness
   c. Body mass index
   d. DEXA
   e. Air displacement

   Correct answers can be found at the back of the book.

Exercise Prescription

Exercise is the closest thing we will ever get to the miracle pill that everyone is seeking. It brings weight loss, appetite control, improved mood and self-esteem, an energy kick, and longer life by decreasing the risk of heart disease, diabetes, stroke, osteoporosis, and chronic disabilities.[1]

OBJECTIVES

- Determine your readiness to start an exercise program
- Learn the factors that govern cardiorespiratory exercise prescription: intensity, mode, duration, and frequency
- Understand the variables that govern development of muscular strength and muscular endurance: mode, resistance, sets, and frequency
- Understand the factors that contribute to the development of muscular flexibility: mode, intensity, repetitions, and frequency

- Learn to write personalized cardiorespiratory, strength, and flexibility exercise programs
- Be introduced to a program for the prevention and rehabilitation of low back pain
- Learn some ways to enhance compliance with exercise
- Be able to write fitness goals

CENGAGENOW Log on to **CengageNOW at academic .cengage.com/login** to find innovative study tools—including pre- and post-tests, personalized study plans, activities, labs, and the personal change planner.

The inspiring story of George Snell from Sandy, Utah, illustrates what fitness can do for a person's health and well-being. At age 45, Snell weighed approximately 400 pounds, his blood pressure was 220/180, he was blind because of diabetes he did not know he had, and his blood glucose (sugar) level was 487. Determined to do something about his physical and medical condition, Snell started a walking/jogging program. After about 8 months of conditioning, he had lost almost 200 pounds, his eyesight had returned, his glucose level was down to 67, and he was taken off medication. Two months later—less than 10 months after initiating his personal exercise program—he completed his first marathon, running a course of 26.2 miles!

Research results have established that being physically active and participating in a lifetime exercise program contribute greatly to good health, physical fitness, and wellness. Nonetheless, too many individuals who exercise regularly are surprised to find, when they take a battery of fitness tests, that they are not as conditioned as they thought they were. Although these people may be exercising regularly, they most likely are not following the basic principles of exercise prescription. Therefore, they do not reap significant benefits.

To obtain optimal results, all programs must be individualized. Our bodies are not all alike, and fitness levels and needs vary among individuals. The information presented in this chapter provides you with the necessary guidelines to write a personalized cardiorespiratory, strength, and flexibility exercise program to promote and maintain physical fitness and wellness. Information on weight management to achieve recommended body composition (the fourth component of physical fitness) is given in Chapter 6.

Monitoring Daily Physical Activity

Almost half of all adults in the United States do not achieve the recommended daily amount of physical activity. The first step toward becoming more active is to carefully monitor daily physical activity. Other than monitoring actual time engaged in activity, an excellent tool to determine daily physical activity is a **pedometer.** Pedometers are small mechanical devices that sense vertical body motion and are used to count footsteps. Wearing a pedometer through-

out the day allows a person to determine the total steps taken in a day. Although with less accuracy, some pedometer brands also record distance, calories burned, speeds, and actual time of activity each day.

A pedometer is a great motivational tool to help increase, maintain, and monitor daily physical activity that involves lower body motion (walking, jogging, running). Pedometer use will most likely increase in the next few years to help promote and quantify daily physical activity.

Before purchasing a pedometer, be sure to verify its accuracy. Many of the free or low-cost pedometers provided by corporations for promotion and advertisement purposes are inaccurate, thus discouraging their use. Pedometers also tend to lose accuracy at very slow walking speeds (30 minutes per mile or less) because the vertical movement of the hip is too small to trigger the spring-mounted lever arm inside the pedometer to properly record the steps taken.

You can obtain a good pedometer for about $25, and ratings are available online. The most accurate pedometer brands are Yamax, Kenz, New Lifestyles, and Walk4Life. To test the accuracy of a pedometer, follow these steps: Clip the pedometer on the waist directly above the knee cap, reset the pedometer to zero, carefully close the pedometer, walk exactly 50 steps at your normal pace, carefully open the pedometer, and look at the number of steps recorded. A reading within 10 percent of the actual steps taken (45 to 55 steps) is acceptable.

The typical male American takes about 6,000 steps per day, whereas women take about 5,300 steps. A general recommendation for adults is 10,000 steps per day, and Table 3.1 provides specific activity ratings based on the number of daily steps taken.

TABLE 3.1

Adult Activity Levels Based on Total Number of Steps Taken per Day

Steps per Day	Category
<5,000	Sedentary lifestyle
5,000–7,499	Low active
7,500–9,999	Somewhat active
10,000–12,499	Active
≥12,500	Highly active

SOURCE: Tudor-Locke, C. and D. R. Basset. "How Many Steps/Day are Enough? Preliminary Pedometer Indices for Public Health," *Sports Medicine* 34:1–8, 2004.

TABLE 3.2

Estimated Number of Steps to Walk or Jog/Run a Mile Based on Gender, Height, and Pace

	Pace (min/mile)							
	Walking				Jogging			
Height	20	18	16	15	12	10	8	6
Women								
5'0"	2371	2244	2117	2054	1997	1710	1423	1136
5'2"	2343	2216	2089	2026	1970	1683	1396	1109
5'4"	2315	2188	2061	1998	1943	1656	1369	1082
5'6"	2286	2160	2033	1969	1916	1629	1342	1055
5'8"	2258	2131	2005	1941	1889	1602	1315	1028
5'10"	2230	2103	1976	1913	1862	1575	1288	1001
6'0"	2202	2075	1948	1885	1835	1548	1261	974
6'2"	2174	2047	1920	1857	1808	1521	1234	947
Men								
5'2"	2310	2183	2056	1993	1970	1683	1396	1109
5'4"	2282	2155	2028	1965	1943	1656	1369	1082
5'6"	2253	2127	2000	1937	1916	1629	1342	1055
5'8"	2225	2098	1872	1908	1889	1602	1315	1028
5'10"	2197	2070	1943	1880	1862	1575	1288	1001
6'0"	2169	2042	1915	1852	1835	1548	1261	974
6'2"	2141	2014	1887	1824	1808	1521	1234	947
6'4"	2112	1986	1859	1795	1781	1494	1207	920

Prediction Equations (pace in min/mile and height in inches):
Walking
Women: Steps/mile = 1949 + [(63.4 × pace) − (14.1 × height)]
Men: Steps/mile = 1916 + [(63.4 × pace) − (14.1 × height)]
Running
Women and Men: Steps/mile = 1084 + [(143.6 × pace) − (13.5 × height)]

SOURCE: Werner W. K. Hoeger et al., "One-Mile Step Count at Walking and Running Speeds." *ACSM's Health & Fitness Journal,* Vol 12(1):14–19, 2008.

All daily steps count, but some of your steps should come in bouts of at least 10 minutes, so as to meet the national physical activity recommendation of accumulating 30 minutes of moderate-intensity physical activity in at least three 10-minute sessions five days per week. A 10-minute brisk walk (a distance of about 1,200 yards at a 15-minute per mile pace) is approximately 1,300 steps. A 15-minute mile (1,770 yards) is about 1,900 steps.[2] Thus, new pedometer brands have an "aerobic steps" function that records steps taken in excess of 60 steps per minute over a 10-minute period of time.

If you do not accumulate the recommended 10,000 daily steps, you can refer to Table 3.2 to determine the additional walking or jogging distance required to reach your goal. For example, if you are 5'8" tall, male, and you typically accumulate 5,200 steps per day, you would need an additional 4,800 daily steps to reach your 10,000-steps goal. You can do so by jogging 3 miles at a 10-minute per mile pace (1,602 steps × 3 miles = 4,806 steps) on some days, and you can walk 2.5 miles at a 15-minute per mile pace (1,908 steps × 2.5 miles = 4,770 steps) on other days. If you do not find a particular speed (pace) that you typically walk or jog at in Table 3.2, you can estimate the number of steps at that speed using the prediction equations at the bottom of this table.

KEY TERMS

Pedometer An electronic device that senses body motion and counts footsteps. Some pedometers also record distance, calories burned, speeds, and time spent being physically active.

The first practical application that you can perform in this course is to determine your current level of daily activity. Activity 3.1 (page 87) will help you keep a four-day log of all physical activities that you do on a daily basis, and a tip sheet is provided in Figure 3.1. On this log, record the time of day, type and duration of the activity/exercise, and, if possible, steps taken while engaged in the activity. The results will provide an indication of how active you are and will serve to monitor changes in the next few months and years.

Readiness for Exercise

The research data on the benefits of regular physical activity and exercise are far too impressive to be ignored. All of the benefits of being active, however, do not help unless people carry out a lifetime program of physical activity. Of greater concern, only a small fraction of the population exercises regularly, and of those who exercise, only about 20 percent are able to achieve a high physical fitness standard. More than half of those who start exercising drop out during the first six months of the program. Sports psychologists are trying to find out why some people exercise habitually and many do not.

If you are not exercising now, are you willing to give exercise a try? The first step is to decide positively that you will try. To help you make this decision, look at Activity 3.2 (page 89). Make a list of the advantages and disadvantages of incorporating exercise into your lifestyle. Your list of advantages may include things such as:

- It will make me feel better.
- My self-esteem will improve.
- I will lose weight.
- I will have more energy.
- It will lower my risk for chronic diseases.

Your list of disadvantages may include:

- I don't want to take the time.
- I'm too out of shape.
- There's no good place to exercise.
- I don't have the willpower to do it.

When the reasons for exercise outweigh the reasons for not exercising, it will become easier to try.

A questionnaire that may provide answers about your readiness to start an exercise program is also included in Activity 3.2, page 89. Read each state-

FIGURE 3.1

Tips to Increase Daily Physical Activity

Everyone can schedule a minimum of 30 minutes for physical activity. With a little creativity and planning, even the person with the busiest schedule can make room for physical activity. Think about your weekly or daily schedule and look for or make opportunities to be more active. Every little bit helps. Consider the following suggestions:

- Walk, cycle, jog, skate, etc., to school, work, the store, or place of worship.
- Use a pedometer to count your daily steps.
- Walk while doing errands.
- Get on or off the bus several blocks away.
- Park the car farther away from your destination.
- At work, walk to nearby offices instead of sending e-mails or using the phone.
- Walk or stretch a few minutes every hour that you are at your desk.
- Take fitness breaks—walking or doing desk exercises—instead of taking cigarette breaks or coffee breaks.
- Incorporate activity into your lunch break (walk to the restaurant).
- Take the stairs instead of the elevator or escalator.
- Play with children, grandchildren, or pets. Everybody wins. If you find it too difficult to be active after work, try it before work.
- Do household tasks.
- Work in the yard or garden.
- Avoid labor-saving devices. Turn off the self-propelled option on your lawnmower or vacuum cleaner.
- Use leg power. Take small trips on foot to get your body moving.
- Exercise while watching TV (for example, use hand weights, stationary bicycle/treadmill/stairclimber, or stretch).
- Spend more time playing sports than sitting in front of the TV or the computer.
- Dance to music.
- Keep a pair of comfortable walking or running shoes in your car and office. You'll be ready for activity wherever you go!
- Make a Saturday morning walk a group habit.
- Learn a new sport or join a sports team.
- Avoid carts when golfing.
- When out of town, stay in hotels with fitness centers.

SOURCE: Adapted from Centers for Disease Control and Prevention, Atlanta, 2007.

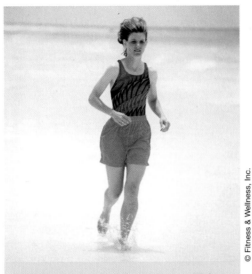

Good cardiorespiratory fitness is essential to enjoy a good quality of life.

© Fitness & Wellness, Inc.

ment carefully and circle the number that best describes your feelings. Be completely honest in your answers. You are evaluated in four categories: mastery (self-control), attitude, health, and commitment. The higher you score in any category—mastery, for example—the more important that reason is for you to exercise.

Scores can vary from 4 to 16. A score of 12 or above is a strong indicator that that factor is important to you, whereas scores of 8 and below are weak indicators. If you score 12 or more points in each category, your chances of initiating and sticking to an exercise program are good. If you do not score at least 12 points in three categories, your chances of succeeding at exercise may be slim. You need to be better informed about the benefits of exercise, and retraining may be helpful. Tips on how to enhance commitment to exercise are provided later in the chapter.

Exercise Prescriptions

To better understand how overall fitness can be developed, we have to be familiar with the guidelines that govern exercise prescriptions for cardiovascular endurance, muscular strength and endurance, and body flexibility. A brief summary of these guidelines is provided in the Physical Activity Pyramid given in Figure 3.2, and they will be explained in detail in the next few sections of this chapter.

Cardiorespiratory Endurance

A sound cardiorespiratory endurance program contributes greatly to enhancing and maintaining good health. Of the four health-related physical fitness components, cardiorespiratory endurance is the single most important—except during older age, when strength seems to be more critical. Even though certain levels of muscular strength and flexibility are necessary to perform **activities of daily living,** a person can get by without a lot of strength and flexibility. A person cannot do without a good cardiorespiratory system, though.

Cardiorespiratory Exercise Prescription

The objective of aerobic exercise is to improve the capacity of the cardiorespiratory system. To accomplish this, the heart muscle has to be overloaded like any other muscle in the human body. Just as the biceps muscle in the upper arm is developed through strength training, the heart muscle is exercised to increase in size, strength, and efficiency.

To better understand how the cardiorespiratory system can be developed, we have to be familiar with four factors involved in aerobic exercise: intensity, mode, duration, and frequency of exercise. The American College of Sports Medicine (ACSM) recommends that a medical exam and a diagnostic exercise stress test be administered prior to **vigorous exercise** by apparently healthy men over age 45 and women over 55.[3]

Intensity of Exercise

Muscles have to be overloaded for them to develop. Just as the training stimulus to develop the biceps muscle can be accomplished with curl-up exercises, the stimulus for the cardiorespiratory system is provided by making the heart pump at a higher rate for a certain period of time.

KEY TERMS

Activities of daily living Everyday behaviors that people normally do to function in life (cross the street, carry groceries, lift objects, do laundry, sweep floors).

Vigorous exercise An exercise intensity that is either above 6 metabolic equivalents (METs) or 60 percent of maximal oxygen uptake or that provides a "substantial" challenge to the individual.

FIGURE 3.2

Physical Activity Pyramid.

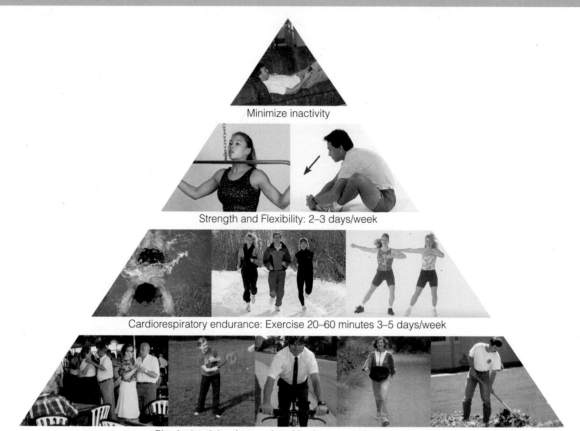

Minimize inactivity

Strength and Flexibility: 2–3 days/week

Cardiorespiratory endurance: Exercise 20–60 minutes 3–5 days/week

Physical activity: Accumulate 60 minutes nearly every day.

Photos © Fitness & Wellness, Inc.

Cardiorespiratory development occurs when the heart is working between 40–50 and 85 percent of **heart rate reserve.**[4,5] The 40–50 percent training intensity should be used by individuals who are quite unfit. Increases in maximal oxygen uptake (VO_{2max}), however, are accelerated when the heart is working closer to 85 percent of heart rate reserve. For this reason, many experts prescribe exercise between 60 and 85 percent. **Intensity of exercise** can be calculated easily, and training can be monitored by checking your pulse. To determine the intensity of exercise or **cardiorespiratory training zone,** follow these steps:

1. Estimate your maximal heart rate (MHR) according to the formula MHR = 220 minus age (220 − age).
2. Check your resting heart rate (RHR) sometime after you have been sitting quietly for 15 to 20 minutes. You may take your pulse for 30 sec-

onds and multiply by 2, or take it for a full minute. As explained in Chapter 2, you can check your pulse on the wrist by placing two or three fingers over the radial artery, or on the neck by placing your fingers over the carotid artery.
3. Determine the heart rate reserve (HRR) by subtracting RHR from MHR (HRR = MHR − RHR).
4. Calculate the training intensities (TIs) at 40, 50, 60, and 85 percent. Multiply HRR by 40, 50, 60, and 85 percent, respectively, and then add the RHR to each of these four values (for example, 85% TI = HRR × .85 + RHR).

Example. The 40, 50, 60, and 85 percent training intensities for a 20-year-old with a resting heart rate of 68 beats per minute (bpm) would be:

MHR: 220 − 20 = 200 bpm
RHR = 68 bpm

HRR: 200 − 68 = 132 beats
40% TI = (132 × .40) + 68 = 121 bpm
50% TI = (132 × .50) + 68 = 134 bpm
60% TI = (132 × .60) + 68 = 147 bpm
85% TI = (132 × .85) + 68 = 180 bpm

Therefore, this person's training zones would be as follows:

Low-intensity cardiorespiratory training zone:
121 to 134 bpm
Moderate-intensity cardiorespiratory training
zone: 134 to 147 bpm
Vigorous-intensity (high) cardiorespiratory
training zone: 147 to 180 bpm

When you exercise to improve the cardiorespiratory system, you should maintain the heart rate between the 60 and 85 percent training intensities to obtain adequate development. If you have been physically inactive, start at 40 to 50 percent intensity and gradually increase to 60 percent during the first six to eight weeks of the exercise program. After that, you may exercise between 60 and 85 percent training intensity.

When determining the training intensity for your own program, you need to consider your personal fitness goals. Individuals who exercise at around the 50 percent training intensity will reap significant health benefits—in particular, improvements in the metabolic profile (see "Health Fitness Standard," pages 29–30, and Chapter 2, Figure 2.1). Training at this lower percentage, however, may place you in only the "average" or moderately fit category (see Table 2.2, page 33). Exercising at this lower intensity does lower the risk for cardiovascular mortality (health fitness) but will not allow you to achieve a "good" or "excellent" cardiorespiratory fitness rating (the physical fitness standard). The latter ratings are obtained by exercising closer to the 85 percent threshold.

Following a few weeks of training, you may have a considerably lower resting heart rate (10 to 20 beats fewer in 8 to 12 weeks). Therefore, you should recompute your target zone periodically. You can compute your own cardiorespiratory training zone by using the form in Activity 3.3, page 91. Once you have reached an ideal level of cardiorespiratory endurance, training in the 60 to 85 percent range will allow you to maintain your fitness level.

Moderate- Versus Vigorous-Intensity Exercise

As fitness programs became popular in the 1970s, vigorous-intensity exercise was routinely prescribed for all fitness participants. Following extensive research in the late 1980s and 1990s, we learned that moderate-intensity physical activity provided substantial health benefits—including decreased risk for cardiovascular mortality, a statement endorsed by the U.S. Surgeon General in 1996.[6] Thus, the emphasis switched from vigorous- to moderate-intensity training in the mid-1990s. In the 1996 report, the Surgeon General also stated that vigorous-intensity exercise would provide even greater benefits than moderate-intensity activity. Limited attention, however, has been paid to this recommendation since the publication of the report.

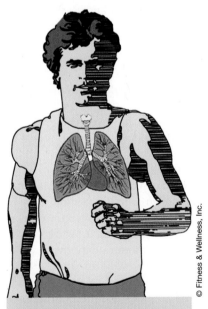

© Fitness & Wellness, Inc.

Cardiorespiratory endurance is the ability of the heart, lungs, and blood vessels to deliver adequate amounts of oxygen to the cells to meet the demands of prolonged physical activity.

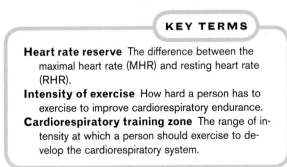

KEY TERMS

Heart rate reserve The difference between the maximal heart rate (MHR) and resting heart rate (RHR).
Intensity of exercise How hard a person has to exercise to improve cardiorespiratory endurance.
Cardiorespiratory training zone The range of intensity at which a person should exercise to develop the cardiorespiratory system.

Vigorous-intensity programs yield higher improvements in VO_{2max} than do moderate-intensity programs. And higher levels of aerobic fitness are associated with lower cardiovascular mortality, even when the duration of moderate-intensity activity is prolonged to match the energy expenditure performed during a shorter vigorous-intensity effort.[7] A recent review of several clinical studies substantiated that vigorous-intensity, as compared with moderate-intensity, activity leads to better improvements in coronary heart disease risk factors, including aerobic endurance, blood pressure, and blood glucose control.[8]

Most recently, a 2007 joint report by the ACSM and the American Heart Association indicated that when feasible, vigorous-intensity physical activity is preferable over moderate-intensity because it provides greater benefits in terms of personal fitness, chronic disease and disability prevention, decreased risk for premature mortality, and lifetime weight management.[9] As a result, the pendulum is again swinging toward vigorous-intensity activity because of the extra benefits and increased chronic disease protection.

Monitoring Exercise Heart Rate

During the first few weeks of an exercise program, you should monitor your exercise heart rate regularly to make sure you are training in the proper zone. Wait until you are about 5 minutes into your exercise session before taking your first reading. When you check your heart rate, count your pulse for 10 seconds and then multiply by 6 to get the per minute pulse rate. Exercise heart rate will remain at the same level for about 15 seconds following exercise. After 15 seconds, your heart rate will drop rapidly. Do not hesitate to stop during your exercise bout to check your pulse. If the rate is too low, increase the intensity of exercise. If the rate is too high, slow down.

To develop the cardiorespiratory system, you do not have to exercise above the 85 percent rate. From a fitness standpoint, training above this percentage will not give extra benefits and actually may be unsafe for some individuals. For unconditioned people and older adults, cardiorespiratory training should be conducted around the 50 percent rate to discourage potential problems associated with high-intensity exercise.

Mode of Exercise

The **mode of exercise** that develops the cardiorespiratory system has to be aerobic in nature.

Aerobic exercise involves the major muscle groups of the body and is rhythmic and continuous in nature. As the amount of muscle mass involved during exercise increases, so does the effectiveness of the activity in providing cardiorespiratory development. Once you have established your cardiorespiratory training zone, any activity or combination of activities that will get your heart rate up to that training zone and keep it there for as long as you exercise will give you adequate development. Examples of these activities are walking, jogging, swimming, water aerobics, cross-country skiing, rope skipping, cycling, racquetball, stair climbing, and stationary running or cycling.

The activity you choose should be based on your personal preferences—what you enjoy doing most—and your physical limitations. Low-impact activities greatly decrease the risk for injuries. Most injuries to beginners are related to high-impact activities. For individuals who have been inactive, general strength conditioning also is recommended prior to initiating an aerobic exercise program. Strength conditioning will reduce the incidence of injuries significantly.

The amount of strength or flexibility a person develops through various activities differs, but in terms of cardiorespiratory development, the heart doesn't know whether you are walking, swimming, or cycling. All the heart knows is that it has to pump at a certain rate, and as long as that rate is in the desired range, your cardiorespiratory fitness will improve. From a health fitness point of view, training in the lower end of the cardiorespiratory zone will yield optimal health benefits. The closer the heart rate is to the higher end of the cardiorespiratory training zone, however, the greater will be the improvements in VO_{2max} (high physical fitness).

Duration of Exercise

In terms of **duration of exercise,** the general recommendation is that a person train between 20 and 60 minutes per session. However, for people who have been successful at losing weight, up to 90 minutes of daily moderate-intensity activity may be required to prevent weight regain.

The duration is based on how intensely a person trains. If the training is done at around 85 percent, 20 minutes of exercise is sufficient. At 40 to 50 percent intensity, the individual should train at least 30 minutes. As mentioned in the discussion of intensity of exercise above, unconditioned people and older adults should train at lower percentages; therefore, the activity should be carried out over a longer time.

Although most experts traditionally have recommended 20 to 60 minutes of continuous aerobic exercise per session, more recent evidence suggests that accumulating 30 minutes or more of moderate-intensity physical activity can provide substantial health benefits.[10] Research further indicates that three 10-minute exercise sessions per day (separated by at least four hours), at approximately 70 percent of maximal heart rate, also produce fitness benefits.[11] Although the increases in VO_{2max} with this program were not as large (57 percent) as those in a group performing one continuous 30-minute bout of exercise per day, the researchers concluded that moderate-intensity exercise, conducted for 10 minutes three times per day, benefits the cardiorespiratory system significantly.

Results of this study are meaningful because people often mention lack of time as the reason for not taking part in an exercise program. Many think they have to exercise at least 20 continuous minutes to get any benefits at all. Even though 20 to 60 minutes are recommended, short, intermittent exercise bouts also are helpful to the cardiorespiratory system.

For people whose goal is weight management, the Institute of Medicine of the National Academy of Sciences recommends accumulating 60 minutes of moderate-intensity physical activity per day,[12] whereas 60 to 90 minutes of daily moderate-intensity activity is necessary to prevent weight regain.[13] These recommendations are based on evidence that people who maintain healthy weight typically accumulate between 1 and 1½ hours of daily physical activity. Exercise duration should be increased gradually to avoid undue fatigue and exercise-related injuries.

If lack of time is a concern, you should exercise daily at a high intensity for 30 minutes, which can burn as many calories as 60 minutes of moderate-intensity exercise (see "Low-Intensity Versus High-Intensity Exercise for Weight Loss," Chapter 6, pages 155–156)—but only 15 percent of adults in the United States typically exercise at a high-intensity level. Novice and overweight exercisers also need proper conditioning prior to high-intensity exercise to avoid injuries or cardiovascular-related problems.

Exercise sessions always should be preceded by a 5- to 10-minute **warm-up** and followed by a 10-minute **cool-down.** The purpose of warm-up is to aid in the transition from rest to exercise. A good warm-up increases muscle and connective tissue extensibility and joint range of motion and enhances muscular activity. A warm-up consists of general calisthenics, mild stretching exercises, and walking/jogging/cycling for a few minutes at a lower intensity level than the actual target zone. The concluding phase of the warm-up is a gradual increase in exercise intensity to the lower end of the target training zone.

In the cool-down, the intensity of exercise is decreased gradually to help the body return to near resting levels, followed by stretching and relaxation activities. Stopping abruptly causes blood to pool in the exercised body parts, diminishing the return of blood to the heart. This reduced blood return can cause a sudden drop in blood pressure, dizziness and faintness, or even the onset of cardiac abnormalities. The cool-down phase also helps dissipate body heat and aid in the removal of lactic acid produced during high-intensity exercise.

Frequency of Exercise

The recommended **frequency of exercise** for aerobic activities is three to five days per week. Initially, only three weekly training sessions of 15 to 20 minutes are recommended to avoid musculoskeletal injuries. You may then increase the frequency so that by the fourth or fifth week you are exercising five times per week for 20 minutes per session in the appropriate heart rate target zone. Thereafter, progressively continue to increase frequency, duration, and intensity of exercise until you have accomplished your goals.

When exercising at 60 to 85 percent of HRR, three 20- to 30-minute exercise sessions per week, performed on nonconsecutive days, are sufficient to improve or maintain VO_{2max}. When training at lower intensities, exercising 30 to 60 minutes more than three days per week is required. If training is conducted more than five days a week, further improvements in VO_{2max} are minimal. Although endurance athletes often train six to seven days per

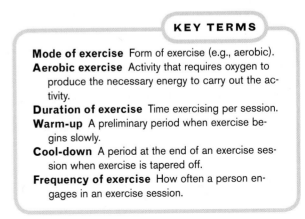

KEY TERMS

Mode of exercise Form of exercise (e.g., aerobic).

Aerobic exercise Activity that requires oxygen to produce the necessary energy to carry out the activity.

Duration of exercise Time exercising per session.

Warm-up A preliminary period when exercise begins slowly.

Cool-down A period at the end of an exercise session when exercise is tapered off.

Frequency of exercise How often a person engages in an exercise session.

week (often twice per day), their training programs are designed to increase training mileage so they can endure long-distance races (6 to 100 miles) at a high percentage of VO_{2max}.

For individuals on a weight-loss program, the recommendation is 60 to 90 minutes of low- to moderate-intensity activity on most days of the week. Longer exercise sessions increase caloric expenditure for faster weight reduction (see Chapter 6, "Exercise: The Key to Successful Weight Management," pages 152–156).

Although three exercise sessions per week will maintain cardiorespiratory fitness, the importance of regular physical activity in preventing disease and enhancing quality of life has been pointed out clearly by the ACSM, the U.S. Centers for Disease Control and Prevention, and the President's Council on Physical Fitness and Sports. These organizations advocate at least 30 minutes of moderate-intensity physical activity almost daily. This routine has been promoted as an effective way to improve health.

These recommendations were subsequently upheld by the U.S. Surgeon General in the 1996 *Report on Physical Activity and Health*. The Surgeon General's report states that people can improve their health and quality of life substantially by including moderate amounts of physical activity on most, preferably all, days of the week. Further, it states that no one (including older adults) is too old to enjoy the benefits of regular physical activity.

To enjoy better health and fitness, physical activity must be pursued regularly. According to Dr. William Haskell, from Stanford University: "Physical activity should be viewed as medication, and, therefore, should be taken on a daily basis." Many of the benefits of exercise and activity diminish within two weeks of substantially decreased physical activity. These benefits are completely lost within two to eight months of inactivity.

A summary of the cardiorespiratory exercise prescription guidelines according to the ACSM is provided in Figure 3.3. Ideally, to reap both the high fitness and the health fitness benefits of exercise, a person needs to exercise a minimum of three times per week in the appropriate target zone for high fitness maintenance, and three to four additional times per week in moderate-intensity activities to enjoy the full benefits of health fitness. All exercise/activity sessions should last about 30 minutes. The form in Activity 3.4, page 95, is provided to help you keep a daily log of your cardiorespiratory (aerobic) activities.

FIGURE 3.3

Cardiorespiratory exercise prescription guidelines.

Activity:	Aerobic (examples: walking, jogging, cycling, swimming, aerobics, racquetball, soccer, stair climbing)
Intensity:	40/50%–85% of heart rate reserve
Duration:	20–60 minutes of continuous aerobic activity
Frequency:	3–5 days per week

American College of Sports Medicine, *Guidelines for Exercise Testing and Prescription* (Philadelphia: Lippincott Williams & Wilkins, 2006).

CRITICAL THINKING

Kate started an exercise program last year as a means to lose weight and enhance her body image. She now runs more than six miles every day, works out regularly on stair-climbers and elliptical machines, strength trains daily, participates in step aerobics three times per week, and plays tennis or racquetball twice a week. Evaluate Kate's program. • What suggestions do you have for improvements?

Muscular Strength and Endurance

The capacity of muscle cells to exert force increases and decreases according to demands placed upon the muscular system. If specific muscle cells are overloaded beyond their normal use, such as in strength-training programs, the cells increase in size (hypertrophy), strength, or endurance, or some combination of these. If the demands on the muscle cells decrease, such as in sedentary living or required rest because of illness or injury, the cells decrease in size (atrophy) and lose strength.

Overload Principle

The **overload principle** states that for strength or endurance to improve, demands placed on the muscle must be increased systematically and progressively over time, and the **resistance** (weight lifted) must be of a magnitude significant enough to produce development. In simpler terms, just like all other organs and systems of the human body, muscles have to be taxed beyond their accustomed loads to increase in physical capacity.

Specificity of Training

Muscular strength is the ability to exert maximum force against resistance. Muscular endurance (also referred to as localized muscular endurance) is the ability of a muscle to exert submaximal force repeatedly over time. Both of these components require **specificity of training.**

As discussed later in this section, a person attempting to increase muscular strength needs a program of few repetitions and near-maximum resistance. To increase muscular endurance, the strength-training program consists primarily of many repetitions at a lower resistance. In like manner, to increase isometric (static) versus dynamic strength (see the section "Mode of Training"), an individual must use the corresponding static or dynamic training procedures to achieve the appropriate results.

Similarly, if a person is trying to improve a specific movement or skill through strength gains, the selected strength-training exercises must resemble the actual movement or skill as closely as possible.

Strength-Training Prescription

As with the prescription of cardiorespiratory exercise, several factors or variables have to be taken into account to improve muscular strength and endurance. These are mode, resistance, sets, and frequency of training.

Mode of Training

Two basic training methods are used to improve strength: isometric and dynamic. **Isometric exercise** involves pushing or pulling against immovable objects. **Dynamic exercise** requires movement with muscle contraction, such as extending the knees with resistance (weight) on the ankles.

Isometric training was used commonly several years ago, but its popularity has waned. Because strength gains with isometric training are specific to the angle of muscle contraction, this type of training remains beneficial in sports such as gymnastics, which require regular static contractions during routines.

Dynamic exercise (previously referred to as **isotonic exercise**) can be conducted without

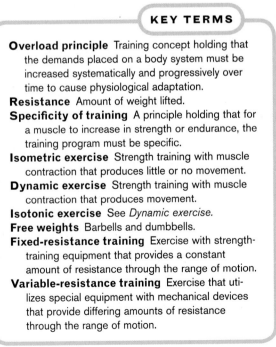

Isometric strength training.

weights or with **free weights** (barbells and dumbbells), **fixed-resistance** machines, **variable-resistance** machines, and isokinetic equipment. When performing dynamic exercises without weights (for example, pull-ups, push-ups), with free weights or with fixed-resistance machines, a constant resistance (weight) is moved through a joint's full range of motion. The greatest resistance that can be lifted equals the maximum weight that can be moved at the weakest angle of the joint,

---

KEY TERMS

Overload principle Training concept holding that the demands placed on a body system must be increased systematically and progressively over time to cause physiological adaptation.

Resistance Amount of weight lifted.

Specificity of training A principle holding that for a muscle to increase in strength or endurance, the training program must be specific.

Isometric exercise Strength training with muscle contraction that produces little or no movement.

Dynamic exercise Strength training with muscle contraction that produces movement.

Isotonic exercise See *Dynamic exercise.*

Free weights Barbells and dumbbells.

Fixed-resistance training Exercise with strength-training equipment that provides a constant amount of resistance through the range of motion.

Variable-resistance training Exercise that utilizes special equipment with mechanical devices that provide differing amounts of resistance through the range of motion.

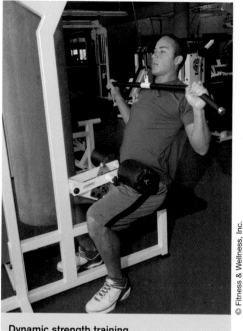

Dynamic strength training.

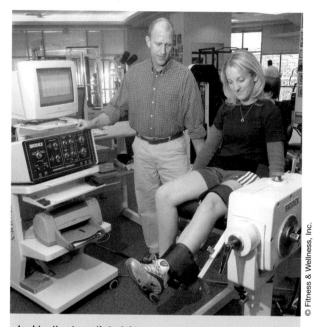

Isokinetic strength training.

because of changes in muscle length and angle of pull as the joint moves through its range of motion.

As strength training became more popular, new strength-training machines were developed. This technology brought about isokinetic and variable-resistance training. These training programs require special machines equipped with mechanical devices that provide differing amounts of resistance, with the intent of overloading the muscle group maximally through the entire range of motion. A distinction of **isokinetic exercise** is that the speed of the muscle contraction is kept constant because the machine provides resistance to match the user's force through the range of motion. Because of the expense of the equipment needed for isokinetic training, this type of program usually is reserved for clinical settings (physical therapy), research laboratories, and certain professional sports.

Dynamic training has two action phases: **concentric** or **positive resistance** and **eccentric** or **negative resistance.** In the concentric phase, the muscle shortens as it contracts to overcome the resistance. For example, during the bench press exercise, when the resistance is lifted from the chest to full arm extension, the triceps muscle on the back of the upper arm contracts and shortens to extend the elbow. During the eccentric phase, the muscle lengthens as it contracts. In the case of the bench press exercise, the same triceps muscle contracts to lower the resistance during elbow flexion, but it lengthens to avoid dropping the resistance.

Eccentric muscle contractions allow us to lower weights in a smooth, gradual, and controlled manner. Without eccentric contractions, weights would be dropped on the way down. Because the same muscles work when you lift and lower a resistance, you should be sure to always execute both actions in a controlled manner. Failure to do so diminishes the benefits of the training program and increases the risk for injuries.

The mode of training depends mainly on the type of equipment available and the specific objective of the training program. Dynamic training is the most popular mode for strength training. Its primary advantage is that strength is gained through the full range of motion. Most daily activities are dynamic in nature. We constantly lift, push, and pull objects, which requires strength through a given range of motion. Another advantage of dynamic exercise is that improvements are measured easily by the amount lifted.

Benefits of isokinetic and variable-resistance training are similar to those of the other dynamic training methods. Theoretically, strength gains should be better because maximum resistance is applied through the entire range of motion. Research, however, has not shown this type of training to be more effective than other modes of dynamic training.

Plate-loaded barbells (free weights) were the most popular weight-training equipment available during the first half of the 20th century. Strength-training machines were developed in the middle of the century but did not become popular until the 1970s. With the advent of, and subsequent technological improvements to, these machines, a stirring debate surfaced over which of the two training modalities was better.

Free weights require that the individual balance the resistance through the entire lifting motion. Thus, a logical assumption could be made that free weights are a better training modality because of the involvement of additional stabilizing muscles needed to balance the resistance as it is moved through its range of motion. Research, nonetheless, has not shown any differences in strength development between the two exercise modalities. Although each modality has pros and cons, the muscles do not know whether the source of a resistance is a barbell, a dumbbell, a universal gym machine, a Nautilus machine, or a simple cinder block. What determines the level of a person's strength development is the quality of the program and the individual's effort during the training program itself—not the type of equipment used.

Resistance

Resistance in strength training is the equivalent of intensity in cardiorespiratory exercise prescription. To stimulate strength development, the general recommendation has been to use a resistance of approximately 80 percent of the maximum capacity (one repetition maximum [1 RM]). For example, a person with a 1 RM of 150 pounds should work with about 120 pounds (150 × .80).

The number of repetitions that one can perform at 80 percent of 1 RM varies among exercises. Data indicate that the total number of repetitions performed at a certain percentage of 1 RM depend on the amount of muscle mass involved (bench press vs. triceps extension) and whether it is a single or multi-joint exercise (leg press vs. leg curl). In both trained and untrained subjects, the number of repetitions is greater with larger muscle mass involvement and multi-joint exercises.[14]

Because of the time factor involved in constantly determining 1 RM on each lift to ensure that the person is indeed working around 80 percent, the accepted rule for many years has been that individuals perform between 3 and 12 repetitions maximum (or 3 to 12 **RM zone**) for adequate strength gains. For example, if a person is training with a resistance of 120 pounds and cannot lift it more than 12 times—that is, the person reaches volitional fatigue at or before 12 repetitions—the training stimulus (weight used) is adequate for strength development. Once the person can lift the resistance more than 12 times, the resistance is increased by 5 to 10 pounds and the person again should build up to 12 repetitions. This is referred to as **progressive resistance training.**

Strength development, however, can also occur when working with less than 80 percent of 1 RM. Although 3 to 12 RM is the most commonly prescribed resistance, benefits do occur when working below 3 or above 12 RM.

At least in the health fitness area, little evidence presently supports the notion that working with a given number of repetitions elicits specific or greater strength, muscular endurance, or **muscular hypertrophy.**[15] Although not precisely to the same extent, muscular strength and endurance are both increased when training within a reasonable amount of repetitions. Thus, the ACSM recommends using a range between 3 and 20 RM. The individual may choose the number of repetitions based on personal preference.

KEY TERMS

Isokinetic exercise Strength training method in which the speed of the muscle contraction is kept constant because the equipment (machine) provides an accommodating resistance to match the user's force through the range of motion.

Concentric Shortening of a muscle during muscle contraction.

Positive resistance The lifting, pushing, or concentric phase of a repetition during the performance of a strength-training exercise.

Eccentric Lengthening of a muscle during muscle contraction.

Negative resistance The lowering or eccentric phase of a repetition during the performance of a strength-training exercise.

RM zone A range of repetitions that are to be performed maximally during one set. For example, an 8 to 12 RM zone implies that the individual will perform anywhere from 8 to 12 repetitions but cannot perform any more (e.g., 9 RM and could not perform a 10th repetition).

Progressive resistance training A gradual increase of resistance over a period of time.

Muscular hypertrophy An increase in muscle mass or size.

Elite strength athletes typically work using a 1 to 6 RM zone but often shuffle training with different numbers of repetitions for selected periods (weeks) of time. Body builders tend to work with moderate resistance levels (60 to 85 percent of 1 RM) and work in an 8 to 20 RM zone. A foremost objective of body building is to increase muscle size. Moderate resistance promotes blood flow to the muscles, "pumping them up" (known as "the pump") and making them look much larger than they do in a resting state.

From a general fitness point of view, working near a 10-repetition threshold seems to improve overall performance most effectively. We live in a dynamic world in which muscular strength and endurance are both required to lead an enjoyable life. Working in an 8 to 12 RM zone produces good results in terms of strength, endurance, and hypertrophy. For older and more frail individuals (50–60 years of age and above), 10 to 15 repetitions of moderate to high intensity of effort are recommended.[16]

We must mention here that a certain resistance (for example, 50 pounds) is seldom the same on two different weight machines, or between free weights and weight machines. The industry has no standard calibration procedure for strength equipment. Consequently, if you lift a certain weight with free weights or a given machine, you may or may not be able to lift the same amount on a different piece of equipment.

Sets

Strength training is done in **sets.** For example, a person lifting 120 pounds eight times performs one set of eight **repetitions** (1/8/120). For general fitness, the recommendation is one to three sets per exercise. Some evidence suggests greater strength gains using multiple sets as opposed to a single set for a given exercise. Other research, however, concludes that similar increases in strength, endurance, and hypertrophy are derived between single- and multiple-set strength training; as long as the single set or at least one of the multiple sets is a heavy (maximum) set performed to volitional exhaustion using an RM zone (for example, 9 RM using an 8 to 12 RM zone).[17] Strength gains may be lessened by performing too many sets.

A recommended program for beginners in their first year of training is one or two light warm-up sets per exercise using about 50 percent of 1 RM (no warm-up sets are necessary for subsequent exercises that use the same muscle group), followed by one to three sets per exercise. Maintaining a resistance and effort that will temporarily fatigue the muscle (volitional exhaustion) in the number of repetitions selected in at least one of the sets is critical to achieve optimal progress. Because of the lower resistances used in body building, four to eight sets can be done for each exercise.

To make the exercise program more time-effective, two or three exercises that require different muscle groups may be alternated. In this way, a person will not have to wait two to three minutes before proceeding to a new set of a different exercise. For example, the bench press, leg extension, and abdominal curl-up exercises may be combined so the person can go almost directly from one set to the next. Body builders should rest no more than a minute to maximize the "pumping" effect.

To avoid muscle soreness and stiffness, new participants ought to build up gradually to the three sets of maximal repetitions. This can be done by performing only one set of each exercise with a lighter resistance on the first day. During the second session, two sets of each exercise can be done: the first light and the second with the regular resistance. During the third session, three sets could be performed—one light and two heavy. After that, a person should be able to do all three heavy sets.

CRITICAL THINKING

What role should strength training have in a fitness program? • Should people be motivated for the health fitness benefits, or should they participate to enhance their body image? • What are your feelings about individuals (male or female) with large body musculature?

Frequency of Training

Strength training should be done either with a total body workout two or three times per week, or more frequently if using a split-body routine (upper body one day and lower body the next). After a maximum strength workout, the muscles should be rested for about 48 hours to allow adequate recovery. If not recovered completely in 2 or 3 days, the person most likely is overtraining and therefore not reaping the full benefits of the program. In that case, a decrease in the total number of sets or exercises, or both, performed during the previous workout is recommended.

A summary of strength-training guidelines for health fitness purposes is provided in Figure 3.4. Significant strength gains require a minimum of eight weeks of consecutive training. After achieving the recommended strength level, one training session per week will be sufficient to maintain the new strength level.

Frequency of strength training for body builders varies from person to person. Because they use moderate resistances, daily or even two-a-day workouts are common. The frequency depends on the amount of resistance, number of sets performed per session, and the person's ability to recover from the previous exercise bout (see Table 3.3). The latter often is dictated by level of conditioning.

Strength-Training Exercises

Two strength-training programs, presented in Appendix A, have been developed to provide a complete body workout. Only a minimum of equipment is required for the first program, "Strength-Training Exercises Without Weights" (Exercises 1 through 15). This program can be conducted within the walls of your own home. Your body weight is used as the primary resistance for most exercises. A few exercises call for a friend's help or basic implements from around your home to provide greater resistance.

"Strength-Training Exercises with Weights" (Exercises 16 through 27) requires machines such as those shown in the various photographs. Some of these exercises can also be performed with free weights.

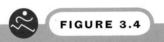

FIGURE 3.4

Strength-training guidelines.

Mode:	8 to 10 dynamic strength-training exercises involving the body's major muscle groups
Resistance:	Sufficient resistance to perform 3 to 20 repetitions to complete or near-complete fatigue (the number of repetitions is optional; you may use 3 to 6, 8 to 12, 12 to 15, or 16 to 20 repetitions)
Sets:	A minimum of 1 set
Frequency:	2 to 3 days per week on nonconsecutive days

American College of Sports Medicine, *Guidelines for Exercise Testing and Prescription* (Philadelphia: Lippincott Williams & Wilkins, 2006).

TABLE 3.3

Guidelines for Various Strength-Training Programs

Strength-Training Program	Resistance	Sets	Rest Between Sets*	Frequency (workouts per week)**
General fitness	3–20 reps max	1–3	2 min	2–3
Strength athletes	1–6 reps max	3–6	3 min	2–3
Body building	8–20 reps near max	3–8	up to 1 min	4–12

*Recovery between sets can be decreased by alternating exercises that use different muscle groups.

**Weekly training sessions can be increased by using a split-body routine.

Strength-Training Exercise Guidelines

As you prepare to design your strength-training program, you should keep several guidelines in mind:

1. Select exercises that will involve all major muscle groups: chest, shoulders, back, legs, arms, hips, and trunk.
2. Never lift weights alone. Always have someone work out with you in case you need a spotter or help with an injury. When using free weights, one to two spotters are recommended for certain exercises (bench press, squats, overhead press).
3. Warm up properly prior to lifting weights by performing a low- to moderate-intensity aerobic activity (5 to 7 minutes) and some gentle stretches for a few minutes.
4. Exercise larger muscle groups first, such as those in the chest, back, and legs. Then proceed to the smaller muscle groups (arms, abdominals, ankles, neck). The bench press exercise works the chest, shoulders, and back of the upper arms (triceps), whereas the triceps extension works the back of the upper arms only.

KEY TERMS

Set The number of repetitions performed for a given exercise.

Repetitions The number of times a movement is performed.

5. Exercise opposing muscle groups for a balanced workout. When you work the chest (bench press), work the back (rowing torso). If you work the biceps (arm curl), work the triceps (triceps extension).

6. Perform all exercises in a controlled manner. Avoid fast and jerky movements, and do not throw the entire body into the lifting motion, which would increase the risk for injury and decrease the effectiveness of the exercise. Do not arch the back when lifting a weight.

7. Perform each exercise through the entire possible range of motion.

8. Breathe naturally, and do not hold your breath as you lift the resistance (weight). Inhale during the eccentric phase (bringing the weight down) and exhale during the concentric phase (lifting or pushing the weight up). Practice proper breathing with lighter weights when you are learning a new exercise.

9. Avoid holding your breath while straining to lift a weight. Holding your breath greatly increases the pressure inside the chest and abdominal cavity, making it nearly impossible for the blood in the veins to return to the heart. Although rare, a sudden high intrathoracic pressure may lead to dizziness, a blackout, a stroke, a heart attack, or a hernia.

10. Based on the program selected, allow adequate recovery time between sets of exercises (see Table 3.3).

11. Discontinue training if you experience unusual discomfort or pain. High-tension loads used in strength training can exacerbate potential injuries. Discomfort and pain are signals to stop and determine what's wrong. Be sure to properly evaluate your condition before you continue training.

12. Stretch out for a few minutes at the end of each strength-training workout to help the muscles return to their normal resting length and to minimize muscle soreness and risk for injury.

Core Strength Training

The trunk (spine) and pelvis are referred to as the "core" of the body. Core muscles include the abdominal muscles (rectus, transversus, and internal and external obliques), hip muscles (front and back), and spinal muscles (lower and upper back muscles). These muscle groups are responsible for maintaining the stability of the spine and pelvis.

Many of the major muscle groups of the legs, shoulders, and arms attach to the core. A strong core allows a person to perform activities of daily living with greater ease, improve sports performance through a more effective energy transfer from large to small body parts, and decrease the incidence of low back pain.

Interest in core strength-training programs has increased recently. A major objective of core training is to exercise the abdominal and lower back muscles in unison. Furthermore, individuals should spend as much time training the back muscles as they do the abdominal muscles. Besides enhancing stability, core training improves dynamic balance, which is often required during participation in physical activity and sports.

Key core-training exercises include the Abdominal Crunch and Bent-Leg Curl-Up, Reverse Crunch, Pelvic Tilt, Lateral Bridge, Prone Bridge, Supine Bridge, Leg Press, Lat Pull-Down, Seated Back, Back Extension (Exercises 4, 11, 12, 13, 14, 15, 19, 21, 25, and 27 in Appendix A), and Pelvic Clock (Exercise 50 in Appendix C, page 270).

When core training is used in athletic conditioning programs, athletes attempt to mimic the dynamic skills used in their sport. To do so, they use special equipment such as balance boards, stability balls, and foam pads. The use of this equipment allows the athletes to train the core while seeking balance and stability in a sport-specific manner.[18]

Designing Your Own Strength-Training Program

The pre-exercise guidelines outlined in the Clearance for Exercise Participation questionnaire (see Activity 1.2, page 25) also apply to strength training. If you have any concerns about whether your present health status will allow you to safely participate in strength training, consult a physician before you start. Strength training is not advised for people with advanced heart disease.

Depending on the facilities available to you, choose one of the two training programs outlined in Appendix A. Once you begin your strength training, you may use the form provided in Activity 3.4, page 95, to keep a record of your training program. The resistance, the number of repetitions, and sets you use with your program should be based on your current strength fitness level and the amount of time that you have for your strength workout. If you are training for reasons other than general health fitness, review Table 3.3 for a summary of the guidelines.

Dietary Recommendations for Strength Development

Individuals who wish to enhance muscle growth and strength during periods of intense strength training should increase protein intake to about 1.5 grams per kilogram of body weight per day. An additional energy intake of 500 daily calories is also recommended to optimize muscle mass gain.

The time when carbohydrates and protein are consumed in relation to the strength-training workout also plays a role in promoting muscle growth. Studies suggest that consuming a pre-exercise snack consisting of a combination of carbohydrates and protein is beneficial to muscle development. The carbohydrates supply energy for training, and the availability of amino acids (the building blocks of protein) in the blood during training enhances muscle building. A peanut butter, turkey, or tuna sandwich, milk or yogurt and fruit, or nuts and fruit consumed 30 to 60 minutes before training are excellent choices for a pre-workout snack.

Consuming a carbohydrate/protein snack immediately following strength training and a second snack an hour thereafter further promotes muscle growth and strength development. Post-exercise carbohydrates help restore muscle glycogen depleted during training and, in combination with protein, induce an increase in blood insulin and growth hormone levels. These hormones are essential to the muscle-building process.

Muscle fibers also absorb a greater amount of amino acids up to 48 hours following strength training. The first hour, nonetheless, seems to be the most critical. A higher level of circulating amino acids in the bloodstream immediately after training is believed to increase protein synthesis to a greater extent than amino acids made available later in the day. A ratio of 4 to 1 grams of carbohydrates to protein is recommended for a post-exercise snack—for example, a snack containing 40 grams of carbohydrates (160 calories) and 10 grams of protein (40 calories).

Flexibility

Improving and maintaining good joint range of motion throughout life is important in enhancing health and quality of life. Nevertheless, fitness participants generally have underestimated and overlooked flexibility fitness.

The most significant detriments to flexibility are sedentary living and lack of physical activity. As physical activity decreases, muscles lose elasticity, and tendons and ligaments tighten and shorten. Aging also reduces the extensibility of soft tissue, decreasing flexibility.

Generally, flexibility exercises to improve range of motion around the joints are conducted following an aerobic workout. Stretching exercises seem to be most effective when a person is warmed up properly. Cool muscle temperatures decrease joint range of motion. Changes in muscle temperature can increase or decrease flexibility by as much as 20 percent. Because of the effects of muscular temperature on flexibility, many people prefer to do their stretching exercises after the aerobic phase of their workout.

Muscular Flexibility Prescription

The overload and specificity of training principles apply to development of muscular flexibility. To increase the total range of motion of a joint, the specific muscles surrounding that joint have to be stretched progressively beyond their accustomed length. The factors of mode, intensity, repetitions, and frequency of exercise also can be applied to flexibility programs.

Mode of Exercise

Three modes of stretching exercises promote flexibility:

1. Ballistic stretching
2. Slow-sustained stretching
3. Proprioceptive neuromuscular facilitation (PNF) stretching

Although all three types of stretching are effective in developing better flexibility, each has certain advantages. **Ballistic** (or **dynamic**) **stretching** exercises provide the necessary force to lengthen the muscles. Although this type of stretching helps to develop flexibility, the ballistic actions may cause muscle soreness and injury as a result of small tears to the soft tissue.

Precautions must be taken not to overstretch ligaments, because they undergo plastic (permanent) elongation. If the stretching force cannot be con-

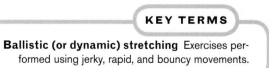

KEY TERMS

Ballistic (or dynamic) stretching Exercises performed using jerky, rapid, and bouncy movements.

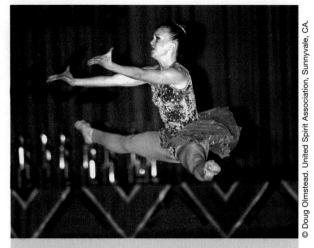

Performance of complex motor skills improves with good flexibility.

© Doug Olmstead. United Spirit Association, Sunnyvale, CA.

trolled, as in fast, jerky movements, ligaments can be overstretched easily. This, in turn, leads to excessively loose joints, increasing the risk for injuries, including joint dislocation and subluxation (partial dislocation). Slow, gentle, and controlled ballistic stretching (instead of jerky, rapid, and bouncy movements), however, is effective in developing flexibility, and most individuals can perform this safely.

Slow-sustained stretching causes the muscles to relax so that greater length can be achieved. This type of stretch causes little pain and has a low risk for injury. Slow-sustained stretching exercises are the most frequently used and recommended for flexibility development programs.

PNF stretching has become more popular in the last few years. This technique, based on a "contract-and-relax" method, requires the assistance of another person. The procedure is as follows:

1. The person assisting with the exercise provides initial force by pushing slowly in the direction of the desired stretch. The initial stretch does not cover the entire range of motion.
2. The person being stretched then applies force in the opposite direction of the stretch, against the assistant, who tries to hold the initial degree of stretch as closely as possible. An isometric contraction is being performed at that angle.
3. After about five or six seconds of isometric contraction, the muscles being stretched are relaxed completely. The assistant then increases the degree of stretch slowly to a greater angle.

4. The isometric contraction is repeated, following which the muscle(s) is relaxed again. The assistant then can increase the degree of stretch slowly one more time.
5. Steps 1 through 4 are repeated two to five times, until the exerciser feels mild discomfort. On the last trial, the final stretched position should be held for 15 to 30 seconds.
6. Theoretically, with the PNF technique, the isometric contraction helps relax the muscle(s) being stretched, which results in longer muscles. Some fitness leaders believe PNF is more effective than slow-sustained stretching.

Another benefit of PNF is an increase in strength of the muscle(s) being stretched. Research has shown approximately 17 and 35 percent increases in absolute strength and muscular endurance, respectively, following 12 weeks of PNF stretching. These increases are attributed to the isometric contractions performed during PNF. The disadvantages are that more pain occurs with PNF, a second person is

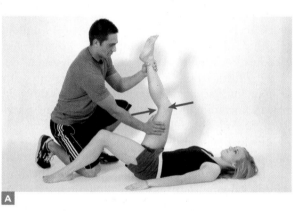

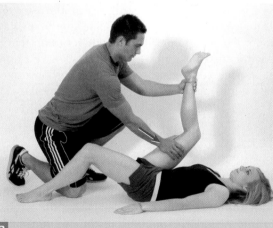

Photos © Fitness & Wellness, Inc.

Proprioceptive neuromuscular facilitation (PNF) stretching technique: (A) isometric phase, (B) stretching phase.

required to assist, and more time is needed to conduct each session.

Intensity of Exercise

When you do flexibility exercises, the **intensity** of each stretch should be only to a point of mild discomfort. Excessive pain is an indication that the load is too high and may lead to injury. All stretching should be done to slightly below the pain threshold. As participants reach this point, they should try to relax the muscle being stretched as much as possible. After completing the stretch, the body part is brought back gradually to the starting point.

Repetitions

The time required for a flexibility exercise session is based on the number of repetitions performed and the length of time each repetition (final stretched position) is held. The general recommendation is that each exercise be done at least four times, holding the final position each time for 15 to 30 seconds. Stretching for 15 to 30 seconds is better to increase range of motion than stretching for shorter periods of time and is just as effective as stretching for longer durations. Individuals who are susceptible to flexibility injuries should limit each stretch to 20 seconds. For these individuals, Pilates exercises are recommended because they increase joint stability (see the discussion on the Pilates exercise system on page 80 in this chapter).

Frequency of Exercise

Flexibility exercises should be conducted a minimum of two or three days per week, but ideally five to seven days per week. After six to eight weeks of almost daily stretching, flexibility can be maintained with only two or three sessions per week, doing about three repetitions of 15 to 30 seconds each. Figure 3.5 summarizes the flexibility development guidelines.

When to Stretch?

Many people do not differentiate a warm-up from stretching. Warming up means starting a workout slowly with walking, cycling, or slow jogging, followed by gentle stretching (not through the entire range of motion). Stretching implies movement of joints through their full range of motion and holding the final degree of stretch according to recommended guidelines.

A warm-up that progressively increases muscle temperature and mimics movement that will occur

FIGURE 3.5

Flexibility development guidelines.

Mode:	A static stretching routine that includes every major joint of the body and focuses on joints that have a decreased range of motion
Intensity:	Stretch to end of range of motion to the point of mild discomfort
Repetitions:	2 to 4 repetitions of each stretch and hold the final stretched position for 15 to 30 seconds
Frequency:	A minimum of 3 days per week (ideally 5 to 7 days per week)

American College of Sports Medicine, *Guidelines for Exercise Testing and Prescription* (Philadelphia: Lippincott Williams & Wilkins, 2006).

during training enhances performance. For some activities, gentle stretching is recommended in conjunction with warm-up routines. Before steady activities (walking, jogging, cycling), a warm-up of 3 to 5 minutes is recommended. The recommendation is up to 10 minutes before stop-and-go activities (for example, racquet sports, basketball, soccer) and athletic participation in general (for example, football, gymnastics). Activities that require abrupt changes in direction are more likely to cause muscle strains if they are performed without proper warm-up that includes mild stretching.

Sport-specific pre-exercise stretching can improve performance in sports that require a greater than average range of motion, such as gymnastics, dance, swimming, diving, hurdling, and figure skating. Some evidence, however, suggests that intense stretching during warm-up can lead to a temporary, short-term (up to 60 minutes) decrease in strength. Thus, extensive stretching conducted prior to participating in

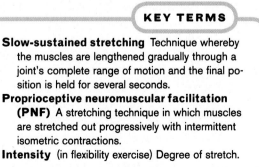

KEY TERMS

Slow-sustained stretching Technique whereby the muscles are lengthened gradually through a joint's complete range of motion and the final position is held for several seconds.

Proprioceptive neuromuscular facilitation (PNF) A stretching technique in which muscles are stretched out progressively with intermittent isometric contractions.

Intensity (in flexibility exercise) Degree of stretch.

athletic events that rely on strength and power for peak performance is not recommended.[19,20]

In terms of preventing injuries, the best time to stretch is controversial. In limited studies on athletic populations, the evidence is unclear as to whether stretching before or after exercise is more beneficial in preventing injury. Additional research is necessary to clarify this issue.

In general, a good time to stretch is after aerobic workouts. Higher body temperature in itself helps to increase the joint range of motion. Muscles also are fatigued following exercise, and a fatigued muscle tends to shorten, which can lead to soreness and spasms. Stretching exercises help fatigued muscles reestablish their normal resting length and prevent unnecessary pain.

Designing a Flexibility Program

To improve body flexibility, each major muscle group should be subjected to at least one stretching exercise. A complete set of exercises for developing muscular flexibility is presented in Appendix B.

You may not be able to hold a final stretched position with some of these exercises (such as lateral head tilts and arm circles), but you still should perform the exercise through the joint's full range of motion. Depending on the number and the length of repetitions, a complete workout will last between 15 and 30 minutes.

CRITICAL THINKING

Carefully consider the relevance of stretching exercises in your personal fitness program throughout the years. • How much importance do you place on these exercises? • Have any conditions improved through your stretching program or have any specific exercises contributed to your health and well-being?

Pilates Exercise System

Pilates exercises have become increasingly popular in recent years. Previously, Pilates training was used primarily by dancers, but now many fitness participants, rehab patients, models, actors, and even professional athletes are embracing this exercise modality. Pilates studios, college courses, and classes at health clubs now are available nationwide.

The Pilates training system was originally developed in the 1920s by German physical therapist Joseph Pilates. The exercises are designed to help strengthen the body's core by developing pelvic stability and abdominal control—coupled with focused breathing patterns. Pilates exercises are performed either on a mat (floor) or with specialized equipment to help increase strength and flexibility of deep postural muscles. The intent is to improve muscle tone and length (providing a limber body), instead of increasing muscle size (hypertrophy). The exercises are performed in a slow, controlled, precise manner. Properly performed, Pilates exercises require intense concentration. Initial Pilates training should be conducted under the supervision of certified instructors with extensive Pilates teaching experience.

Fitness goals of Pilates programs include improved flexibility, muscle tone, posture, spinal support, body balance, low back health, sports performance, and mind-body awareness. The Pilates program also is used to help lose weight, increase lean tissue, and manage stress. Although Pilates programs are popular, research is required to corroborate the benefits attributed to this training system.

Preventing and Rehabilitating Low Back Pain

Few people make it through life without having low back pain at some point. An estimated 60 to 80 percent of all Americans will suffer from chronic back pain in their lives. On a yearly basis, more than 75 million people report having chronic low back pain.

Back pain is considered chronic if it persists longer than three months. About 80 percent of the time, backache syndrome is preventable and is caused by (a) physical inactivity, (b) poor postural habits and body mechanics, (c) excessive body weight, and/or (d) psychological stress. Data also indicate that back injuries are more common among smokers.

Although people tend to think of back pain as a skeletal problem, the spine's curvature, alignment, and movement are controlled by surrounding muscles. Lack of physical activity is the most common reason for chronic low back pain. A major contributor to back pain is sitting for long periods, which causes back muscles to shorten, stiffen, and become weaker.

Deterioration or weakening of the abdominal and gluteal muscles, along with tightening of the lower back (erector spinae) muscles, brings about an unnatural forward tilt of the pelvis (see Figure 3.6). This tilt puts extra pressure on the spinal vertebrae, causing pain in the lower back. Accumulation of fat around the midsection of the body contributes to the forward tilt of the pelvis, which further aggravates the condition.

Low back pain is frequently associated with faulty posture and improper body mechanics or body positions in all of life's daily activities, including sleeping, sitting, standing, walking, driving, working, and exercising. Incorrect posture and poor mechanics, as explained in Figure 3.7, increase strain on the lower back as well as many other bones, joints, muscles, and ligaments.

Back pain can be reduced greatly by including some specific stretching and strengthening exercises in the regular fitness program. In most cases, back pain is present only with movement and physical activity. If the pain is severe and persists even at rest, the first step is to consult a physician, who can rule out any disc damage and may prescribe proper bed rest using several pillows under the knees for leg support (see Figure 3.7). This position helps release muscle spasms by stretching the muscles involved. In addition, a physician may prescribe a muscle relaxant or anti-inflammatory medication (or both) and some type of physical therapy.

In most cases of low back pain, even with severe pain, people feel better within days or weeks without treatment from health care professionals.[21] To relieve symptoms, you may use over-the-counter pain relievers and hot or cold packs. You should also stay active to avoid further weakening of the back muscles. Low-impact activities like walking, swimming, water aerobics, and cycling are recommended. Once you are pain free in the resting state, you need to start correcting the muscular imbalance by stretching the tight muscles and strengthening the weak ones. Stretching exercises always are performed first.

If there is no indication of disease or injury, such as leg numbness or pain, a herniated disc, or fractures, spinal manipulation by a chiropractor or other health care professional can provide pain relief. Spinal manipulation as a treatment modality for low back pain has been endorsed by the Federal Agency for Health Care Policy and Research. The guidelines suggest that spinal manipulation may help to alleviate discomfort and pain during the first few weeks of an acute episode of low back pain. Generally, benefits are seen within 10 treatments. People who have had chronic pain for more than six months should avoid spinal manipulation until they have been thoroughly examined by a physician.

Back pain can be reduced greatly through aerobic exercise, muscular flexibility exercise, and muscular strength and endurance training that includes specific exercises to strengthen the spine-stabilizing muscles. Exercise requires effort by the patient, and it may create discomfort initially, but exercise promotes circulation, healing, muscle size, and muscle strength and endurance. Many patients abstain from aggressive physical therapy because they are unwilling to commit the time required for the program.

Aerobic exercise is beneficial because it helps decrease body fat and psychological stress. During an episode of back pain, however, people often avoid activity and cope by getting more rest. Rest is recommended if the pain is associated with a herniated disc, but if your physician rules out a serious problem, exercise is a better choice of treatment. Exercise helps restore physical function, and individuals who start and maintain an aerobic exercise program have back pain less frequently. Individuals who exercise also are less likely to require surgery or other invasive treatments.

FIGURE 3.6

Incorrect (left) and correct (right) pelvic alignment.

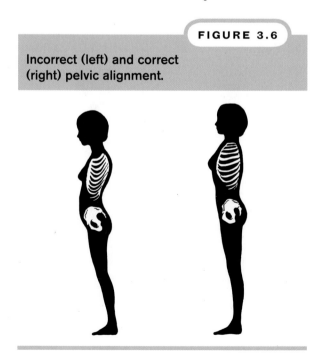

KEY TERMS

Pilates Exercises that help strengthen the body's core by developing pelvic stability and abdominal control coupled with focused breathing patterns.

FIGURE 3.7

Your back and how to care for it.

HOW TO STAY ON YOUR FEET WITHOUT TIRING YOUR BACK

To prevent strain and pain in everyday activities, it is restful to change from one task to another before fatigue sets in. You can lie down between chores; you should check body position frequently, drawing in the abdomen, flattening the back, bending the knees slightly.

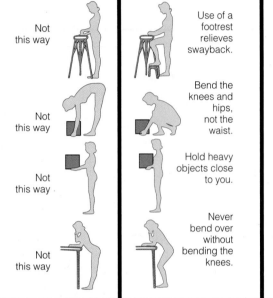

Not this way

Not this way

Not this way

Not this way

Use of a footrest relieves swayback.

Bend the knees and hips, not the waist.

Hold heavy objects close to you.

Never bend over without bending the knees.

HOW TO PUT YOUR BACK TO BED

For proper bed posture, a firm mattress is essential. Bedboards, sold commercially, or devised at home, may be used with soft mattresses. Bedboards, preferably, should be made of ¾-inch plywood. Faulty sleeping positions intensify swayback and result not only in backache but in numbness, tingling, and pain in arms and legs.

Incorrect:
Lying flat on back makes swayback worse.
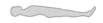

Use of high pillow strains neck, arms, shoulders.

Sleeping face down exaggerates swayback, strains neck and shoulders.

Bending one hip and knee does not relieve swayback.

Correct:
Lying on side with knees bent effectively flattens the back. Flat pillow may be used to support neck, especially when shoulders are broad.

Sleeping on back is restful and correct when knees are properly supported.
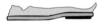

Raise the foot of the mattress eight inches to discourage sleeping on the abdomen.
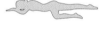

Proper arrangement of pillows for resting or reading in bed.

HOW TO SIT CORRECTLY

A back's best friend is a straight, hard chair. If you can't get the chair you prefer, learn to sit properly on whatever chair you get. To correct sitting position from forward slump: Throw head well back, then bend it forward to pull in the chin. This will straighten the back. Now tighten abdominal muscles to raise the chest. Check position frequently.

Use of footrest relieves swayback. Aim is to have knees higher than hips.

Correct way to sit while driving, close to pedals. Use seat belt or hard backrest, available commercially.

TV slump leads to "dowager's hump," strains neck and shoulders.

If chair is too high, swayback is increased.

Keep neck and back in as straight a line as possible with the spine. Bend forward from hips.

Driver's seat too far from pedals emphasizes curve in lower back.

Strained reading position. Forward thrusting strains muscles of neck and head.

In terms of flexibility, regular stretching exercises that help the hip and trunk go through a functional range of motion, rather than increasing the range of motion, are recommended. That is, for proper back care, stretching exercises should not be performed to the extreme range of motion. Individuals with a greater spinal range of motion also have a higher incidence of back injury. Spinal stability, instead of mobility, is desirable for back health.[22]

Several exercises for preventing and rehabilitating the backache syndrome are given in Appendix C, pages 269–270. These exercises can be done twice or more daily when a person has back pain. Under normal circumstances, doing these exercises three to four times a week is enough to prevent the syndrome.

Psychological stress may also lead to back pain. Excessive stress causes muscles to contract. In the case of the lower back, frequent tightening of the muscles can throw the back out of alignment and constrict blood vessels that supply oxygen and nutrients to the back. If you suffer from excessive stress and back pain at the same time, proper stress management (see Chapter 7) should be a part of your comprehensive back-care program.

Contraindicated Exercises

Most strength and flexibility exercises are relatively safe to perform, but even safe exercises can be hazardous if they are done incorrectly. Some exercises may be safe for you to perform occasionally but, when executed repeatedly, could cause trauma and injury. Preexisting muscle or joint conditions (old sprains or injuries) can further increase the risk of harm when performing certain exercises. As you develop your exercise program, you are encouraged to follow the exercise descriptions and guidelines given in this book.

A few exercises are not recommended because they pose a potentially high risk for injury. These exercises are sometimes performed in videotaped workouts and some fitness classes. **Contraindicated exercises** may cause harm because of the excessive strain placed on muscles and joints—in particular, the spine, lower back, knees, neck, and shoulders.

Illustrations of contraindicated exercises are presented in Appendix D. Safe alternative exercises are listed below each contraindicated exercise and are illustrated in Appendix A (strength exercises) pages 258–266, and Appendix B (flexibility exercises),

pages 267–268. In isolated instances, a qualified physical therapist may select one or a few of the contraindicated exercises to treat a certain injury or disability in a carefully supervised setting. Unless you are instructed specifically to use one of these exercises, it is best that you select safe exercises from this book.

Getting Started

Introducing new behaviors into one's daily routine takes most people months or longer to accomplish. A fitness program is no exception. Adding exercise to a person's lifestyle may require retraining (behavior modification).

Different things motivate different people to start and remain in a fitness program. Regardless of your initial reason for initiating an exercise program, you now need to plan for ways to make your workout fun. The psychology behind it is simple: If you enjoy an activity, you will continue to do it.

The first few weeks probably will be the most difficult, but where there's a will, there's a way. Once you begin to see positive changes, it won't be as hard. Soon you will develop a habit for exercise that will be deeply satisfying and will bring about a sense of self-accomplishment. The suggestions in the Behavior Modification Planning box have been used by people to help them change behavior and adhere to a lifetime exercise program.

While fitness evaluation is important to assess changes in physical capacity, attention must be given to actual program compliance. Regular physical activity is the key to better health and quality of life (see "Health Fitness Standard" in Chapter 2, pages 29–30). Exercise logs provide the means to carefully document your participation in fitness programs and allow you to monitor your progress and compare it against previous months and years. Activity 3.4, pages 95–98, contains exercise log sheets to monitor your cardiorespiratory endurance, muscular strength, and muscular flexibility programs. You are strongly encouraged to keep a detailed record of all of your activities.

KEY TERMS

Contraindicated exercises Exercises that are not recommended because they pose potentially high risk for injury.

Tips to Enhance Compliance with Your Fitness Program

1. Set aside a regular time for exercise. If you don't plan ahead, it is a lot easier to skip. On a weekly basis, using red ink, schedule your exercise time into your day planner. Next, hold your exercise hour "sacred." Give exercise priority equal to the most important school or business activity of the day.

   If you are too busy, attempt to accumulate 30 to 60 minutes of daily activity by doing separate 10-minute sessions throughout the day. Try reading the mail while you walk, taking stairs instead of elevators, walking the dog, or riding the stationary bike as you watch the evening news.

2. Exercise early in the day, when you will be less tired and the chances of something interfering with your workout are minimal; thus, you will be less likely to skip your exercise session.

3. Select aerobic activities you enjoy. Exercise should be as much fun as your favorite hobby. If you pick an activity you don't enjoy, you will be unmotivated and less likely to keep exercising. Don't be afraid to try out a new activity, even if that means learning new skills.

4. Combine different activities. You can train by doing two or three different activities the same week. This **cross-training** may reduce the monotony of repeating the same activity every day. Try lifetime sports. Many endurance sports, such as racquetball, basketball, soccer, badminton, roller skating, cross-country skiing, and body surfing (paddling the board), provide a nice break from regular workouts.

5. Use the proper clothing and equipment for exercise. A poor pair of shoes, for example, can make you more prone to injury, discouraging you from the beginning.

6. Find a friend or group of friends to exercise with. Social interaction will make exercise more fulfilling. Besides, exercise is harder to skip if someone is waiting to go with you.

7. Set goals and share them with others. Quitting is tougher when someone else knows what you are trying to accomplish. When you reach a targeted goal, reward yourself with a new pair of shoes or a jogging suit.

8. Purchase a pedometer (step counter) and build up to 10,000 steps per day. These 10,000 steps may in-clude all forms of daily physical activity combined. Pedometers motivate people toward activity because they track daily activity, provide feedback on activity level, and remind the participant to enhance daily activity.

9. Don't become a chronic exerciser. Overexercising can lead to chronic fatigue and injuries. Exercise should be enjoyable, and in the process you should stop and smell the roses.

10. Exercise in different places and facilities. This will add variety to your workouts.

11. Exercise to music. People who listen to fast-tempo music tend to exercise more vigorously and longer. Using headphones when exercising outdoors, however, can be dangerous. Even indoors, it is preferable not to use headphones so you still can be aware of your surroundings.

12. Keep a regular record of your activities. Keeping a record allows you to monitor your progress and compare it against previous months and years (see Activity 3.4, page 96).

13. Conduct periodic assessments. Improving to a higher fitness category is often a reward in itself, and creating your own rewards is even more motivating.

14. Listen to your body. If you experience pain or unusual discomfort, stop exercising. Pain and aches are an indication of potential injury. If you do suffer an injury, don't return to your regular workouts until you are fully recovered. You may cross-train using activities that don't aggravate your injury (for instance, swimming instead of jogging).

15. If a health problem arises, see a physician. When in doubt, it's better to be safe than sorry.

Try It

The most difficult challenge about exercise is to keep going once you start. The above behavioral change tips will enhance your chances for exercise adherence. In your Online Journal or class notebook, describe which suggestions were most useful in helping you stick to your exercise program and why they are so effective for you.

Setting Fitness Goals

Before you leave this chapter, consider your fitness goals. In the last few decades we have become accustomed to "quick fixes," with everything from super fast foods to one-hour dry cleaning. Fitness, however, has no quick fix. Fitness takes time and dedication, and only those who are committed and persistent will reap the rewards. As described in Chapter 1, setting realistic fitness goals will guide your program. Activity 3.4, page 95, offers a goal-setting form that will help you determine your fit-ness goals. Take the time, either by yourself or with your instructor's help, to fill it out.

As you prepare to write realistic fitness goals, base them on the results of your initial fitness test (pre-test). For instance, if your cardiorespiratory fitness category was "poor" on the pre-test, you should not expect to improve to the "excellent" category in a little more than three months. Whenever possible, your fitness goals should be measurable and time specific. A goal that simply states "to improve my cardiorespiratory endurance" is not as good as a goal that states "to improve to the 'good' fitness

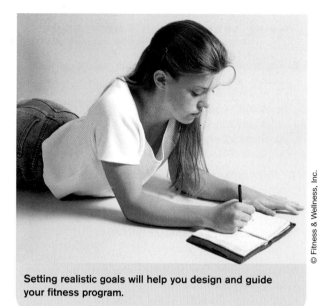

Setting realistic goals will help you design and guide your fitness program.

© Fitness & Wellness, Inc.

your goal. A sample of objectives to accomplish the previously stated goal for development of cardiorespiratory endurance could be:

1. Use jogging as the mode of exercise.
2. Jog at 10:00 a.m. five times per week.
3. Jog around the track in the field house.
4. Jog for 30 minutes each exercise session.
5. Monitor heart rate regularly during exercise.
6. Take the 1.5-Mile Run Test once a month.

You will not always meet your specific objectives. If this happens often, your goal may be out of reach. Reevaluate your objectives and make adjustments accordingly. If you set unrealistic goals at the beginning of your exercise program, be flexible with yourself and reconsider your plan of action, but do not quit. Reconsidering your plan of action does not mean that you have failed. Failure comes only to those who stop trying, and success comes to those who are committed and persistent.

category in cardiorespiratory endurance by April 15" or "to run the 1.5-mile course in less than 11 minutes the week of final exams."

After determining each goal, monitor your progress toward it regularly. You also will need to write measurable objectives to accomplish it. These objectives will be the actual plan of action to accomplish

KEY TERMS

Cross-training Using a combination of different aerobic activities to develop or maintain cardiorespiratory endurance.

www WEB INTERACTIVE

Strength Training Muscle Map & Explanation. This site provides an anatomical map of the body's muscles. Click on the muscle for exercises designed to specifically strengthen that particular muscle, complete with a video and safety information.
http://www.global-fitness.com/strength/s_musclemap.php

Sport-Fitness Advisor. This site provides a battery of fitness tests. Click on "Flexibility Tests" for the Sit-and-Reach Test, Trunk Rotation Test, or Groin Flexibility Test.
http://www.sport-fitness-advisor.com/fitnesstests.html

ASSESS YOUR BEHAVIOR

CENGAGENOW

*Log on to **academic.cengage.com/login** and take a wellness inventory to assess the behaviors that might benefit most from healthy change.*

1. Do you accumulate at least 30 minutes of moderate- (or high-)intensity physical activity a minimum of five days per week?

2. Do you participate in a vigorous-intensity aerobic exercise program for a minimum of 20 minutes at least three times per week?

3. Do you engage in an overall strength-training program in which you perform at least one set of 3 to 20 repetitions to near fatigue, using 8 to 10 dynamic exercises that involve the major muscle groups of the body, a minimum of two times per week?

4. Does your exercise program include stretching all major joints of the body a minimum of three times per week?

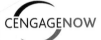

*Log on to **academic.cengage.com/login** to assess your understanding of this chapter's topics by taking the chapter pre-test and exploring the modules recommended in your Personalized Study Plan.*

1. The optimal or high-intensity cardiorespiratory training zone for a 22-year-old individual with a resting heart rate of 68 bpm is
   a. 120 to 148.
   b. 132 to 156.
   c. 138 to 164.
   d. 146 to 179.
   e. 154 to 188.

2. Which of the following activities does *not* contribute to the development of cardiorespiratory endurance?
   a. Low-impact aerobics
   b. Jogging
   c. 400-yard dash
   d. Racquetball
   e. All of the activities contribute to its development.

3. The recommended duration for each cardiorespiratory training session is
   a. 10 to 20 minutes.
   b. 15 to 30 minutes.
   c. 20 to 60 minutes.
   d. 45 to 70 minutes.
   e. 60 to 120 minutes.

4. During an eccentric muscle contraction,
   a. the muscle shortens as it overcomes the resistance.
   b. there is little or no movement during the contraction.
   c. a joint has to move through the entire range of motion.
   d. the muscle lengthens as it contracts.
   e. the speed is kept constant throughout the range of motion.

5. The training concept that states that the demands placed on a system must be increased systematically and progressively over time to cause physiological adaptation is referred to as
   a. the overload principle.
   b. positive-resistance training.
   c. specificity of training.
   d. variable-resistance training.
   e. progressive resistance.

6. For health fitness during strength training, each set should be performed between
   a. 1 and 6 reps maximum.
   b. 4 and 10 reps maximum.
   c. 3 and 20 reps maximum.
   d. 8 and 20 reps maximum.
   e. 10 and 30 reps maximum.

7. Which of the following is *not* a mode of stretching?
   a. Proprioceptive neuromuscular facilitation
   b. Elastic elongation
   c. Ballistic stretching
   d. Slow-sustained stretching
   e. All are modes of stretching.

8. When you perform stretching exercises, the degree of stretch should be
   a. through the entire arc of movement.
   b. to about 80 percent of capacity.
   c. to the point of mild discomfort.
   d. applied until the muscle(s) start shaking.
   e. progressively increased until the desired stretch is attained.

9. Low back pain is associated with
   a. physical inactivity.
   b. faulty posture.
   c. excessive body weight.
   d. improper body mechanics.
   e. All are correct choices.

10. A goal is effective when it is
    a. written.
    b. measurable.
    c. time specific.
    d. monitored.
    e. All are correct choices.

Correct answers can be found at the back of the book.

Daily Physical Activity Log

Name _____ Date _____

Course _____ Section _____

Date: [_____] Day of the Week: [_____]

Time of Day	Exercise/Activity	Duration	Number of Steps	Comments
[ ]	[ ]	[ ]	[ ]	[ ]
[ ]	[ ]	[ ]	[ ]	[ ]
[ ]	[ ]	[ ]	[ ]	[ ]
[ ]	[ ]	[ ]	[ ]	[ ]
[ ]	[ ]	[ ]	[ ]	[ ]
[ ]	[ ]	[ ]	[ ]	[ ]
[ ]	[ ]	[ ]	[ ]	[ ]
Totals:			[ ]	[ ]

Activity category based on steps per day (use Table 3.1, page 62): [_____]

Date: [_____] Day of the Week: [_____]

Time of Day	Exercise/Activity	Duration	Number of Steps	Comments
[ ]	[ ]	[ ]	[ ]	[ ]
[ ]	[ ]	[ ]	[ ]	[ ]
[ ]	[ ]	[ ]	[ ]	[ ]
[ ]	[ ]	[ ]	[ ]	[ ]
[ ]	[ ]	[ ]	[ ]	[ ]
[ ]	[ ]	[ ]	[ ]	[ ]
[ ]	[ ]	[ ]	[ ]	[ ]
Totals:			[ ]	[ ]

Activity category based on steps per day (use Table 3.1, page 62): [_____]

Date: _____ Day of the Week: _____

Time of Day	Exercise/Activity	Duration	Number of Steps	Comments
Totals:				

Activity category based on steps per day (use Table 3.1, page 62): _____

Date: _____ Day of the Week: _____

Time of Day	Exercise/Activity	Duration	Number of Steps	Comments
Totals:				

Activity category based on steps per day (use Table 3.1, page 62): _____

Briefly evaluate your current activity patterns, discuss your feelings about the results, and provide a goal for the weeks ahead.

_____

_____

_____

_____

Exercise Readiness

Name _____ Date _____

Course _____ Section _____

List advantages of starting an exercise program.

1. _____

2. _____

3. _____

4. _____

5. _____

6. _____

7. _____

8. _____

9. _____

10. _____

List disadvantages of starting an exercise program.

1. _____

2. _____

3. _____

4. _____

5. _____

6. _____

7. _____

8. _____

9. _____

10. _____

Instructions

Carefully read each statement and circle the number that best describes your feelings in each statement. Please be completely honest with your answers.

	Strongly Agree	Mildly Agree	Mildly Disagree	Strongly Disagree
1. I can walk, ride a bike (or a wheelchair), swim, or walk in a shallow pool.	4	3	2	1
2. I enjoy exercise.	4	3	2	1
3. I believe exercise can help decrease the risk for disease and premature mortality.	4	3	2	1
4. I believe exercise contributes to better health.	4	3	2	1
5. I have previously participated in an exercise program.	4	3	2	1
6. I have experienced the feeling of being physically fit.	4	3	2	1
7. I can envision myself exercising.	4	3	2	1
8. I am contemplating an exercise program.	4	3	2	1
9. I am willing to stop contemplating and give exercise a try for a few weeks.	4	3	2	1
10. I am willing to set aside time at least three times a week for exercise.	4	3	2	1
11. I can find a place to exercise (the streets, a park, a YMCA, a health club).	4	3	2	1
12. I can find other people who would like to exercise with me.	4	3	2	1
13. I will exercise when I am moody, fatigued, and even when the weather is bad.	4	3	2	1
14. I am willing to spend a small amount of money for adequate exercise clothing (shoes, shorts, leotards, or swimsuit).	4	3	2	1
15. If I have any doubts about my present state of health, I will see a physician before beginning an exercise program.	4	3	2	1
16. Exercise will make me feel better and improve my quality of life.	4	3	2	1

Scoring Your Test:

This questionnaire allows you to examine your readiness for exercise. You have been evaluated in four categories: mastery (self-control), attitude, health, and commitment. Mastery indicates that you can be in control of your exercise program. Attitude examines your mental disposition toward exercise. Health provides evidence of the wellness benefits of exercise. Commitment shows dedication and resolution to carry out the exercise program. Write the number you circled after each statement in the corresponding spaces below. Add the scores on each line to get your totals. Scores can vary from 4 to 16. A score of 12 and above is a strong indicator that that factor is important to you, and 8 and below is low. If you score 12 or more points in each category, your chances of initiating and adhering to an exercise program are good. If you fail to score at least 12 points in three categories, your chances of succeeding at exercise may be slim. You need to be better informed about the benefits of exercise, and a retraining process may be required.

Mastery: 1. _____ + 5. _____ + 6. _____ + 9. _____ = _____

Attitude: 2. _____ + 7. _____ + 8. _____ + 13. _____ = _____

Health: 3. _____ + 4. _____ + 15. _____ + 16. _____ = _____

Commitment: 10. _____ + 11. _____ + 12. _____ + 14. _____ = _____

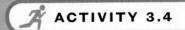

Goal-Setting Form and Exercise Logs

Name _____ Date _____

Course _____ Section _____

I. Instructions

Indicate your general goal for the four health-related components of fitness and write the specific objectives you will use to accomplish these goals in the next few weeks.

Cardiorespiratory endurance goal: _____

Specific objectives:

1. _____

2. _____

3. _____

Muscular strength/endurance goal: _____

Specific objectives:

1. _____

2. _____

3. _____

Muscular flexibility goal: _____

Specific objectives:

1. _____

2. _____

3. _____

Body composition goal: _____

Specific objectives:

1. _____

2. _____

3. _____

_____ _____

My signature   Witness signature

_____ _____

Today's date   Date of completion

II. Aerobic Exercise Log

Date	Body Weight	Exercise Heart Rate	Type of Exercise	Distance in Miles	Time Hrs./Min.	Daily Steps*
1						
2						
3						
4						
5						
6						
7						
8						
9						
10						
11						
12						
13						
14						
15						
16						
17						
18						
19						
20						
21						
22						
23						
24						
25						
26						
27						
28						
29						
30						
31						
			Total			

*Daily steps can be determined using a pedometer.

Exercise Logs CONTINUED

Name _____ Course _____ Section _____

III. Strength-Training Log

Date Exercise	St/Reps/Res*	St/Reps/Res*	St/Reps/Res*	St/Reps/Res*	St/Reps/Res*	St/Reps/Res*	St/Reps/Res*

*St/Reps/Res = Sets, Repetitions, and Resistance (e.g., 1/6/125 = 1 set of 6 repetitions with 125 pounds)

Name _____   Course _____   Section _____

III. Strength-Training Log

Date							
Exercise	St/Reps/Res*	St/Reps/Res*	St/Reps/Res*	St/Reps/Res*	St/Reps/Res*	St/Reps/Res*	St/Reps/Res*

*St/Reps/Res = Sets, Repetitions, and Resistance (e.g., 1/6/125 = 1 set of 6 repetitions with 125 pounds)

Evaluating Fitness Activities

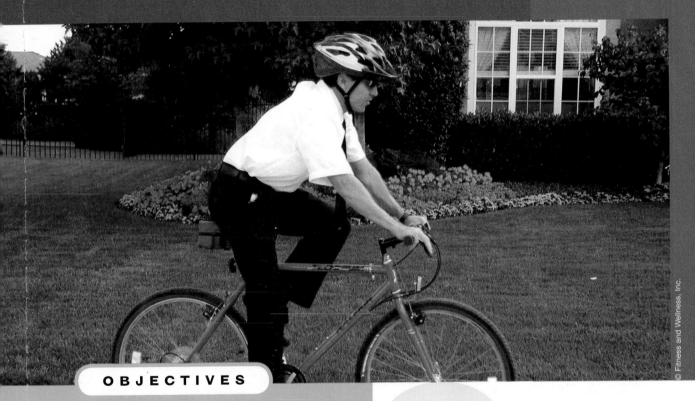

OBJECTIVES

- Learn the benefits and advantages of selected aerobic activities
- Learn to rate the fitness benefits of aerobic activities
- Evaluate the contributions of skill-related fitness activities
- Understand the sequence of a standard aerobic workout
- Learn ways to enhance your aerobic workouts

CENGAGENOW Log on to **CengageNOW** at academic .cengage.com/login to find innovative study tools—including pre- and post-tests, personalized study plans, activities, labs, and the personal change planner.

One of the fun aspects of exercise is the sheer variety of activities promoting fitness that are available to you. You can select one or a combination of activities for your program—your choice should be based on personal enjoyment, convenience, and availability. A summary of the most popular physical activities in the United States and the percentage of adults who participate in them is presented in Figure 4.1.

Aerobic Activities

Most people who exercise pick and adhere to a single mode, such as walking, swimming, or jogging. Yet, no single activity develops total fitness. Many activities contribute to cardiorespiratory development, but the extent of contribution to other fitness components is limited and varies among the activities. For total fitness, aerobic activities should be supplemented with strength and flexibility exercises. Cross-training can add enjoyment to the program, decrease the risk for incurring injuries from overuse, and keep exercise from becoming monotonous.

Exercise sessions should be convenient. To enjoy exercise, you should select a time when you will not be rushed and a location that is nearby. People do not enjoy driving across town to get to the gym, health club, track, or pool. If parking is a problem, you may get discouraged quickly and quit. All of these factors can supply excuses not to stick to an exercise program.

Walking

The most natural, easiest, safest, and least expensive form of aerobic exercise is walking. For years, many fitness practitioners believed that walking was not vigorous enough to improve cardiorespiratory functioning, but brisk walking at speeds of 4 miles per hour or faster does improve cardiorespiratory fitness. From a health fitness viewpoint, a regular walking program can prolong life significantly (see the discussion of cardiovascular diseases in Chapter 8). Although walking obviously takes longer than jogging, the caloric cost of brisk walking is only about 10 percent lower than jogging the same distance.

Walking is perhaps the best activity to start a conditioning program for the cardiorespiratory system.

FIGURE 4.1

Most popular adult physical activities in the United States.

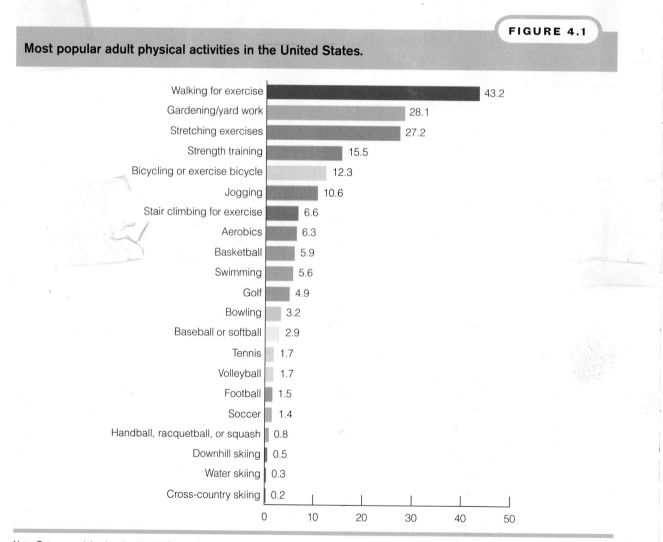

Note: Data are weighted to the 1998 U.S. population and age-adjusted to the year 2000 population standard. "Participation" = activity reported as being done at least once during the past 2 weeks.

SOURCE: Centers for Disease Control and Prevention, National Health Interview Survey (NHIS), 1998, Atlanta.

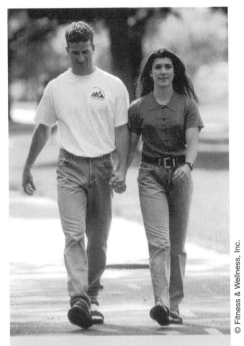

Walking is the most natural aerobic physical activity.

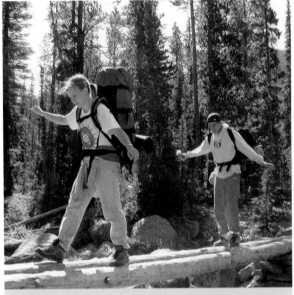

An 8-hour hike can burn as many calories as a 20-mile walk or jog.

Inactive people should start with 1-mile walks four or five times per week. Walk times can be increased gradually by 5 minutes each week. Following three to four weeks of conditioning, a person should be able to walk 2 miles at a 4-mile-per-hour pace, five times per week. Greater aerobic benefits accrue from walking longer and swinging the arms faster than normal. Light handweights, a backpack (4 to 6 pounds), or tension belts that add load to the upper body (arms) also add to the intensity of walking. Because of the additional load on the cardiorespiratory system, extra weights or loads are not recommended for people who have or are at risk for cardiovascular disease.

Walking in chest-deep water is an excellent form of aerobic activity, particularly for people who have leg and back problems. Because of the buoyancy of water, individuals submerged in water to armpit level weigh only about 10 to 20 percent of their weight outside the water. The resistance the water creates as a person walks in the pool adds to the intensity of the activity and provides a good cardiorespiratory workout.

Hiking

Hiking is an excellent activity for the entire family, especially during the summer and on summer vacations. Many people feel guilty if they are unable to continue their exercise routine during vacations.

The intensity of hiking over uneven terrain is greater than walking. An eight-hour hike can burn as many calories as a 20-mile walk or jog.

Another benefit of hiking is the relaxing effects of beautiful scenery. This is an ideal activity for highly stressed people who live near woods and hills. A rough day at the office can fade quickly in the peacefulness and beauty of the outdoors.

Jogging

Next to walking, jogging is one of the most accessible forms of exercise. A person can find places to jog almost everywhere. The lone requirement to prevent injuries is a good pair of jogging shoes.

The popularity of jogging in the United States started shortly after publication of Dr. Kenneth Cooper's first *Aerobics* book in 1968. Jim Fixx's *Complete Book of Running* in the mid-1970s contributed further to the phenomenal growth of jogging as a fitness activity in the United States.

Jogging three to five times a week is one of the fastest ways to improve cardiorespiratory fitness. The risk for injury, however—especially in beginners—is higher with jogging than walking. For proper conditioning, jogging programs should start with one to two weeks of walking. As fitness improves, walking and jogging can be combined, gradually increasing the jogging segment until it fills the full 20 to 30 minutes.

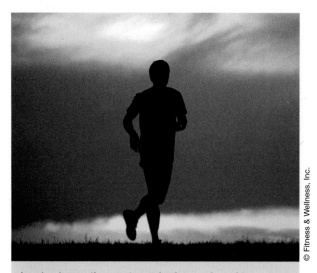

Jogging is one the most popular forms of aerobic exercise.

© Fitness & Wellness, Inc.

Many people abuse this activity. People run too fast and too long. Some joggers think that if a little is good, more is better. Not so with cardiorespiratory endurance. As indicated under "Frequency of Exercise" on page 69 in Chapter 3, the aerobic benefit of training more than 30 minutes five times per week is minimal. Furthermore, the risk for injury increases greatly as speed (running instead of jogging) and mileage go up. Jogging approximately 15 miles per week is sufficient to reach an excellent level of cardiorespiratory fitness.

A good pair of shoes is a must for joggers. Many foot, knee, and leg problems originate from improperly fitted or worn-out shoes. A good pair of shoes should offer lateral stability and not lean to either side when placed on a flat surface. The shoe also should bend at the ball of the foot, not at midfoot. Worn-out shoes should be replaced. After 500 miles of use, jogging shoes lose about a third of their shock absorption capabilities. If you suddenly have problems, check your shoes first. It may be time for a new pair.

An alternative form of jogging, especially for injured people, those with chronic back problems, and overweight individuals, is deep-water running. This entails running in place while treading water and is almost as strenuous as jogging on land. The running motions used on land are accentuated by pumping the arms and legs hard through the full range of motion. The participant usually wears a flotation vest to help maintain the body in an upright position. Many elite athletes train in water to lessen the wear and tear on the body caused by long-

distance running. These athletes have been able to maintain high oxygen uptake values through rigorous water running programs.

For safety reasons, joggers (and walkers) should follow these precautions:

1. Stay away from high-speed roads.
2. Do not wear headphones, so that you can be aware of your surroundings. Using headphones may keep you from hearing a car horn, a voice, or a potential attacker.
3. Go against the traffic so that you can spot and avoid all oncoming traffic.
4. Do not wear dark clothes. Reflective clothing or fluorescent material worn on different parts of the body is highly recommended. A flashlight, particularly an LED light, not only alerts drivers to your presence, but also helps illuminate the street. Motorists can see a light from a greater distance than they can spot the reflective material.
5. Wear a billed cap and clear glasses in the dark. The billed cap will hit a branch or other object before such hits your head. Clear glasses can protect your eyes from unseen objects or insects.
6. Run behind vehicles at intersections. Drivers often look only in the direction of oncoming traffic and do not look in the opposite direction before proceeding onto the street.
7. Select different routes. A potential attacker may lie in wait if you are predictable in your running route. Running with a partner is also preferable because there is always strength in numbers. And do not wear your hair in a ponytail, as such provides an easy grip for a potential attacker.
8. Avoid walking or jogging in unfamiliar areas. When visiting a new area, always inquire as to safe areas to walk or jog.

Aerobics

Aerobics, formerly known as **aerobic dance**, consists of a combination of stepping, walking, jogging, skipping, kicking, and arm swinging movements performed to music. It is a fun way to exercise and promote cardiorespiratory development at the same time.

High-impact aerobics (HIA) is the traditional form of aerobics. The movements exert a great amount of vertical force on the feet as they contact the floor. Proper leg conditioning through other forms of weight-bearing aerobic exercises (brisk walking and jogging), as well as strength training, is recommended prior to participating in HIA.

HIA is an intense activity, and it produces the highest rate of aerobics injuries. Shin splints, stress fractures, low back pain, and tendinitis are all too common in HIA enthusiasts. These injuries are caused by the constant impact of the feet on firm surfaces. As a result, several alternative forms of aerobics have been developed.

In **low-impact aerobics (LIA),** the impact is reduced because each foot contacts the surface separately, but the recommended intensity of exercise is more difficult to maintain than with HIA. To help elevate the exercise heart rate, all arm movements and weight-bearing actions that lower the center of gravity should be accentuated. Sustained movement throughout the program is also crucial to keep the heart rate in the target cardiorespiratory zone.

A third aerobics modality is **step aerobics (SA),** in which participants step up and down from a bench. Benches range in height from 2 to 10 inches. SA adds another dimension to the aerobics program. As noted previously, variety adds enjoyment to aerobic workouts. SA is considered a high-intensity but low-impact activity. The intensity of the activity can be controlled easily by the height of the bench. Aerobic benches or plates can be stacked together safely to adjust the height of the steps. Beginners are encouraged to use the lowest stepping height and then advance gradually to a higher bench. This will decrease the risk for injury. Even though one foot is always in contact with the floor or bench during step aerobics, this activity is not recommended for individuals with ankle, knee, or hip problems.

Other forms of aerobics include a combination of HIA and LIA, as well as **moderate-impact aerobics (MIA).** MIA incorporates **plyometric training.** This type of training is used frequently by jumpers (high, long, and triple jumpers) and athletes in sports that require quick jumping ability, such as basketball and gymnastics.

With MIA, one foot is in contact with the ground most of the time. Participants, however, continually try to recover from all lower-body flexion actions. This is done by extending the hip, knee, and ankle joints quickly without allowing the foot (or feet) to leave the ground. These quick movements make the exercise intensity of MIA quite high.

Swimming

Swimming, another excellent form of aerobic exercise, uses many of the major muscle groups in the body. This provides a good training stimulus for the heart and lungs. Swimming is a great exercise option for individuals who cannot jog or walk for extended periods.

Compared with other activities, the risk for injuries from swimming is low. The aquatic medium helps to support the body, taking pressure off bones and joints in the lower extremities and the back. Maximal heart rates during swimming are approximately 10 to 13 beats per minute (bpm) lower than during running. The horizontal position of the body is thought to aid blood flow distribution throughout the body, decreasing the demand on the cardiorespiratory system. Direct contact with cool water seems to help dissipate body heat more

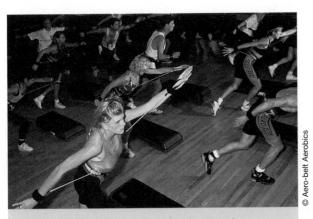
© Aero-belt Aerobics

Step aerobics using a resistive-cord belt to enhance upper body work.

KEY TERMS

Aerobic dance A series of exercise routines performed to music; more commonly termed "aerobics" now.

High-impact aerobics (HIA) Exercises incorporating movements in which both feet are off the ground at the same time momentarily.

Low-impact aerobics (LIA) Exercises in which at least one foot is in contact with the ground or floor at all times.

Step aerobics (SA) A form of exercise that combines stepping up and down from a bench with arm movements.

Moderate-impact aerobics (MIA) Aerobics that include plyometric training.

Plyometric training A form of exercise that requires forceful jumps or springing off the ground immediately after landing from a previous jump.

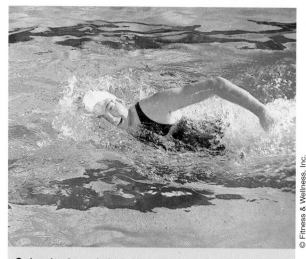

Swimming is a relatively injury-free activity.

© Fitness & Wellness, Inc.

land-based walk/jog test. This is because most of the work with swimming is done by the upper body musculature.

Although the heart's ability to pump more blood improves significantly with any type of aerobic activity, the primary increase in the ability of cells to utilize oxygen (oxygen uptake [VO_2]) with swimming occurs in the upper body and not the lower extremities. Therefore, fitness improvements with swimming are best attained by comparing changes in distance a person swims in a given time; say, 12 minutes.

> ### CRITICAL THINKING
>
> Participation in sports is a good predictor of adherence to exercise later in life. • What previous experiences have you had with participation in sports? • Were these experiences positive, and what effect do they have on your current physical activity patterns?

Water Aerobics

Water aerobics is fun and safe for people of all ages. Besides developing fitness, it provides an opportunity for socialization and fun in a comfortable, refreshing setting. Water aerobics incorporates a combination of rhythmic arm and leg actions performed in a vertical position while submerged in waist-to-armpit-deep water. The vigorous limb movements against the water's resistance during water aerobics provide the training stimuli for cardiorespiratory development.

The popularity of water aerobics as an exercise modality to develop the cardiorespiratory system can be attributed to several factors:

efficiently, further decreasing the strain on the heart.

Some exercise specialists recommend that this difference in maximal heart rate (10 to 13 bpm) be subtracted prior to determining cardiorespiratory training intensities. For example, the estimated maximal swimming heart rate for a 20-year-old would be approximately 187 bpm (220 − 20 − 13). Studies are inconclusive as to whether this decrease in heart rate in water also occurs at submaximal intensities below 70 percent of maximal heart rate.[1] One can argue, nonetheless, that apparently healthy people are able to achieve higher work capacities during land-based activities; thus, the same exercise intensity can be given for water activities. If a lower intensity is used, training benefits may be decreased.

To produce better training benefits during swimming, swimmers should minimize gliding periods such as those in the breast stroke and side stroke. Achieving proper training intensities with these strokes is difficult. The forward crawl is recommended for better aerobic results.

Overweight individuals have to swim fast enough to achieve an adequate training intensity. Excessive body fat makes the body more buoyant, and often the tendency is to float along. This may be good for reducing stress and relaxing, but it does not greatly increase caloric expenditure to aid with weight loss. Walking or jogging in waist- or armpit-deep water is a better choice for overweight individuals who cannot walk or jog on land for an extended period of time.

With reference to the principle of specificity of training, cardiorespiratory improvements from swimming cannot be measured adequately with a

1. Water buoyancy reduces weight-bearing stress on joints and thereby lessens the risk for injuries.
2. Water aerobics is a more feasible type of exercise for overweight individuals and those with arthritic conditions who may not be able to participate in weight-bearing activities such as walking, jogging, and aerobics.
3. Water aerobics is an excellent exercise modality to improve functional fitness in older adults (see Chapter 9, pages 246–248).
4. Heat dissipation in water is beneficial to obese participants, who seem to undergo a higher heat strain than average-weight individuals.
5. Water aerobics is available to swimmers and nonswimmers alike.

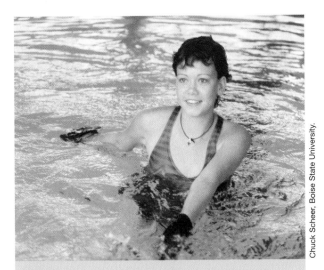

Water aerobics offers fitness and fun in an environment relatively low in risk for injury.

Chuck Scheer, Boise State University.

The exercises used during water aerobics are designed to elevate the heart rate, which contributes to cardiorespiratory development. In addition, the aquatic medium provides increased resistance for strength improvement with virtually no impact. Because of this resistance to movement, strength gains with water aerobics seem to be better than with land-based aerobic activities. Water exercises also help the joints move through their range of motion, promoting flexibility.

Another benefit is that weight can be reduced without the pain and fear of injuries experienced by many who initiate exercise programs. Water aerobics provides a relatively safe environment for injury-free participation in exercise. The cushioned environment of the water allows patients recovering from leg and back injuries, individuals with joint problems, injured athletes, pregnant women, and obese people to benefit from water aerobics. In water, these people can exercise to develop and maintain cardiorespiratory endurance while limiting or eliminating the potential for further injury.

Similar to swimming, maximal heart rates achieved during water aerobics are lower than during running. The difference between water aerobics and running is about 10 bpm.[2] Further, research comparing physiological differences between self-paced treadmill running and self-paced water aerobics exercise showed that even though individuals work at a lower heart rate intensity in water, the VO_2 level was the same for both treadmill and water exercise modalities.[3] Apparently healthy people, therefore, can sustain land-based exercise intensities during a water aerobics workout and experience fitness benefits similar to or greater than during land aerobics.[4]

Cycling

Most people learn cycling in their youth. Because it is a non-weight-bearing activity, cycling is a good exercise modality for people with lower-body or lower-back injuries. Cycling helps to develop the cardiorespiratory system, as well as muscular strength and endurance in the lower extremities. With the advent of stationary bicycles, this activity can be performed year-round.

Raising the heart rate to the proper training intensity is more difficult with cycling. As the amount of muscle mass involved during aerobic exercise decreases, so does the demand placed on the cardiorespiratory system. The thigh muscles do most of the work in cycling, making it harder to achieve and maintain a high cardiorespiratory training intensity.

Maintaining a continuous pedaling motion and eliminating coasting periods helps the participant achieve a faster heart rate. Exercising for longer periods also helps to compensate for the lower heart rate intensity during cycling. Comparing cycling with jogging, similar aerobic benefits take roughly three times the distance at twice the speed of jogging. Cycling, however, puts less stress on muscles and joints than jogging does, making cycling a good exercise modality for people who cannot walk or jog.

The height of the bike seat should be adjusted so the knee is flexed at about 30 degrees when the foot is at the bottom of the pedaling cycle. The body should not sway from side to side as the person rides. The cycling cadence also is important for maximal efficiency. Bike tension or gears should be set at a moderate level so the rider can achieve about 60 to 100 revolutions per minute.

Safety is a key issue in road cycling. More than a million bicycle injuries occur each year. Proper equipment and common sense are necessary. A well-designed and well-maintained bike is easier to maneuver. Toe clips are recommended to keep feet from sliding and to maintain equal upward and downward force on the pedals.

Skill is important in both road and mountain cycling. Cyclists must be in control of the bicycle at all times. They have to be able to maneuver the bike in traffic, maintain balance at slow speeds, switch gears, apply the brakes, watch for pedestrians and stop lights, ride through congested areas, and overcome a variety of obstacles in the mountains. Stationary cycling, in contrast, does not require special skills. Nearly everyone can do it.

Bike riders must follow the same rules as motorists. Many accidents happen because cyclists run traffic lights and stop signs. Some further suggestions are as follows:

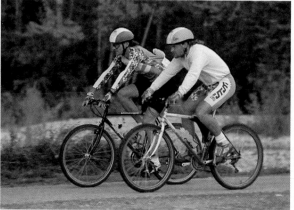

Road cycling requires skill for safety and enjoyment.

© Fitness & Wellness, Inc.

1. Select the right bike. Frame size is important. The size is determined by standing flatfooted while straddling the bike. Regular bikes (road bikes) should have a 1″ to 2″ clearance between the groin and the top tube of the frame. On mountain bikes, the clearance should be about 3″. The recommended height of the handlebars is about 1″ below the top of the seat. Upright handlebars are available for individuals with neck or back problems. Hard, narrow seats on road or racing bikes tend to be especially uncomfortable for women. To avoid saddle soreness, use wider and more cushioned seats such as gel-filled saddles.

2. Use bike hand signals to let the traffic around you know of your intended actions.

3. Don't ride side by side with another rider; single file is safer.

4. Be aware of turning vehicles and cars backing out of alleys and parking lots; always yield to motorists in these situations.

5. Be on the lookout for storm drains, railroad tracks, and cattle guards, which can cause unpleasant surprises. Front wheels can get caught and riders may be thrown from the bike if these hazards are not crossed at the proper angle (preferably 90 degrees).

6. Wear a good helmet, certified by the Snell Memorial Foundation or the American National Standards Institute. Many serious accidents and even deaths have been prevented by the use of helmets. Fashion, aesthetics, comfort, or price should not be a factor when selecting and using a helmet for road cycling. Health and life are too precious to give up because of vanity and thriftiness.

7. Wear appropriate clothes and shoes. Clothing should be bright, very visible, and lightweight and not restrict movement. Cycling shorts are recommended to prevent skin irritation. For greater comfort, the shorts have extra padding sewn into the seat and crotch areas. They do not tend to wrinkle and they wick away perspiration from the skin. Shorts should be long enough to keep the skin from rubbing against the seat. Experienced cyclists also wear special shoes with a cleat that snaps directly onto the pedal.

8. Take extra warm clothing in a backpack during the winter months in case you have a breakdown and have to walk a long distance for assistance.

9. Watch out for ice in cold weather. If you see ice on car windows, expect ice on the road. Be especially careful on and under bridges, because they tend to have ice even when the roads elsewhere are dry.

10. Use the brightest bicycle lights you can when riding in the dark, and always keep the batteries well charged. For additional safety, wear reflectors on the upper torso, arms, and legs, so passing motorists are alerted to you. Stay on streets that have good lighting and plenty of room on the side of the road, even if that means riding an extra few minutes to get to your destination.

11. Take a cell phone if you have one, and let someone else know where you are going and when to expect you back.

Before buying a stationary bike, be sure to try the activity for a few days. If you enjoy it, you may want to purchase one. Invest with caution. If you opt to buy a lower-priced model, you may be disappointed. Good stationary bikes have comfortable seats, are stable, and provide a smooth and uniform pedaling motion. A sticky bike that is hard to pedal leads to discouragement and ends up being stored in the corner of a basement.

Spinning®

Spinning is a vigorous-intensity/low-impact activity typically performed in a room or studio with dim lights and motivational music, under the direction of

Tips for People Who Have Been Inactive for a While

- Take the sensible approach by starting slowly.
- Begin by choosing moderate-intensity activities you enjoy the most. By choosing activities you enjoy, you'll be more likely to stick with them.
- Gradually build up the time spent exercising by adding a few minutes every few days or so until you can comfortably perform a minimum recommended amount of exercise (20 minutes per day).
- As the minimum amount becomes easier, gradually increase either the length of time exercising or the intensity of the activity, or both.
- Vary your activities, both for interest and to broaden the range of benefits.
- Explore new physical activities.
- Reward and acknowledge your efforts.

SOURCE: Adapted from Centers for Disease Control and Prevention, Atlanta, 2005.

Try It
Fill out the cardiorespiratory exercise prescription in Activity 3.3. In your Online Journal or class notebook, describe how well you implement the above suggestions.

a certified instructor and with the noise of many bikes working together. This exercise modality gained immediate popularity upon its introduction in the 1980s. Sometimes referred to as studio or indoor cycling, spinning is performed on stationary bicycles developed by world-class cyclist Johnny Goldberg. To bring his rigorous workouts indoors, Goldberg modified his stationary bike into the first Spinner bike.

Participants now use specially designed Spinner bikes available at sports equipment stores. The bikes include racing handlebars, pedals with clips, adjustable seats, and a resistance knob to control the intensity of the workout. Use of an exercise heart rate monitor is encouraged to track the intensity at various stages of the workout. The intensity of training is modulated by changing the resistance on the bike (flywheel), changing the cadence, and by sitting or standing in various positions.

As presently designed, the Spinning program combines five basic movements and five workout stages, with the understanding that participants' exercise needs and goals vary. The five exercise movements are:

1. Seated flat—pedaling in the basic seated bike position
2. Seated hill climb—pedaling in the basic seated position but with increased resistance applied
3. Standing running—pedaling while standing up
4. Standing hill climb—pedaling standing up but with a more challenging resistance level
5. Jumping—surging out of the saddle using either controlled movements and a constant speed or at a fast pace, as during a breakaway in a bike race

The five workout stages, also known as energy zones, are used to simulate actual cycling training and racing. The workouts are divided into endurance, all-terrain, strength, recovery, and advanced training. Cadence, exercise movements, and exercise heart rate dictate the differences among the various zones. Workouts are planned according to each person's fitness level and selected percentages of maximal heart rate during each stage. These workouts provide a challenging program for people of all ages and fitness levels. The social aspect of this activity makes Spinning appealing to many exercisers.

Cross-Training

Cross-training combines two or more activities. This type of training is designed to enhance fitness, provide needed rest for tired muscles, decrease injuries, and eliminate the monotony and burnout of single-activity programs. Cross-training may combine aerobic and nonaerobic activities such as moderate jogging, speed training, and strength training.

Cross-training can produce better workouts than a single activity. For example, jogging develops the lower body, and swimming builds the upper body. Rowing contributes to upper-body development, and cycling builds the legs. Combining activities such as these provides good overall conditioning and at the same time helps to improve or maintain fitness. Cross-training also offers an opportunity to develop skill and have fun with differing activities.

Speed training often is coupled with cross-training. Faster performance times in aerobic activities (running, cycling) are generated with speed or **interval training.** People who want to improve their running times often run shorter intervals at faster speeds than the actual racing pace.

KEY TERMS

Interval training A repeated series of exercise work bouts (intervals) interspersed with low-intensity or rest intervals.

For example, a person wanting to run a 6-minute mile may run four 440-yard intervals at a speed of 1 minute and 20 seconds per interval. A 440-yard walk/jog can become a recovery interval between fast runs.

Strength training is used commonly with cross-training. It helps to condition muscles, tendons, and ligaments. Improved strength enhances overall performance in many activities and sports. For example, although road cyclists in one study who trained with weights showed no improvement in aerobic capacity, the cyclists' riding time to exhaustion improved 33 percent when they exercised at 75 percent of their maximal capacity.[5]

Rope Skipping

Rope skipping contributes to cardiorespiratory fitness and also helps to increase reaction time, coordination, agility, dynamic balance, and muscular strength in the lower extremities. At first, rope skipping may seem to be a highly strenuous form of aerobic exercise. Beginners often reach maximal heart rates after only two or three minutes of jumping. As skill improves, however, the energy demands decrease considerably.

Some people have claimed training benefits equal to a 30-minute jog in only 10 minutes of skipping. Although differences in strength and flexibility development are observed in different activities, 10 minutes of rope skipping at a certain heart rate provides similar cardiorespiratory benefits, regardless of the nature of the activity. To obtain an adequate aerobic workout, the duration of exercise must be at least 20 minutes.

As with high-impact aerobics, a major concern of rope skipping is the stress placed on the lower extremities, increasing the risk for injuries. Fitness experts recommend that skipping be used sparingly, and primarily as a supplement to an aerobic exercise program.

Cross-Country Skiing

Many people consider cross-country skiing the ultimate aerobic exercise because it requires vigorous lower- and upper-body movements. The large amount of muscle mass involved in cross-country skiing makes the intensity of the activity high, yet it places little strain on muscles and joints. One of the highest maximal oxygen uptakes ever measured (85 mL/kg/min) was found in an elite cross-country skier.

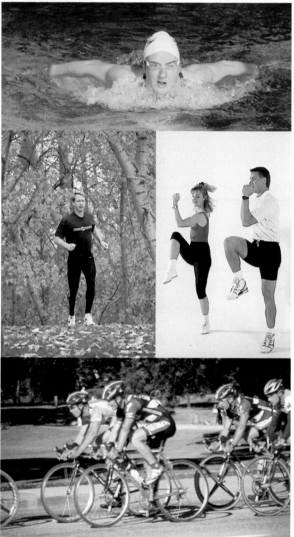

Cross-training enhances fitness, decreases the rate of injuries, and eliminates the monotony of single-activity programs.

Photos © Fitness & Wellness, Inc.

In addition to being an excellent aerobic activity, cross-country skiing is soothing. Skiing through the beauty of the snow-covered countryside can be highly enjoyable. Although the need for snow is an obvious limitation, simulation equipment for year-round cross-country training is available at many sporting goods stores.

Some skill is necessary to be proficient at cross-country skiing. Poorly skilled individuals are not able to elevate the heart rate enough to cause adequate aerobic development. Individuals contemplating this activity should seek instruction to be able to fully enjoy and reap the rewards of cross-country skiing.

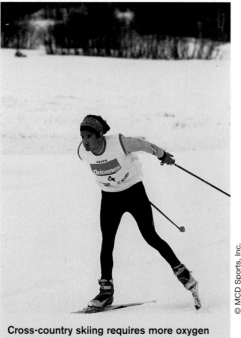

Cross-country skiing requires more oxygen and energy than most other aerobic activities.

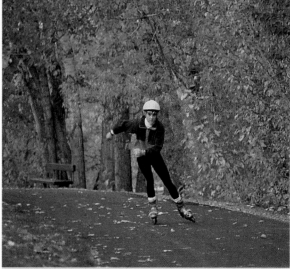

In-line skating is a low-impact fitness activity.

In-Line Skating

Frequently called blading, in-line skating is also a highly popular fitness activity. Millions of children and adults participate in this activity. In the early 1990s, stores could not keep up with the demand for in-line skates.

In-line skating has its origin in ice skating. Because warm-weather ice skating was not feasible, wheels replaced blades for summertime participation. Although four-wheel roller skates were invented in the mid-1700s, the activity did not really catch on until the late 1800s. The first in-line skate with five wheels in a row attached to the bottom of a shoe was developed in 1823. The in-line concept took hold in the United States in 1980, when hockey skates were adapted for road-skating.

In-line skating is an excellent activity to develop cardiorespiratory fitness and lower body strength. Intensity of the activity is regulated by how hard you blade. The key to effective cardiorespiratory training is to maintain a constant and rhythmic pattern, using arms and legs, and to minimize the gliding phase of blading. Because blading is a weight-bearing activity, participants also develop superior leg strength.

Instruction is necessary to achieve a minimum level of proficiency in this sport. Bladers commonly encounter hazards—potholes, cracks, rocks, gravel, sticks, oil, street curbs, and driveways. Unskilled bladers are more prone to falls and injuries.

Good equipment will make the activity safer and more enjoyable. Blades range in price from $40 to $500. Recreational participants need not purchase the more costly competitive skates. An adequate blade should provide strong ankle support; soft and flexible boots do not provide enough support. Small wheels offer more stability, and larger wheels enable greater speed. Blades should be purchased from stores that understand the sport and can provide sound advice according to skill level and needs.

Protective equipment is a must for in-line skating. Similar to road cycling, a good helmet that meets the safety standards set by the Snell Memorial Foundation or the American National Standards Institute is important to protect yourself in case of a fall. Wrist guards and knee and elbow pads also are recommended, because the kneecap and the elbows are easily injured in a fall. Nighttime bladers should wear light-colored clothing and reflective tape.

Rowing

Rowing is a low-impact activity that provides a complete body workout. It mobilizes most major muscle groups, including those in the arms, legs, hips, abdomen, trunk, and shoulders. Rowing is a good form of aerobic exercise and, because of the nature of the activity (constant pushing and pulling against resistance), promotes strength development.

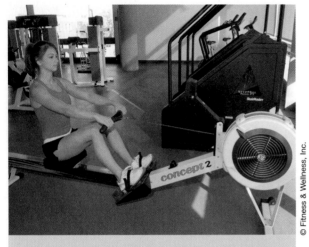

In addition to aerobic development, rowing also contributes to good strength development.

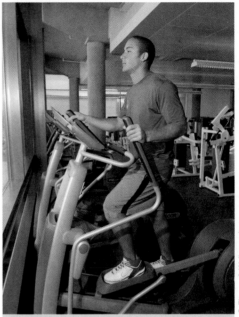

Stair climbing provides a rigorous aerobic workout.

To accommodate different fitness levels, workloads can be regulated on most rowing machines. Stationary rowing, however, is not among the most popular forms of aerobic exercise. As they would on stationary bicycles, people should try the activity for a few weeks before purchasing a unit.

Stair Climbing

If sustained for at least 20 minutes, stair climbing is a very efficient form of aerobic exercise. Precisely because of the high intensity of climbing stairs, many people prefer to take escalators and elevators. They may even dislike living in two-story homes because they have to climb the stairs frequently.

Not too many places have enough flights of stairs to climb continuously for 20 minutes. Stair-climbing machines offer an alternative. In terms of injuries, stair climbing seems to be a relatively safe exercise modality. Because the feet never leave the climbing surface, it is considered a low-impact activity. Joints and ligaments are not strained during climbing. The intensity of exercise is controlled easily, because most stair-climbing equipment can be programmed to regulate the workload.

Racquet Sports

In racquet sports such as tennis, racquetball, squash, and badminton, the aerobic benefits are dictated by players' skill, the intensity of the game, and the length of time spent playing. Skill is necessary to participate effectively in these sports and is crucial

to sustain continuous play. Frequent pauses during play do not allow people to maintain the heart rate in the appropriate target zone to stimulate cardiorespiratory development.

Many people participate in racquet sports for reasons of enjoyment, social fulfillment, and relaxation.

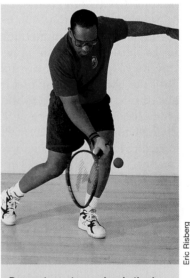

Racquet sports require rhythmic and continuous activity to provide cardiorespiratory benefit.

To develop cardiorespiratory fitness, these people supplement the sport with other forms of aerobic exercise such as jogging, cycling, or swimming. If a racquet sport is the main form of aerobic exercise, participants must try to run hard, fast, and as constantly as possible during play—and avoid spending a lot of time retrieving balls, birds, or shuttlecocks. Just as in low-impact aerobics, all movements should be accentuated by reaching out and bending more than usual, for better cardiorespiratory development.

CRITICAL THINKING

In your own experience with personal fitness programs throughout the years, what factors have motivated you and helped you the most to stay with a program?
• What factors have kept you from being physically active, and what can you do to change these factors?

Rating the Fitness Benefits of Aerobic Activities

The fitness contributions of the aerobic activities discussed in this chapter vary according to the specific activity and the individual. As noted previously, the health-related components of physical fitness are cardiorespiratory endurance, muscular strength and endurance, muscular flexibility, and body composition. Although accurately assessing the contributions to each fitness component is difficult, a summary of likely benefits of these activities is provided in Table 4.1. Instead of a single rating or number, ranges are given for some of the categories because the benefits derived are based on the person's effort while participating in the activity.

Regular participation in aerobic activities provides notable health benefits, including an increase in cardiorespiratory endurance, quality of life, and longevity. The extent of cardiorespiratory development (improvement in maximal oxygen uptake [VO_{2max}]) depends on the intensity, duration, and frequency of the activity. The nature of the activity often dictates potential aerobic development. For example, jogging is much more strenuous than walking.

The effort during exercise also influences the amount of physiological development. The training benefits of just going through the motions of a low-impact aerobics routine are less than those of accentuating all motions (see earlier discussion of low-impact aerobics). Table 4.1 includes a starting

fitness level for each aerobic activity. Beginners should start with low-intensity activities that have a minimum risk for injuries. In some cases, such as in high-impact aerobics and rope skipping, the risk for injuries remains high despite adequate conditioning. These activities should be used only to supplement training and are not recommended for beginners or as the sole mode of exercise.

Physicians who work with cardiac patients frequently use *metabolic equivalents* (METs) to measure activity levels. One **MET** represents the body's energy requirement at rest, or the equivalent of a VO_2 of 3.5 mL/kg/min. A 10 MET activity requires a tenfold increase in the resting energy requirement, or approximately 35 mL/kg/min. MET levels for a given activity vary according to the individual's effort. The harder a person exercises, the higher the MET level. The range of METs for the various activities is included in Table 4.1, as is the various aerobic activities' effectiveness in aiding weight management. As a rule, the greater the muscle mass involved during exercise, the better the results. Rhythmic and continuous activities that involve considerable muscle mass are most effective in burning calories.

Higher-intensity activities burn more calories as well. Increasing exercise time will compensate for lower intensities. If carried out long enough (60 to 90 minutes, five to six times per week), even brisk walking can be a good exercise mode to lose weight. Additional information on a comprehensive weight management program is given in Chapter 6.

Skill-Related Fitness

Skill-related fitness is needed for success in athletics and effective performance of lifetime sports and activities. The components of skill-related fitness, defined in Chapter 1, are agility, balance, coordination, power, speed, and reaction time. All of these are important, to varying degrees, in sports and athletics.

For example, outstanding gymnasts must achieve good skill-related fitness in all components. Significant agility is necessary to perform a double back somersault with a full twist—a skill in which the athlete must rotate simultaneously around one axis and

---

KEY TERMS

MET Short for *metabolic equivalent*, the rate of energy expenditure at rest, or the equivalent of a VO_2 of 3.5 mL/kg/min.

TABLE 4.1

Ratings of Selected Aerobic Activities

Activity	Recommended Starting Fitness Level[1]	Injury Risk[2]	Potential Cardiorespiratory Endurance Development (VO_{2MAX})[3,4]	Upper Body Strength Development[3]	Lower Body Strength Development[3]	Upper Body Flexibility Development[3]	Lower Body Flexibility Development[3]	Weight Management[3]	MET Level[4,5,6]	Caloric Expenditure (cal/hour)[4,6]
Aerobics										
High-Impact Aerobics	A	H	3–4	2	4	3	2	4	6–12	450–900
Moderate-Impact Aerobics	I	M	2–4	2	3	3	2	3	6–12	450–900
Low-Impact Aerobics	B	L	2–4	2	3	3	2	3	5–10	375–750
Step Aerobics	I	M	2–4	2	3–4	3	2	3–4	5–12	375–900
Cross-Country Skiing	B	M	4–5	4	4	2	2	4–5	10–16	750–1,200
Cross-Training	I	M	3–5	2–3	3–4	2–3	1–2	3–5	6–15	450–1,125
Cycling										
Road	I	M	2–5	1	4	1	1	3	6–12	450–900
Stationary	B	L	2–4	1	4	1	1	3	6–10	450–750
Hiking	B	L	2–4	1	3	1	1	3	6–10	450–750
In-Line Skating	I	M	2–4	2	4	2	2	3	6–10	450–750
Jogging	I	M	3–5	1	3	1	1	5	6–15	450–1,125
Jogging, Deep Water	A	L	3–5	2	2	1	1	5	8–15	600–1,125
Racquet Sports	I	M	2–4	3	3	3	2	3	6–10	450–750
Rope Skipping	I	H	3–5	2	4	1	2	3–5	8–15	600–1,125
Rowing	B	L	3–5	4	2	3	1	4	8–14	600–1,050
Spinning	I	L	4–5	1	4	1	1	4	8–15	600–1,125
Stair Climbing	B	L	3–5	1	4	1	1	4–5	8–15	600–1,125
Swimming (front crawl)	B	L	3–5	4	2	3	1	3	6–12	450–900
Walking	B	L	1–2	1	2	1	1	3	4–6	300–450
Walking, Water, Chest-Deep	I	L	2–4	2	3	1	1	3	6–10	450–750
Water Aerobics	B	L	2–4	3	3	3	2	3	6–12	450–900

[1] B = Beginner, I = Intermediate, A = Advanced

[2] L = Low, M = Moderate, H = High

[3] 1 = Low, 2 = Fair, 3 = Average, 4 = Good, 5 = Excellent

[4] Varies according to the person's effort (intensity) during exercise.

[5] 1 MET represents the rate of energy expenditure at rest (3.5 mL/kg/min). Each additional MET is a multiple of the resting value. For example, 5 METs represents an energy expenditure equivalent to five times the resting value, or about 17.5 mL/kg/min.

[6] Varies according to body weight.

twist around a different one. Static balance is essential for maintaining a handstand or a scale. Dynamic balance is needed to perform many of the gymnastics routines (for example, balance beam, parallel bars, pommel horse).

Coordination is important to successfully integrate into one routine various skills requiring varying degrees of difficulty. Power and speed are needed to propel the body into the air, such as when tumbling or vaulting. Quick reaction time is necessary in determining when to end rotation upon a visual clue, such as spotting the floor on a dismount.

As with the health-related fitness components, the principle of specificity of training applies to skill-related components. According to this principle, the training program must be specific to the type of skill the individual is trying to achieve.

Development of agility, balance, coordination, and reaction time is highly task specific. To attain a certain skill, the individual must practice the same task many times. There is little crossover learning effect from one skill to another.

For instance, proper practice of a handstand (balance) eventually will lead to successful performance of that skill, but complete mastery of the skill does not ensure that the person will immediately be able to transfer this mastery to other static balance positions in gymnastics. Power and speed may be improved with a specific strength-training program or frequent repetition of the specific task to be improved, or both.

The rate of learning in skill-related fitness varies from person to person, mainly because these components seem to be determined to a large extent by hereditary factors. Individuals with good skill-related fitness tend to do better and learn faster when performing a wide variety of skills. Nevertheless, few individuals enjoy complete success in all skill-related components. Furthermore, though skill-related fitness can be enhanced with practice, improvements in reaction time and speed are limited and seem to be related primarily to genetic endowment.

Although we do not know how much skill-related fitness is desirable, everyone should attempt to develop and maintain a better than average level. This type of fitness is not only crucial for athletes but is important for everyone who wants to lead a better and happier life. Improving skill-related fitness affords an individual more enjoyment and success in a wider variety of lifetime sports (for instance, basketball, tennis, and racquetball) and can help a person cope more effectively in emergency situations. For example:

1. Good reaction time, balance, coordination, and agility can help you avoid a fall or break a fall and thereby minimize injury.
2. The ability to generate maximum force in a short time (power) may be crucial to ameliorate injury or even preserve life in a situation in which you may be called upon to move a person out of danger or lift a heavy object that has fallen.
3. In our society, with an expanding average lifespan and residential sprawl to wider streets, maintaining foot speed can be especially important for older adults. Many of them and, for that matter, many unfit and overweight young people, no longer have the fleetness they need to cross an intersection safely before the light changes for oncoming traffic.

Regular participation in a health-related fitness program can heighten performance of skill-related components, and vice versa. For example, significantly overweight people do not have good agility or speed. Because participating in aerobic and strength-training programs helps take off body fat, an overweight individual who loses weight through an exercise program may also improve agility and speed. A sound flexibility program decreases resistance to motion around body joints, which may increase agility, balance, and overall coordination. Improvements in strength definitely help develop power.

Similar to the fitness benefits of the aerobic activities discussed previously in this chapter and given in Table 4.1, the contributions of skill-related activities also vary among activities and individuals. The extent to which an activity helps develop each skill-related component varies by the effort the indi-

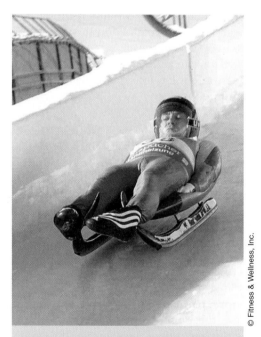

A 54-year-old athlete with a high level of skill fitness competing in the sport of luge at the world-class level.

© Fitness & Wellness, Inc.

vidual makes and, most important, by proper execution (technique) of the skill (correct coaching is highly recommended) and the individual's potential based on genetic endowment. A summary of potential contributions to skill-related fitness for selected activities is provided in Table 4.2.

Team Sports

Choosing activities that you enjoy will greatly enhance your adherence to exercise. People tend to repeat things they enjoy doing. Enjoyment by itself is a reward. Therefore, combining individual activities (such as jogging or swimming) with team sports can deepen your commitment to fitness.

People with good skill-related fitness usually participate in lifetime sports and games, which in turn helps develop health-related fitness. Individuals who enjoyed basketball or soccer in their youth

tend to stick to those activities later in life. The availability of teams and community leagues may be all that is needed to stop contemplating and start participating. The social element of team sports provides added incentive to participate. Team sports offer an opportunity to interact with people who share a common interest. Being a member of a team creates responsibility—another incentive to exercise, because you are expected to be there. Furthermore, team sports foster lifetime friendships, strengthening the social and emotional dimensions of wellness.

For those who were not able to participate in youth sports, it's never too late to start (see the discussion of behavior modification and motivation in Chapter 1). Don't be afraid to select a new activity, even if that means learning new skills. The fitness and social rewards will be ample.

Tips to Enhance Your Aerobic Workout

A typical aerobic workout is divided into three parts (see Figure 4.2):

1. A 5- to 10-minute warm-up phase during which the heart rate is increased gradually to the target zone
2. The actual aerobic workout, during which the heart rate is maintained in the target zone for 20 to 60 minutes
3. A 10-minute aerobic cool-down, when the heart rate is lowered gradually toward the resting level

To monitor the target training zone, you will have to check your exercise heart rate. As described in Chapter 2, the pulse can be checked on the radial or the carotid artery. When you check the heart rate, begin with zero and count the number of beats in a 10-second period, then multiply by 6 to get the per-minute pulse rate. You should take your exercise heart rate for 10 seconds rather than a full minute because the heart rate begins to slow down 15 seconds after you stop exercising.

Feeling the pulse while exercising is difficult. Therefore, participants should stop during exercise to check the pulse. If the heart rate is too low, increase the intensity of the exercise. If the rate is too high, slow down. You may want to practice taking your pulse several times during the day to become familiar with the technique.

TABLE 4.2

Contributions of Selected Activities to Skill-Related Components

Activity	Agility	Balance	Coordination	Power	Reaction Time	Speed
Alpine Skiing	4	5	4	2	3	2
Archery	1	2	4	2	3	1
Badminton	4	3	4	2	4	3
Baseball	3	2	4	4	5	4
Basketball	4	3	4	3	4	3
Bowling	2	2	4	1	1	1
Cross-Country Skiing	3	4	3	2	2	1
Football	4	4	4	4	4	3
Golf	1	2	5	3	1	3
Gymnastics	5	5	5	4	3	3
Ice Skating	5	5	5	3	3	3
In-Line Skating	4	4	4	3	2	4
Judo/Karate	5	5	5	4	5	4
Racquetball	5	4	4	4	5	4
Soccer	5	3	5	5	3	4
Table Tennis	5	3	5	3	5	3
Tennis	4	3	5	3	5	3
Volleyball	4	3	5	4	5	3
Water Skiing	3	4	3	2	2	1
Wrestling	5	5	5	4	5	4

1 = Low, 2 = Fair, 3 = Average, 4 = Good, 5 = Excellent

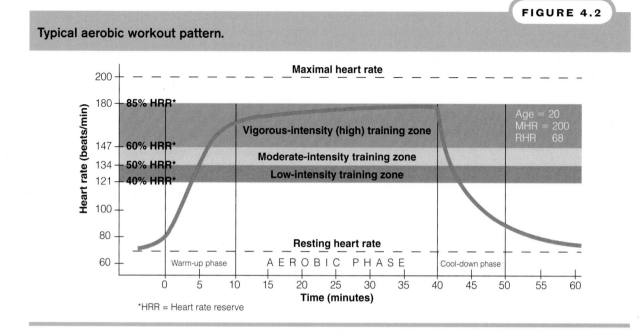

FIGURE 4.2

Typical aerobic workout pattern.

For the first few weeks of your program, you should monitor your heart rate several times during the exercise session. As you become familiar with your body's response to exercise, you may have to monitor the heart rate only twice—at 5 to 7 minutes into the exercise session and then a second time near the end of the workout.

Another technique sometimes used to determine your exercise intensity is simply to talk during exercise and then take your pulse immediately after that. Learning to associate the amount of difficulty when talking with the actual exercise heart rate will allow you to develop a sense of how hard you are working. Generally, if you can talk easily, you are not working hard enough. If you can talk but are slightly breathless, you should be close to the target range. If you cannot talk at all, you are working too hard.

If you have difficulty keeping up with your exercise program, you may need to reconsider your objectives and start much more slowly. Behavior modi-

fication is a process. From a physiological and psychological point of view, you may not be able to carry out an exercise session for a full 20 to 30 minutes. For the first two to three weeks, therefore, you may just want to take a few 10-minute daily walks. As your body adapts physically and mentally, you may increase the length and intensity of the exercise sessions gradually.

Most important, learn to listen to your body. At times you will feel unusually fatigued or have much discomfort. Pain is the body's way of letting you know that something is wrong. If you have pain or undue discomfort during or after exercise, you need to slow down or discontinue your exercise program and notify the course instructor. The instructor may be able to pinpoint the reason for the discomfort or recommend that you consult your physician. You also will be able to prevent potential injuries by paying attention to pain signals and making adjustments accordingly.

www WEB INTERACTIVE

Let's Get Physical Challenge. This site describes an eight-week, interactive program designed to help individuals participate in regular, moderate physical activity.

This is a fun, noncompetitive program designed to educate people of all ages and abilities. You can do it!
http://www.physicalfitness.org/lgp.html

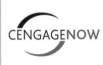

*Log on to **academic.cengage.com/login** and take a wellness inventory to assess the behaviors that might benefit most from healthy change.*

1. Are you able to incorporate a variety of activities into your exercise program?

2. Do you participate in recreational sports as a means to further enhance fitness and add enjoyment to your exercise program?

3. Do you have an alternate plan in case of inclement weather (rain/cold) or injury that would keep you from your regular training program (jogging, cycling)?

*Log on to **academic.cengage.com/login** to assess your understanding of this chapter's topics by taking the chapter pre-test and exploring the modules recommended in your Personalized Study Plan.*

1. Using a combination of aerobic activities to develop overall fitness is known as
   a. health-related fitness.
   b. circuit training.
   c. plyometric exercise.
   d. cross-training.
   e. skill-related fitness.

2. The best aerobic activity choice for individuals with leg or back injuries is
   a. walking in chest-deep water.
   b. jogging.
   c. step aerobics.
   d. rope skipping.
   e. cross-country skiing.

3. The approximate jogging mileage to reach the "excellent" cardiorespiratory fitness classification is
   a. 5 miles.
   b. 10 miles.
   c. 15 miles.
   d. 25 miles.
   e. 50 miles.

4. To help elevate the exercise heart rate during low-impact aerobics, a person should
   a. accentuate arm movements.
   b. sustain movement throughout the program.
   c. accentuate weight-bearing actions.
   d. All of the above.
   e. None of the above.

5. Achieved maximal heart rates during swimming are approximately _____ bpm lower than during running.
   a. 2–4
   b. 5–9
   c. 10–13
   d. 14–20
   e. 20–25

6. Which of the following is *not* a basic movement in Spinning?
   a. Seated running
   b. Standing hill climb
   c. Seated flat
   d. Jumping
   e. All of the above are exercise movements in Spinning.

7. Cross-country skiing
   a. is a high-impact activity.
   b. is primarily an anaerobic activity.
   c. places great strain on muscles and joints.
   d. is a low-intensity activity.
   e. All are incorrect choices.

8. A MET represents
   a. the symbol used to indicate that the exercise goal has been met.
   b. a unit of measure that is used to express the value achieved during the Metabolic Exercise Test.
   c. the maximal exercise time achieved.
   d. the rate of energy expenditure at rest.
   e. All choices are incorrect.

9. Which of the following is *not* a component of skill-related fitness?
   a. Mobility
   b. Coordination
   c. Reaction time
   d. Agility
   e. All are skill-related components.

10. When checking exercise heart rate, one should
    a. continue to exercise at the prescribed rate while checking the heart rate.
    b. stop exercising and take the pulse for no longer than 15 seconds.
    c. exercise at a low-to-moderate intensity.
    d. stop exercise and take the heart rate for a full minute.
    e. All choices are valid ways to check exercise heart rate.

Correct answers can be found at the back of the book.

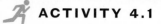

My Personal Fitness Program

Name _____   Date _____

Course _____   Section _____

I. In the spaces below, provide a list of five activities in which you have participated during the last 6 months. In addition to fitness activities (jogging, aerobics, swimming, strength training), you may list other activities in which you frequently participate that require physical effort (for example, walking, cycling, sweeping, vacuuming, gardening).

    According to your own effort of participation, rate each activity for its health-related and motor skill-related benefits (1 = low, 2 = fair, 3 = average, 4 = good, 5 = excellent). Also indicate the frequency and duration of participation (list times per week, month, or 6 months) and add comments regarding your personal feelings related to your participation in the respective activity (liked it, was fun, too hard, got hurt, need more skill, could do it forever, etc.).

	Cardiorespiratory Endurance	Muscular Strength	Muscular Flexibility	Weight Management	Agility	Balance	Coordination	Power	Reaction Time	Speed
1.										
Comments										
2.										
Comments										
3.										
Comments										
4.										
Comments										

	Cardiorespiratory Endurance	Muscular Strength	Muscular Flexibility	Weight Management	Agility	Balance	Coordination	Power	Reaction Time	Speed
5.										

Comments

II. On a separate sheet of paper, keep a 7-day log of all physical activities that you perform. On a daily basis, keep a record of the exact minutes throughout the day that you are active and rate each activity according to its intensity (moderate- or high-intensity). Total your minutes for each day and compute a daily average for all activities. Attach the log to this activity and then answer the following questions:

A. Did you exercise aerobically at least 3 times per week for 20 to 30 minutes each session?

_____ Yes   _____ No

B. Did you accumulate an average of 60 minutes of daily physical activity?

_____ Yes   _____ No

C. What percentage of your total physical activity was moderate intensity,

_____ %

and what percentage was vigorous intensity?

_____ %

III. According to items I and II above, evaluate your current level of physical activity. State how you feel about your results and indicate if your program is primarily conducive to health fitness or physical fitness (or neither). Do you deem any changes necessary to meet previously stated goals (see Activity 3.4, page 95)?

_____

_____

_____

_____

_____

_____

_____

_____

_____

Nutrition for Wellness

© Kayte M. Deioma/PhotoEdit

OBJECTIVES

- Define nutrition and describe its relationship to health and well-being
- Learn the functions of nutrients in the human body
- Become familiar with nutrients, food groups, and nutrient standards, and learn how to achieve a balanced diet through the use of the USDA MyPyramid guidelines
- Become familiar with eating disorders and with their associated medical problems and behavior patterns
- Identify myths and fallacies regarding nutrition
- Learn the 2005 Dietary Guidelines for Americans

Good nutrition is clearly linked by scientific studies to overall health and well-being. Proper nutrition means that one's diet supplies all the essential **nutrients** to carry out normal tissue growth, repair, and maintenance. It also implies that the diet will provide enough **substrates** to produce the energy necessary for work, physical activity, and relaxation.

Too much or too little of any nutrient can precipitate serious health problems. The typical U.S. diet is too high in calories, sugar, saturated fat, trans fat, and sodium, and not high enough in whole grains, fruits, and vegetables—factors that undermine good health. Food availability is not the problem. The problem is overconsumption.

According to a report on nutrition and health issued by the U.S. Surgeon General, diseases of dietary excess and imbalance are among the leading causes of death in the United States. Similar trends are observed in developed countries throughout the world. In the report, based on more than 2,000 scientific studies, the Surgeon General said that dietary changes can bring better health to all Americans. Other surveys reveal that on a given day, nearly half of the people in the United States eat no fruit and almost a fourth eat no vegetables.

Diet and nutrition often play a crucial role in the development and progression of chronic diseases. A diet high in saturated fat, trans fat, and cholesterol increases the risk for atherosclerosis and coronary heart disease. In sodium-sensitive individuals, high salt intake has been linked to high blood pressure. As many as 30 percent to 50 percent of all cancers may be diet related. Obesity, diabetes mellitus, and osteoporosis also have been associated with faulty nutrition.

The Essential Nutrients

The **essential nutrients** the human body requires are carbohydrates, fats, proteins, vitamins, minerals, and water. Carbohydrates, fats, proteins, and water are termed **macronutrients** because people need to take in proportionately large amounts daily. Nutritionists refer to vitamins and minerals as **micronutrients** because the body requires them in relatively small amounts.

Depending on the amount of nutrients and calories they contain, foods can be classified as high-nutrient density or low-nutrient density. Foods with high-nutrient density contain a low or moderate amount of **calories** but are packed with nutrients. Foods that are high in calories but contain few nutrients are of low-nutrient density and commonly are called "junk food."

Carbohydrates

Carbohydrates are the major source of calories the body uses to provide energy for work, cell maintenance, and heat. They also help regulate fat and metabolize proteins. Each gram of carbohydrates provides the human body with 4 calories. The major sources of carbohydrates are breads, cereals, fruits, vegetables, and milk and other dairy products. Carbohydrates are classified as simple carbohydrates and complex carbohydrates.

Simple Carbohydrates

Simple carbohydrates (such as candy, soda, and cakes), commonly denoted as sugars, have little nutritive value. These carbohydrates are divided into two groups:

- Monosaccharides (glucose, fructose, and galactose)
- Disaccharides (sucrose, lactose, and maltose)

Simple carbohydrates often take the place of more nutritive foods in the diet.

Complex Carbohydrates

Complex carbohydrates are formed when simple carbohydrate molecules are linked together. Three types of complex carbohydrates are:

- Starches, found commonly in seeds, corn, nuts, grains, roots, potatoes, and legumes
- Dextrins, formed from the breakdown of large starch molecules exposed to dry heat, such as when bread is baked or cold cereals are manufactured
- Glycogen, the animal polysaccharide synthesized from glucose and found in only small amounts in meats. Glycogen constitutes the body's reservoir of glucose. Many hundreds to thousands of glucose molecules are linked to be stored as glycogen in the liver and muscles. When a surge of energy is needed, enzymes in the muscle and the liver break down glycogen and thus make glucose readily available for energy transformation.

Complex carbohydrates provide many valuable nutrients and also are an excellent source of fiber (also called roughage).

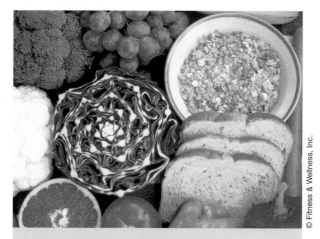

High-fiber foods are essential in a healthy diet.

© Fitness & Wellness, Inc.

Fiber

Fiber is a form of complex carbohydrate. A high-fiber diet gives a person a feeling of fullness without added calories. Dietary fiber is present mainly in plant leaves, skins, roots, and seeds. Processing and refining foods removes almost all of the natural fiber.

In the American diet, the main sources of fiber are whole-grain cereals and breads, fruits, vegetables, and legumes. Fiber is important in the diet because it decreases the risk for cardiovascular disease and cancer. Increased fiber intake also may lower the risk for coronary heart disease because saturated fats often take the place of fiber in the diet, thus increasing the formation of cholesterol. Other health disorders that have been tied to low intake of fiber are constipation, diverticulitis, hemorrhoids, gallbladder disease, and obesity.

The daily recommended amount of fiber intake for adults 50 years and younger is 25 grams for women and 38 grams for men. Most people in the United States eat only 15 grams of fiber per day, putting them at increased risk for disease. A person can increase fiber intake by eating more fruits, vegetables, legumes, grains, and cereals. A six-year study provided strong evidence linking increased fiber intake of 30 grams per day to a significant reduction in heart attacks, cancer of the colon, breast cancer, diabetes, and diverticulitis.[1] Table 5.1 provides the fiber content of selected foods.

Fibers are typically classified according to their solubility in water. Soluble fiber dissolves in water and forms a gel-like substance that encloses food particles. This property allows soluble fiber to bind and excrete fats from the body. Soluble fiber has been shown to decrease blood cholesterol and blood sugar levels. Soluble fiber is found primarily in oats, fruits, barley, and legumes.

Insoluble fiber is not easily dissolved in water, and the body cannot digest it. This fiber is important because it binds water, resulting in a softer and bulkier stool that increases peristalsis (involuntary muscle contractions of intestinal walls), forcing the stool onward, and allows food residues to pass through the intestinal tract more quickly. Speeding the passage of food residues through the intestines seems to lower the risk for colon cancer, mainly because cancer-causing agents are not in contact as long with the intestinal wall. Insoluble fiber also is thought to bind with carcinogens (cancer-producing substances), and more water in the stool may dilute the cancer-causing agents, lessening their potency. Sources of insoluble fiber include wheat, cereals, vegetables, and skins of fruits.

A practical guideline to obtain your fiber intake is to eat at least five daily servings of fruits and vegetables and three servings of whole-grain foods (whole-grain bread, cereal, and rice).

KEY TERMS

Nutrition The science that studies the relationship of foods to optimal health and performance.

Nutrients Substances found in food that provide energy, regulate metabolism, and help with growth and repair of body tissues.

Substrates Foods that are used as energy sources (carbohydrates, fats, proteins).

Essential nutrients Carbohydrates, fats, proteins, vitamins, minerals, and water—the nutrients the human body requires for survival.

Macronutrients The nutrients the body needs in proportionately large amounts: Carbohydrates, fats, proteins, and water.

Micronutrients The nutrients the body needs in small quantities—vitamins and minerals—that serve specific roles in transformation of energy and body tissue synthesis.

Calorie The amount of heat necessary to raise the temperature of 1 gram of water 1 degree centigrade; used to measure the energy value of food and the cost of physical activity.

Carbohydrates Compounds composed of carbon, hydrogen, and oxygen that the body uses as its major source of energy.

Fiber Plant material that human digestive enzymes cannot digest.

TABLE 5.1

Fiber Content of Selected Foods

Food (gm)	Serving Size	Dietary Fiber
Almonds, shelled	¼ cup	3.9
Apple	1 medium	3.7
Banana	1 small	1.2
Beans (red, kidney)	½ cup	8.2
Blackberries	½ cup	4.9
Beets, red, canned (cooked)	½ cup	1.4
Brazil nuts	1 oz	2.5
Broccoli (cooked)	½ cup	3.3
Brown rice (cooked)	½ cup	1.7
Carrots (cooked)	½ cup	3.3
Cauliflower (cooked)	½ cup	5.0
Cereal		
All Bran	1 oz	8.5
Cheerios	1 oz	1.1
Cornflakes	1 oz	0.5
Fruit and Fibre	1 oz	4.0
Fruit Wheats	1 oz	2.0
Just Right	1 oz	2.0
Wheaties	1 oz	2.0
Corn (cooked)	½ cup	2.2
Eggplant (cooked)	½ cup	3.0
Lettuce (chopped)	½ cup	0.5
Orange	1 medium	4.3
Parsnips (cooked)	½ cup	2.1
Pear	1 medium	4.5
Peas (cooked)	½ cup	4.4
Popcorn (plain)	1 cup	1.2
Potato (baked)	1 medium	4.9
Strawberries	½ cup	1.6
Summer squash (cooked)	½ cup	1.6
Watermelon	1 cup	0.1

Fats

Fats, or **lipids,** are the most concentrated source of energy. Each gram of fat supplies 9 calories to the body. Fats, also part of the cell structure, are used as stored energy and as an insulator to preserve body heat. They absorb shock, supply essential fatty acids, and carry the fat-soluble vitamins A, D, E, and K. The main sources of dietary fat are milk and other dairy products, and meats and alternatives. Fats are classified into simple, compound, and derived fats.

Simple Fats

Simple fats consist of a glyceride molecule linked to one, two, or three units of fatty acids. According to the number of fatty acids attached, simple fats are divided into monoglycerides (one fatty acid), diglycerides (two fatty acids), and triglycerides (three fatty acids). More than 90 percent of the weight of fat in foods and more than 95 percent of the stored fat in the human body is in the form of triglycerides.

The length of the carbon atom chain and the amount of hydrogen saturation in fatty acids vary. Based on the extent of saturation, fatty acids are said to be saturated or unsaturated. Unsaturated fatty acids are classified further into monounsaturated and polyunsaturated fats. Saturated fatty acids are mainly of animal origin. Unsaturated fats are found mostly in plant products.

In saturated fatty acids, the carbon atoms are fully saturated with hydrogen; only single bonds link the carbon atoms on the chain. These saturated fatty acids are more commonly known as saturated fats. Examples of foods high in saturated fatty acids are meats, meat fat, lard, whole milk, cream, butter, cheese, ice cream, coconut oil, and palm oils. Satu-

---

BEHAVIOR MODIFICATION PLANNING

Tips to Increase Fiber in Your Diet

- Eat more vegetables, either raw or steamed
- Eat salads daily that include a wide variety of vegetables
- Eat more fruit, including the skin
- Choose whole-wheat and whole-grain products
- Choose breakfast cereals with more than 3 grams of fiber per serving
- Sprinkle a teaspoon or two of unprocessed bran or 100 percent bran cereal on your favorite breakfast cereal
- Add high-fiber cereals to casseroles and desserts
- Add beans to soups, salads, and stews
- Add vegetables to sandwiches: sprouts, green and red pepper strips, diced carrots, sliced cucumbers, red cabbage, onions
- Add vegetables to spaghetti: broccoli, cauliflower, sliced carrots, mushrooms
- Experiment with unfamiliar fruits and vegetables— collards, kale, broccoflower, asparagus, papaya, mango, kiwi, starfruit
- Blend fruit juice with small pieces of fruit and crushed ice
- When increasing fiber in your diet, drink plenty of fluids

Try It

Do you know your average daily fiber intake? If you do not know, keep a 3-day record of daily fiber intake. How do you fare against the recommended guidelines? If your intake is low, how can you change your diet to increase your daily fiber intake?

rated fats tend to be solids that typically do not melt at room temperature. Coconut and palm oils are exceptions. In general, saturated fats raise the blood cholesterol level. The jury on coconut and palm oils is still out, because recent research indicates that these oils may be neutral in terms of their effects on cholesterol and may actually provide some health benefits.

In unsaturated fatty acids (unsaturated fats), double bonds form between the unsaturated carbons. Monounsaturated fatty acids (MUFA) have only one double bond along the chain. Examples are olive, canola, rapeseed, peanut, and sesame oils. Polyunsaturated fatty acids (PUFA) contain two or more double bonds between unsaturated carbon atoms along the chain. Corn, cottonseed, safflower, walnut, sunflower, and soybean oils are high in polyunsaturated fatty acids. Unsaturated fats are usually liquid at room temperature.

Another type of fat, trans fatty acids, are receiving a lot of attention. Hydrogen often is added to monounsaturated and polyunsaturated fats to increase shelf life and to solidify them so they are more spreadable. During this process, called "partial hydrogenation," the position of hydrogen atoms may be changed along the carbon chain, transforming the fat into a trans fatty acid. Margarine and spreads, shortening, some nut butters, crackers, cookies, dairy products, meats, processed foods, and fast foods often contain trans fatty acids.

Trans fatty acids are not essential and provide no known health benefit. In truth, health-conscious people minimize their intake of these types of fats because diets high in trans fatty acids increase rigidity of the coronary arteries, elevate cholesterol, and contribute to the formation of blood clots that may lead to heart attacks and strokes.

Trans fats are found in about 40 percent of supermarket foods, including almost all cookies, 80 percent of frozen breakfast foods, 75 percent of snacks and chips, most cake mixes, and almost 50 percent of all cereals. Doughnuts, french fries, stick margarine, vegetable shortening, and cookies and crackers are all high in trans fatty acid content.

Paying attention to food labels is important, because the words "partially hydrogenated" and "trans fatty acids" indicate that the product carries a health risk just as high or higher than that of saturated fat.

Compound Fats

Compound fats are a combination of simple fats and other chemicals. Examples are phospholipids, glucolipids, and lipoproteins.

Derived Fats

Derived fats combine simple and compound fats. Sterols are an example. Although sterols contain no fatty acids, they are considered lipids because they do not dissolve in water. The most often mentioned sterol is cholesterol, which is found in many foods and is manufactured from saturated fats in the body.

Proteins

Proteins are used to build and repair tissues, including muscles, blood, internal organs, skin, hair, nails, and bones. They are a part of hormones, enzymes, and antibodies and help maintain a normal balance of body fluids. Proteins can also be used as a source of energy, but only if not enough carbohydrates are available. The primary sources are meats, meat alternates, milk, and other dairy products.

Proteins are composed of **amino acids,** containing nitrogen, carbon, hydrogen, and oxygen. Nine of the 20 amino acids are called essential amino acids because the body cannot produce them. The other 11, termed nonessential amino acids, can be manufactured in the body if food proteins in the diet provide enough nitrogen. For normal body function, all amino acids must be present in the diet.

A deficiency in protein is not a problem in the usual American diet. Two glasses of skim milk combined with about 4 ounces of poultry or fish meet the daily protein requirement. Protein deficiency, however, could be a concern in some vegetarian diets (see discussion on vegetarianism, pages 130–131).

Vitamins

Vitamins function as **antioxidants** and as coenzymes (primarily the B complex), which regulate the work of enzymes; and vitamin D even functions as a hormone. Based on their solubility, vitamins are

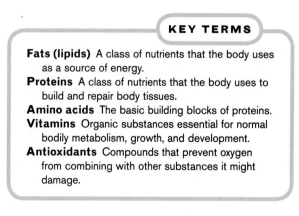

KEY TERMS

Fats (lipids) A class of nutrients that the body uses as a source of energy.

Proteins A class of nutrients that the body uses to build and repair body tissues.

Amino acids The basic building blocks of proteins.

Vitamins Organic substances essential for normal bodily metabolism, growth, and development.

Antioxidants Compounds that prevent oxygen from combining with other substances it might damage.

classified into two types: fat-soluble vitamins (A, D, E, and K) and water-soluble vitamins (B complex and C). The body cannot manufacture vitamins; they can be obtained only through a well-balanced diet. Additional information on the importance of vitamins is presented later in this chapter.

Minerals

Minerals serve several important functions. They are constituents of all cells, especially those in hard parts of the body (bones, nails, teeth); are crucial in maintaining water balance and the acid-base balance; are essential components of respiratory pigments, enzymes, and enzyme systems; and regulate muscular and nervous tissue excitability.

Water

Water, the most important nutrient, is involved in almost every vital body process. Water is used in digesting and absorbing food, in the circulatory process, in removing waste products, in building and rebuilding cells, and in transporting other nutrients.

Water is contained in almost all foods, but primarily in liquid foods, fruits, and vegetables. Although for decades the recommendation was to consume at least eight cups of water per day, a panel of scientists of the Institute of Medicine of the National Academy of Sciences (NAS) has indicated that people are getting enough water from the liquids (milk, juices, sodas, coffee) and the moisture

TABLE 5.2

Recommended Dietary Allowances and Adequate Intakes for Selected Nutrients

	Recommended Dietary Allowances (RDAs)													Adequate Intakes (AIs)					
	Thiamin (mg)	Riboflavin (mg)	Niacin (mg NE)	Vitamin B₆ (mg)	Folate (mcg DFE)	Vitamin B₁₂ (mcg)	Phosphorus (mg)	Magnesium (mg)	Vitamin A (mcg)	Vitamin C (mg)	Vitamin E (mg)	Selenium (mcg)	Iron (mcg)	Calcium (mg)	Vitamin D (mcg)	Fluoride (mg)	Pantothenic acid (mg)	Biotin (mg)	Choline (mg)
Males																			
14–18	1.2	1.3	16	1.3	400	2.4	1,250	410	900	75	15	55	11	1,300	5	3	5.0	25	550
19–30	1.2	1.3	16	1.3	400	2.4	700	400	900	90	15	55	8	1,000	5	4	5.0	30	550
31–50	1.2	1.3	16	1.3	400	2.4	700	420	900	90	15	55	8	1,000	5	4	5.0	30	550
51–70	1.2	1.3	16	1.7	400	2.4	700	420	900	90	15	55	8	1,200	10	4	5.0	30	550
>70	1.2	1.3	16	1.7	400	2.4	700	420	900	90	15	55	8	1,200	15	4	5.0	30	550
Females																			
14–18	1.0	1.0	14	1.2	400	2.4	1,250	360	700	65	15	55	15	1,300	5	3	5.0	25	400
19–30	1.1	1.1	14	1.3	400	2.4	700	310	700	75	15	55	18	1,000	5	3	5.0	30	425
31–50	1.1	1.1	14	1.3	400	2.4	700	320	700	75	15	55	18	1,000	5	3	5.0	30	425
51–70	1.1	1.1	14	1.5	400	2.4	700	320	700	75	15	55	8	1,200	10	3	5.0	30	425
>70	1.1	1.1	14	1.5	400	2.4	700	320	700	75	15	55	8	1,200	15	3	5.0	30	425
Pregnant	1.4	1.4	18	1.9	600	2.6	*	+40	750	85	15	60	27	*	*	3	6.0	30	450
Lactating	1.5	1.6	17	2.0	500	2.8	*	*	1,300	120	19	70	10	*	*	3	7.0	35	550

*Values for these nutrients do not change with pregnancy or lactation. Use the value listed for women of comparable age.

SOURCE: Adapted with permission from *Recommended Dietary Allowances,* 10th Edition, and the *Dietary Reference Intakes* series. Copyright © 1989 and 2002, respectively, by the National Academy of Sciences. Courtesy of the National Academies Press, Washington, DC.

content of solid foods. Caffeine-containing drinks are also acceptable as a water source because data indicate that people who regularly consume such beverages do not have a greater 24-hour urine output than those who don't.

Most Americans and Canadians remain well hydrated simply by using thirst as their guide. An exception to this practice, however, is when an individual exercises in the heat or does so for an extended time. Water lost under these conditions must be replenished regularly, without waiting for the onset of thirst.

Nutrition Standards

Nutritionists use a variety of standards. The most widely known is the **Recommended Dietary Allowance (RDA).** This is not the only standard, though. Nutrition standards include the **Dietary Reference Intakes (DRIs)** and the Daily Values on food labels. Each standard has a different purpose and utilization in dietary planning and assessment.

Dietary Reference Intakes

To help people meet dietary guidelines, the NAS has developed the DRIs as nutrition standards for healthy people in the United States and Canada. The DRIs are based on a review of the most current research on adequate amounts and maximum safe nutrient intakes of healthy people. The DRI reports are written by the Food and Nutrition Board of the Institute of Medicine in cooperation with scientists from Canada.

Within the umbrella of the DRIs are four types of reference values for planning and assessing diets:

1. Estimated Average Requirements (EARs)
2. Recommended Dietary Allowances (RDAs)
3. Adequate Intakes (AIs)
4. Tolerable Upper Intake Levels (ULs).

The type of reference value used for a given nutrient and a specific age/gender group is determined according to available scientific information and the intended use of the dietary standard.

The **Estimated Average Requirement (EAR)** is the amount of nutrient that is estimated to meet the nutrient requirement of half the healthy people in specific age and gender groups. At this nutrient intake level, the nutritional requirements of the upper 50 percent of the people are not met.

The RDAs set forth the daily amount of a nutrient considered adequate to meet the known nutrient needs of nearly all healthy people in the United States. The RDAs for selected nutrients are presented in Table 5.2. Because the committee must decide what level of intake to recommend for everybody, the RDA is set well above the EAR and covers about 98 percent of the population. Stated another way, the RDA recommendation for any nutrient is well above almost everyone's actual requirement.

The RDA could be considered a goal for adequate intake. The process for determining the RDA depends on being able to set an EAR. RDAs are statistically determined from the EAR values. If an EAR cannot be set, no RDA can be established.

When data are insufficient or inadequate to set an EAR, an **Adequate Intake (AI)** value is determined instead of the RDA. The AI value is derived from approximations of observed nutrient intakes by a group or groups of healthy people. The AI value for children and adults is expected to meet or exceed the nutritional requirements of a specific healthy population.

The **Tolerable Upper Intake Level (UL),** which eventually will be available for all nutrients, establishes the highest level of nutrient intake that seems to be safe for most healthy people and be-

---

> **KEY TERMS**
>
> **Minerals** Inorganic elements needed by the body.
> **Recommended Dietary Allowance (RDA)** The daily amount of a nutrient (statistically determined from the EARs) considered adequate to meet the known nutrient needs of almost 98 percent of all healthy people in the United States.
> **Dietary Reference Intakes (DRIs)** Four types of nutrient standards that are used to establish adequate amounts and maximum safe nutrient intakes in the diet: Estimated Average Requirements (EARs), Recommended Dietary Allowances (RDAs), Adequate Intakes (AIs), and Tolerable Upper Intake Levels (ULs).
> **Estimated Average Requirement (EAR)** The amount of a nutrient that meets the dietary needs in half the people.
> **Adequate Intake (AI)** The recommended amount of a nutrient intake when sufficient evidence is not available to calculate the EAR and subsequent RDA.
> **Tolerable Upper Intake Level (UL)** The highest level of nutrient intake that appears to be safe for most healthy people without an increased risk for adverse effects.

yond which there is an increased risk of adverse effects. As intakes increase above the UL, so does the risk for adverse effects. Generally speaking, the optimum nutrient range for healthy eating is between the RDA and the UL. The established ULs for selected nutrients are presented in Table 5.3.

Daily Values

The **Daily Values (DVs)** are reference values for nutrients and food components for use on commercial food labels. The DVs are based on a 2,000-calorie diet and may therefore require adjustments depending on an individual's daily **Estimated Energy Requirement (EER)** in calories.

For example, on a 2,000-calorie diet (EER), recommended carbohydrate intake is about 300 grams (about 60 percent of EER), and fat is less than 65 grams (about 30 percent of EER) (see Figure 5.1). The vitamin, mineral, and protein DVs were adapted from the RDAs. The DVs are also not as specific for age and gender groups as are the DRIs.

The food label is a good guide for planning a daily diet. For example, if the DV for carbohydrates in a given meal adds up to only 35 percent, you know that several additional high-carbohydrate food items are required throughout that day to reach the 100 percent DV. Further, if the DV for fat from another food item is 60 or 70 percent, you should limit your fat intake during the rest of that day.

TABLE 5.3

Tolerable Upper Intake Levels (UL) of Selected Nutrients for Adults (19–70 years)

Nutrient	UL per Day
Calcium	2.5 gr
Phosphorus	4.0 gr*
Magnesium	350 mg
Vitamin D	50 mcg
Fluoride	10 mg
Niacin	35 mg
Iron	45 mg
Vitamin B_6	100 mg
Folate	1,000 mcg
Choline	3.5 gr
Vitamin A	3,000 mcg
Vitamin C	2,000 mg
Vitamin E	1,000 mg
Selenium	400 mcg

*3.5 gr per day for pregnant women.

Both the DRIs and the DVs apply only to healthy adults. They are not intended for people who are ill and may require additional nutrients or dietary adjustments.

CRITICAL THINKING

What do the nutrition standards mean to you? • How much of a challenge would it be to apply those standards in your daily life?

FIGURE 5.1

Food label using Daily Values.

Nutrition Facts

Serving Size 1 cup (240 ml)
Servings Per Container 4

Amount Per Serving

Calories 120 Calories from Fat 45

	% Daily Value*
Total Fat 5g	**8%**
Saturated Fat 3g	**15%**
Trans Fat 1g	
Cholesterol 20mg	**7%**
Sodium 120mg	**5%**
Total Carbohydrate 12g	**4%**
Dietary Fiber 0g	**0%**
Sugars 12g	
Protein 8g	

Vitamin A 10% • Vitamin C 4%
Calcium 30% • Iron 0%

* Percent Daily Values are based on a 2,000 calorie diet. Your daily values may be higher or lower depending on your calorie needs:

	Calories	2,000	2,500
Total Fat	Less than	65g	80g
Sat Fat	Less than	20g	25g
Cholesterol	Less than	300mg	300mg
Sodium	Less than	2,400mg	2,400mg
Total Carbohydrate		300g	375g
Fiber		25g	30g

Calories per gram:
Fat 9 • Carbohydrate 4 • Protein 4

Dietary Guidelines

Most people would like to live life to its fullest, have good health, and lead a productive life. One of the ways to do this is through a well-balanced diet. As illustrated in Table 5.4, the recommended guidelines by the NAS state that daily caloric intake should be distributed so that 45 to 65 percent of the total calories come from carbohydrates (mostly complex carbohydrates and less than 25 percent from sugar), 20 to 35 percent from fat, and 10 to 35 percent from proteins.[2] These ranges offer greater flexibility in planning diets according to individual health and physical activity needs.

In addition to the macronutrients, the diet must include all of the essential vitamins and minerals. The source of fat calories is also critical. The National Cholesterol Education Program recommends that saturated fat constitute less than 7 percent, polyunsaturated fat up to 10 percent, and monounsaturated fat up to 20 percent of total calories. Rating a given diet accurately is difficult without a complete nutrient analysis. You have an opportunity to perform this analysis in Activity 5.1, pages 143–144.

The NAS guidelines are in sharp contrast to those of major national health organizations, which recommend 50 to 60 percent of total calories from carbohydrates, less than 30 percent from fat, and about 15 percent from protein. The most drastic difference appears in the NAS-allowed range of fat intake, up to 35 percent of total calories. This

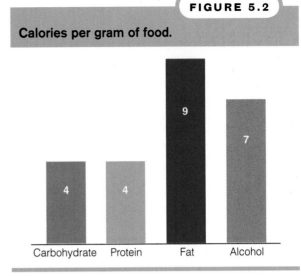

FIGURE 5.2

Calories per gram of food.

higher percentage was included to accommodate individuals with metabolic syndrome (see Chapter 8, page 205), who have an abnormal insulin response to carbohydrates and may need additional fat in the diet.

The NAS recommendations will be effective only if people consistently replace saturated and trans fatty acids with unsaturated fatty acids. The latter will require dramatic changes in the typical "unhealthy" American diet, which is generally high in red meats, whole dairy products, and fast foods—all of which are high in saturated and/or trans fatty acids.

Determining Fat Content in the Diet

As illustrated in Figure 5.2, each gram of carbohydrate and protein supplies the body with 4 calories, and fat provides 9 calories per gram consumed (alcohol yields 7 calories per gram). In this regard, just

TABLE 5.4

Current and Recommended Intake of Carbohydrate, Fat, and Protein Expressed as a Percentage of Total Calories

	Current	Recommended*
Carbohydrates	50%	45–65%
Simple	26%	Less than 25%
Complex	24%	20–40%
Fat	34%	20–35%**
Monounsaturated	11%	Up to 20%
Polyunsaturated	10%	Up to 10%
Saturated	13%	Less than 7%
Protein	16%	10–35%

*2002 recommended guidelines by the National Academy of Sciences.

**Less than 30% recommended by most health organizations. A higher amount may be indicated for people with metabolic syndrome.

FIGURE 5.3

Determining percent calories from fat in food.

Serving = 120 calories   Fat = 5 g

Percent Fat Calories = (g of fat × 9)
÷ calories per serving × 100

5 g of fat × 9 calories per g of fat =
45 calories from fat

45 calories from fat ÷ 120 calories per
serving × 100 = 38% fat

looking at the total amount of grams consumed for each type of food can be misleading.

For example, a person who consumes 160 grams of carbohydrates, 100 grams of fat, and 70 grams of protein has a total intake of 330 grams of food. This indicates that 30 percent of the total grams of food is in the form of fat (100 grams of fat ÷ 330 grams of total food × 100).

Almost half of this diet, however, consists of fat calories. In the diet, 640 calories are derived from carbohydrates (160 grams × 4 calories/gram), 280 calories from protein (70 grams × 4 calories/gram), and 900 calories from fat (100 grams × 9 calories/gram), for a total of 1,820 calories. If 900 calories are derived from fat, you can see that almost half of the total caloric intake is in the form of fat (900 ÷ 1,820 × 100 = 49.5 percent).

Realizing that each gram of fat provides 9 calories is a useful guideline when figuring the fat content of individual foods. As shown in Figure 5.3, all you have to do is multiply the grams of fat by 9 and divide by the total calories in that specific food. Multiply that number by 100 to get the percentage. For example, if a food label lists a total of 120 calories and 7 grams of fat, the fat content is 53 percent of total calories (7 × 9 ÷ 120 × 100). This simple guideline can help you decrease fat in your diet.

KEY TERMS

Phytonutrients Compounds found in vegetables and fruits with cancer-fighting properties.

Balancing the Diet

Achieving and maintaining a balanced diet is not as difficult as most people think. The MyPyramid healthy eating guide in Figure 5.4 contains five major food groups and oils. The food groups are grains, vegetables, fruits, milk, and meats and beans.

Whole grains, vegetables, fruits, and low-fat milk (and by-products) provide the nutritional base for a healthy diet. If you increase the intake of these food groups, remember to decrease the intake of low-nutrient density foods to effectively balance caloric intake with energy needs.

Whole grains are a major source of fiber as well as other nutrients. Whole grains contain the entire grain kernel (the bran, germ, and endosperm). Examples include whole-wheat flour, whole cornmeal, oatmeal, cracked wheat (bulgur), and brown rice.

Refined grains have been milled, a process that removes the bran and germ. The process also removes fiber, iron, and many B vitamins. Refined grains include white flour, white bread, white rice, and degermed cornmeal. Refined grains are often enriched to add back B vitamins and iron. Fiber, however, is not added back.

In addition to providing nutrients crucial to health, fruits and vegetables are the sole source of **phytonutrients** ("phyto" comes from the Greek word for plant). The main function of phytonutrients in plants is to protect them from sunlight. In humans, phytonutrients seem to have a powerful ability to block the formation of cancerous tumors. Their actions are so diverse that at almost every stage of cancer, phytonutrients have the ability to block, disrupt, slow down, or even reverse the process (also see Chapter 8).

These compounds are not found in pills. The message here is to eat a diet with ample fruits and vegetables. The daily recommended amount of fruits and vegetables has absolutely no substitute. People can't expect to eat a poor diet, pop a few pills, and derive the same benefits.

Milk and milk products (select low-fat or nonfat) can decrease the risk of low bone mass (osteoporosis) throughout life. Besides calcium, milk is also a good source of potassium, vitamin D, and protein, and may aid with body weight management.

The recommendation for poultry, fish, or meat is to eat 3 ounces—and no more than 6 ounces—daily. All visible fat and skin should be trimmed off meats and poultry before cooking.

FIGURE 5.4

MyPyramid: Steps to a healthier you.

The colors of the pyramid illustrate variety: each color represents one of the five food groups, plus one for oils. Different band widths suggest the proportional contribution of each food group to a healthy diet.

A person climbing steps reminds consumers to be physically active each day.

The narrow slivers of color at the top imply moderation in foods rich in solid fats and added sugars.

The broad bases at the bottom represent nutrient-dense foods that should make up the bulk of the diet.

Greater intakes of grains, vegetables, fruit, and milk are encouraged by the broad bases of orange, green, red, and blue.

SOURCE: USDA, 2005.

GRAINS
In general, 1 slice of bread, 1 cup of ready-to-eat cereal, ½ cup of cooked rice, cooked pasta, or cooked cereal can be considered as 1 oz equivalent of grains. Look for "whole" before the grain name on the list of ingredients and make at least half your grains whole.

VEGETABLES
In general, 1 cup of raw or cooked vege-tables or vegetable juice, or 2 cups of raw leafy greens can be considered as 1 cup from the vegetable group. Try to eat more dark green and orange veggies, as well as dry beans and peas.

FRUITS
In general, 1 cup of fruit or 100% fruit juice, or ½ cup of dried fruit can be considered as 1 cup from the fruit group. Eat a variety of fruit, including fresh, frozen, canned, or dried fruit. Go easy on fruit juices.

OILS
Measured in teaspoons of either oils or solid fats. Most sources should come from fish, nuts, and vegetable oils. Limit solid fats such as butter, stick margarine, shortening, and lard.

MILK
In general, 1 cup of milk or yogurt, 1½ oz of natural cheese, or 2 oz of processed cheese can be con-sidered as 1 cup from the milk group. Go low-fat or fat free. If you can't consume milk, choose lactose-free products or other calcium sources.

MEATS & BEANS
In general: 1 oz of meat, poultry, or fish, ¼ cup cooked dry beans, 1 egg, 1 tbsp of peanut butter, or ½ oz of nuts or seeds can be consid-ered as 1 oz equivalent from the Meats & Beans group.

Recommended Daily Amounts from Each Food Group

FOOD GROUP	1600 cal	1800 cal	2000 cal	2200 cal	2400 cal	2600 cal	2800 cal	3000 cal
Fruits	1½ c	1½ c	2 c	2 c	2 c	2 c	2½ c	2½ c
Vegetables	2 c	2½ c	2½ c	3 c	3 c	3½ c	3½ c	4 c
Grains	5 oz	6 oz	6 oz	7 oz	8 oz	9 oz	10 oz	10 oz
Meat and legumes	5 oz	5 oz	5½ oz	6 oz	6½ oz	6½ oz	7 oz	7 oz
Milk	3 c	3 c	3 c	3 c	3 c	3 c	3 c	3 c
Oils	5 tsp	5 tsp	6 tsp	6 tsp	7 tsp	8 tsp	8 tsp	10 tsp
Discretionary calorie allowance	132 cal	195 cal	267 cal	290 cal	362 cal	410 cal	426 cal	512 cal

*Discretionary calorie allowance: At each calorie level, people who consistently choose calorie-dense foods may be able to meet their nutrient needs without consuming their full allotment of calories. The difference between the calories needed to supply nutrients and those needed for energy is known as the *discretionary calorie allowance.*

The difficult part for most people is retraining themselves to adopt a lifetime healthy nutrition plan. You can achieve a balanced diet if you (a) avoid excessive fats, oils, sweets, sodium (salt), and alcohol; (b) increase your fiber intake; and (c) eat the minimum number of servings recommended for each of the five major groups in MyPyramid.

Nutrient Analysis

To aid you in balancing your diet, Activity 5.1, pages 143–144, provides a form for you to record your daily food intake. First, make as many copies as the number of days you wish to analyze. Whenever you eat something, record the food and the amount eaten. Doing this immediately after each meal will enable you to keep track of your actual food intake more easily.

At the end of each day, consult the list of foods in Appendix E and record the number of calories for all foods consumed. Referring to Activity 5.1, pages 143–144, record the amount and calories under the respective food groups. If you eat twice the amount of a standard serving, double the calories and the amount.

You can evaluate the diet by comparing your food intake against MyPyramid guidelines (see Figure 5.4) according to your age, gender, and activity level. If you meet the minimum daily amounts for each food group at the end of each day, you are doing quite well in balancing your diet.

In addition to meeting the daily amount guidelines, a complete nutrient analysis is recommended to rate your diet accurately. A nutrient analysis can pinpoint potential problem areas in your diet, such as too much fat, saturated fat, cholesterol, and sodium. A complete nutrient analysis can be an educational experience, because most people do not realize how detrimental and non-nutritious many common foods are.

You can also do the analysis by logging on to academic.cengage.com/login and using the information you have recorded already on the form provided in Activity 5.1. Up to seven days may be analyzed when using the software. Before running the software, fill out the information at the top of the form (age, weight, height, gender, and activity rating), and make sure the foods are recorded by the standard amounts given in the list of selected foods in Appendix E. The analysis also accommodates vegetarianism.

Vegetarianism

More than 12 million people in the United States follow vegetarian diets. **Vegetarians** rely primarily on foods from the bread, cereal, rice, pasta, and fruit and vegetable groups and avoid foods from animal sources, including the milk, yogurt, and cheese and meat groups.

The five basic types of vegetarians are:

1. Vegans: those who eat no animal products at all
2. Ovovegetarians: those who allow eggs in the diet
3. Lactovegetarians: those who allow foods from the milk group
4. Ovolactovegetarians: those who include egg and milk products in the diet
5. Semivegetarians: those who do not eat red meat but include fish and poultry in addition to milk products and eggs in their diets

Well-planned vegetarian diets are healthful and consistent with the Dietary Guidelines for Americans, and can meet the DRIs for nutrients. Vegetarians who do not select their food combinations properly, however, can develop nutritional deficiencies of protein, vitamins, minerals, and even calories. Even more attention should be paid when planning vegetarian diets for infants and children. Without careful planning, a strictly plant-based diet will prevent proper growth and development.

Protein deficiency is a concern in some vegetarian diets. Vegans in particular must be careful to eat foods that provide a balanced distribution of essential amino acids, such as grain products and legumes. Strict vegans also need a supplement of vitamin B_{12}. This vitamin is not found in plant foods; its only source is animal foods. A deficiency of this vitamin can lead to anemia and nerve damage.

The key to a healthful vegetarian diet is to eat foods with complementary proteins. Most plant-based products lack one or more essential amino acids in adequate amounts. For example, both grains and legumes are good protein sources, but neither provides all the essential amino acids. Grains and cereals are low in the amino acid lysine, and legumes lack methionine. When combined, foods from these two groups, such as tortillas and beans, rice and beans, rice and soybeans, or wheat bread and peanuts, complement each other. These complementary proteins may be consumed over the course of the day, but it is best if they are consumed during the same meal.

MyPyramid can also be used as a guide for vegetarians. The key is food variety. Most vegetarians today consume dairy products and eggs. Meat can be replaced with legumes, nuts, seeds, eggs, and meat substitutes (tofu, tempeh, soy milk, and commercial meat replacers such as veggie burgers and soy hot dogs). For additional MyPyramid healthy eating tips for vegetarians and ways to get enough of the previously mentioned nutrients, go to http://mypyramid.gov/.

Consumption of nuts and soy foods, commonly used in vegetarian diets, has received considerable attention in recent years. Although nuts are 70 to 90 percent fat, most of it is unsaturated fat. And research indicates that people who eat nuts several times a week have a lower incidence of heart disease. Eating 2 to 3 ounces (about one-half cup) of almonds, walnuts, or macadamia nuts a day may decrease high blood cholesterol by about 10 percent.

Heart-health benefits are attributed to the unsaturated fats and also to other nutrients found in nuts, such as vitamin E and folic acid. Nuts are also packed with additional B vitamins, calcium, copper, potassium, magnesium, fiber, and phytonutrients. Many of these nutrients are cancer-protective and cardioprotective.

Nuts do have a drawback: They are high in calories. A handful of nuts provides as many calories as a piece of cake. Therefore, you should avoid using nuts as a snack. Nuts are recommended for use in place of high-protein foods such as meats, bacon, and eggs, or as part of a meal in fruit or vegetable salads, homemade bread, pancakes, casseroles, yogurt, and oatmeal. Peanut butter is also healthier than cheese or some cold cuts in sandwiches.

The increasing popularity of soy foods is attributed primarily to Asian research that points to less heart disease and fewer hormone-related cancers in people who regularly consume soy foods. The benefits of soy lie in its high protein content and plant chemicals, known as isoflavones, that act as antioxidants and may protect against estrogen-related cancers (breast, ovarian, and endometrial). Soy consumption also has been linked to a lower risk for prostate cancer.

In addition, soy protein can lower blood cholesterol to a greater extent than would be expected just from its low-fat and high-fiber content. The evidence of heart-protecting benefits from soy foods is so strong that the Food and Drug Administration allows the following claim on food labels: "25 grams of soy proteins a day, as part of a diet low in saturated fat and cholesterol, may reduce the risk of heart disease." One to two cups of soy milk, ½ cup of tofu, 1½ tablespoons of soy protein isolate, or ¼ cup of soy flour provide about 10 grams of soy protein.

Those who are interested in vegetarian diets should consult other resources. A thorough discussion on such diets cannot be covered adequately in a few paragraphs.

Nutrient Supplementation

Approximately half of all adults in the United States take daily nutrient **supplements.** Nutrient requirements for the body normally can be met by consuming as few as 1,200 calories per day, as long as the diet contains the recommended amounts of food from the different food groups.

Most supplements do not seem to provide additional benefits for healthy people who eat a balanced diet. They do not help people run faster, jump higher, relieve stress, improve their sexual prowess, cure a common cold, or boost energy levels. Some of the special cases are discussed below.

People should not take **megadoses** of vitamins and minerals. For some nutrients, a dose of five times the RDA taken over several months may create problems. For others, such a dose may not pose any threat to human health. Vitamin and mineral intake should not exceed the ULs. For nutrients that do not have an established UL, a person should not take a dosage higher than three times the RDA.

Among the populations that may benefit from supplementation are those with nutrient deficiencies (including low calcium intake), alcoholics and street-drug users who do not have a balanced diet, smokers, vegans (strict vegetarians), individuals on

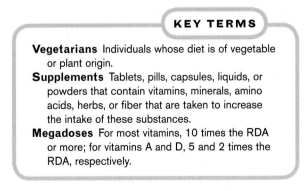

KEY TERMS

Vegetarians Individuals whose diet is of vegetable or plant origin.

Supplements Tablets, pills, capsules, liquids, or powders that contain vitamins, minerals, amino acids, herbs, or fiber that are taken to increase the intake of these substances.

Megadoses For most vitamins, 10 times the RDA or more; for vitamins A and D, 5 and 2 times the RDA, respectively.

extremely low calorie diets (fewer than 1,200 calories per day), older adults who don't eat balanced meals regularly, newborn infants (usually given a single dose of vitamin K to prevent abnormal bleeding), and people who have disease-related disorders or who are taking medications that interfere with proper absorption of nutrients.

Iron deficiency (determined through blood testing) is more common in women than men. Iron supplementation is frequently recommended for women who have a heavy menstrual flow. Some pregnant and lactating women also may require supplements. The average pregnant woman who eats an adequate amount of a variety of foods should take a low dose of iron supplement daily. Women who are pregnant with more than one baby may need additional supplements.

Antioxidants

Much research and discussion is taking place regarding the effectiveness of antioxidants in thwarting several chronic diseases. Although foods probably contain more than 4,000 antioxidants, the four most studied antioxidants are vitamins C, E, and beta-carotene (a precursor to vitamin A) and the mineral selenium (see Table 5.5).

Oxygen is utilized during metabolism to change carbohydrates and fats into energy. During this process, oxygen is transformed into stable forms of water and carbon dioxide. A small amount of oxygen, however, ends up in an unstable form, referred to as oxygen free radicals.

Free radicals attack and damage proteins and lipids, in particular cell membranes and DNA. This damage is thought to contribute to the development of conditions such as cardiovascular disease, cancer, emphysema, cataracts, Parkinson's disease, and premature aging. Environmental factors that seem to encourage the formation of free radicals include solar radiation, cigarette smoke, air pollution, radiation, some drugs, injury or infection, and chemicals (such as pesticides), among others.

The body's own defense systems typically neutralize free radicals so they don't cause any damage. When free radicals are produced faster than the body can neutralize them, however, they can damage the cells.

Antioxidants work best in the prevention and progression of disease, but they cannot repair damage that has already occurred or cure people with disease. The benefits are obtained primarily from food sources themselves, and controversy surrounds the benefits of antioxidants taken in supplement form.

For years people believed that taking antioxidant supplements could further prevent free-radical damage, but adding to the controversy, a report published in 2007 in the *Journal of the American Medical Association* indicated that antioxidant supplements actually increase the risk for death.[3] Vitamin E, beta-carotene, and vitamin A increased the risk for mortality by 4, 7, and 16 percent, respectively. Vitamin C had no effect on mortality, while selenium decreased risk by 9 percent. Some researchers, however, have questioned the design and conclusions of this report. More research is definitely required to settle the controversy.

Antioxidant Nutrients

Antioxidants are found abundantly in food, especially in fruits and vegetables (see Table 5.6). Un-

TABLE 5.5

Antioxidant Nutrients, Sources, and Functions

Nutrient	Good Sources	Antioxidant Effect
Vitamin C	Citrus fruit, kiwi fruit, cantaloupe, strawberries, broccoli, green or red peppers, cauliflower, cabbage	Appears to inactivate oxygen free radicals.
Vitamin E	Vegetable oils, yellow and green leafy vegetables, margarine, wheat germ, oatmeal, almonds, whole-grain breads, cereals	Protects lipids from oxidation.
Beta-carotene	Carrots, squash, pumpkin, sweet potatoes, broccoli, green leafy vegetables	Soaks up oxygen free radicals.
Selenium	Seafood, Brazil nuts, meat, whole grains	Helps prevent damage to cell structures.

TABLE 5.6

Antioxidant Content of Selected Foods

Beta-Carotene	IU
Apricot (1 medium)	675
Broccoli (½ cup, frozen)	1,740
Broccoli (½ cup, raw)	680
Cantaloupe (1 cup)	5,160
Carrot (1 medium, raw)	20,255
Green peas (½ cup, frozen)	535
Mango (1 medium)	8,060
Mustard greens (½ cup, frozen)	3,350
Papaya (1 medium)	6,120
Spinach (½ cup, frozen)	7,395
Sweet potato (1 medium, baked)	24,875
Tomato (1 medium)	1,395
Turnip greens (½ cup, boiled)	3,960

Vitamin C	mg
Acerola (1 cup, raw)	1,640
Acerola juice (8 oz)	3,864
Cantaloupe (½ melon, medium)	90
Cranberry juice (8 oz)	90
Grapefruit (½, medium, white)	52
Grapefruit juice (8 oz)	92
Guava (1 medium)	165
Kiwi (1 medium)	75
Lemon juice (8 oz)	110
Orange (1 medium)	66
Orange juice (8 oz)	120
Papaya (1 medium)	85
Pepper (½ cup, red, chopped, raw)	95
Strawberries (1 cup, raw)	88

Vitamin E	IU	mg*
Almond oil (1 tbsp)		5.3
Almonds (1 oz)	10.1	
Canola oil (1 tbsp)		9.0
Cottonseed oil (1 tbsp)		5.2
Hazelnuts (1 oz)	4.4	
Kale (1 cup)	15.0	
Margarine (1 tbsp)		2.0
Peanuts (1 oz)	3.0	
Shrimp (3 oz, boiled)	3.1	
Sunflower seeds (1 oz, dry)	14.2	
Sunflower seed oil (1 tbsp)		6.9
Sweet potato (1 medium, baked)	7.2	
Wheat germ oil (1 tbsp)		20.0

Selenium	mcg
Brazil nuts (1)	100
Bread, whole-wheat enriched (1 slice)	15
Beef (3 oz)	33
Cereals (3½ oz)	20
Chicken breast, roasted, no skin (3 oz)	24
Cod, baked (3 oz)	57
Egg, hard boiled (1 large)	15
Fruits (3½ oz)	1
Noodles, enriched, boiled (1 cup)	50
Oatmeal, cooked (1 cup)	23
Red snapper (3 oz)	150
Rice, long grain, cooked (1 cup)	20
Salmon, baked (3 oz)	35
Spaghetti w/meat sauce (1 cup)	36
Tuna, canned, water, drained (3 oz)	68
Turkey breast, roasted, no skin (3 oz)	28
Walnuts, black, chopped (¼ cup)	5
Vegetables (3½ oz)	1

*Vitamin E values for oils are commonly expressed in milligrams (mg). One mg is almost equal to 1 IU (international unit). ,

fortunately, most Americans do not eat the minimum daily recommended amounts of fruits and vegetables.

Vitamin E belongs to a group of eight compounds (four tocopherols and four tocotrienols) of which alpha-tocopherol is the most active form. The RDA for vitamin E is 15 mg or 22 IU (international units). Vitamin E is found primarily in oil-rich seeds and vegetable oils.

Vitamin E supplements from natural sources contain d-alpha tocopherol, which is better absorbed by the body than dl-alpha tocopherol, a synthetic form composed of a variety of E compounds. Vitamin E is fat soluble, thus a supplement should be taken with a meal that has some fat in it.

Although no evidence indicates that vitamin E supplementation below the upper limit of 1,000 mg per day is harmful, little or no clinical research supports any health benefits. Foods high in vitamin E include almonds, hazelnuts, peanuts, canola oil, sawflower oil, cottonseed oil, kale, sunflower seeds, shrimp, wheat germ, sweet potato, avocado, and tomato sauce. You should incorporate some of these foods regularly in the diet to obtain the RDA.

Studies have shown that vitamin C may offer benefits against heart disease, cancer, and cataracts. People who consume the recommended amounts of daily fruits and vegetables, however, need no supplementation because they obtain their daily vitamin C requirements through their diet alone.

Vitamin C is water soluble, and the body eliminates it in about 12 hours. For best results, consume vitamin C–rich foods twice a day. High intake of a vitamin C supplement, above 500 mg per day, is not recommended. The body absorbs very little vitamin C beyond the first 200 mg per serving or dose. Foods high in vitamin C include oranges and other citrus fruit, kiwi fruit, cantaloupe, guava, bell peppers, strawberries, broccoli, kale, cauliflower, and tomatoes.

Beta-carotene supplementation was encouraged in the early 1990s, but obtaining the daily recommended dose of beta-carotene (20,000 IU) from food sources rather than supplements is preferable. Clinical trials have found that beta-carotene supplements do not offer protection against heart disease or cancer and do not provide any other health benefits. Therefore, the recommendation is to "skip the pill and eat the carrot." One medium raw carrot contains about 20,000 IU of beta-carotene. Other foods high in beta-carotene include sweet potatoes, pumpkin, cantaloupe, squash, kale, broccoli, tomatoes, peaches, apricots, mangoes, papaya, turnip greens, and spinach.

Adequate intake of the mineral selenium is encouraged. Individuals who take 200 micrograms (mcg) of selenium daily seem to decrease their risks for prostate cancer by 63 percent, colorectal cancer by 58 percent, and lung cancer by 46 percent.[4] Data also point to decreased risks for cancers of the breast, liver, and digestive tract. According to Dr. Edward Giovannucci of the Harvard Medical School, the evidence for benefits of selenium in reducing prostate cancer risk is so strong that public health officials should recommend that people increase selenium intake now.[5]

One Brazil nut (unshelled) that you crack yourself provides about 100 mcg of selenium. Shelled nuts found in supermarkets average only about 20 mcg each. Based on the current body of research, a dose of 100 to 200 mcg per day seems to provide the necessary amount of antioxidant for this nutrient. There is no reason to take more than 200 mcg daily. In fact, the UL for selenium has been set at 400 mcg. Too much selenium can damage cells rather than protect them. If you choose to take supplements, take an organic form of selenium from yeast and not selenium selenite.

Multivitamins

Although much interest has been generated by the previously mentioned supplements, multivitamins are still the preferred supplement of the American people. A multivitamin complex that provides 100 percent of the DV for most nutrients can help fill in certain dietary deficiencies.[6] Some evidence suggests that regular intake decreases the risk for cardiovascular disease and colon cancer and improves immune function. Multivitamins, however, are not magic pills. They may help, but they are not a license to eat carelessly. Multivitamins don't provide energy, fiber, or phytonutrients.

Vitamin D

Vitamin D is attracting a lot of attention because current research suggests that it possesses anticancer properties (especially against breast, colon, and prostate cancers and possibly lung and digestive cancers), decreases inflammation (fighting cardiovascular disease, periodontal disease, and arthritis), strengthens the immune system, controls blood pressure, helps maintain muscle strength, and may help deter diabetes and fight depression. Vitamin D is also necessary for absorption of calcium, a nutrient critical for building and maintaining bones and teeth.

The theory that vitamin D protects against cancer is based on studies showing that people who live farther north (who have less sun exposure during the winter months) have a higher incidence of cancer. Evidence suggests that we should get between 1,000 and 2,000 IU (25 to 50 mcg) per day.[7] Good sources of vitamin D in the diet include salmon, mackerel, tuna, and sardines. Fortified milk, yogurt, orange juice, margarines, and cereals are also good sources.

To obtain 1,000 to 2,000 IU per day from food sources alone, however, is difficult. The best source of vitamin D is sunshine. Ultraviolet rays lead to the production in the skin of an inactive form of vitamin D (D_3). The inactive form is then transformed by the liver, and subsequently the kidneys, into the active form of vitamin D. Sun-generated vitamin D is also better than that obtained from foods or supplements.

Although excessive sun exposure can lead to skin damage, you should strive for daily "safe sun" exposure; that is, up to 15 minutes of unprotected sun exposure of the face, arms, and hands during peak daylight hours a few times a week (10:00 a.m. and 4:00 p.m.). Such exposure will generate between

1,000 and 2,000 IU of vitamin D. And even though the UL has been set at 2,000 IU, experts believe that this figure needs revision because there are no data implicating toxic effects up to 10,000 IU a day.[8]

Generating too much vitamin D from the sun is impossible because the body generates only what it needs. Most people are not getting enough vitamin D. The current recommended daily intake ranges between 200 and 600 IU (5–15 mcg), based on your age. People at the highest risk for low vitamin D levels are older adults, those with dark skin (they make less vitamin D), and individuals who spend most of their time indoors and get little sun exposure. In the United States and Canada, most of the population cannot make vitamin D from the sun during the winter months. During periods of limited sun exposure, you should consider a daily vitamin D_3 supplement of up to 2,000 IU per day (some vitamins contain vitamin D_2, which is a less potent form of the vitamin).

Folate

Supplementation of folate (a B vitamin) has been recommended for all premenopausal women. In particular, folate supplements are encouraged prior to and during pregnancy. This also applies to women who might become pregnant. Studies have shown that high folate intake (400 mcg per day) during early pregnancy can prevent serious birth defects. Folate also seems to offer protection against colon and cervical cancers. In all the above instances, supplements should be taken under a physician's supervision.

Increasing evidence indicates that taking 400 mcg of folate along with vitamins B_6 and B_{12} prevents heart attacks by reducing homocysteine levels in the blood (see Chapter 8). High concentrations of homocysteine accelerate the process of plaque formation (atherosclerosis) in the arteries. Five servings of fruits and vegetables per day usually meet the needs for these nutrients. Currently, close to 9 in 10 adults in the United States do not meet the recommended 400 mcg of folate per day. Because of the critical role of folate in preventing heart disease, some experts also recommend a daily vitamin B complex that includes 400 mcg of folate.

Benefits of Foods

Even though you may consider taking some supplements, fruits and vegetables are the richest sources of antioxidants and phytonutrients. Researchers at

the U.S. Department of Agriculture compared the antioxidant effects of vitamins C and E with those of various common fruits and vegetables. The results indicated that ¾ cup of cooked kale (which contains only 11 IU of vitamin E and 76 mg of vitamin C) neutralized as many free radicals as approximately 800 IU of vitamin E or 600 mg of vitamin C supplements. Other excellent sources of antioxidants found by these researchers include blueberries, strawberries, spinach, Brussels sprouts, plums, broccoli, beets, oranges, and grapes.

Many people who eat unhealthy diets think they need supplementation for balance. This is a fallacy about nutrition. The problem here is not necessarily a lack of vitamins and minerals, but a diet too high in calories, saturated fat, and sodium. Vitamin, mineral, and fiber supplements do not supply all of the nutrients and other beneficial substances present in food and needed for good health.

Wholesome foods contain vitamins, minerals, carbohydrates, fiber, proteins, fats, phytonutrients, and other substances not yet discovered. Researchers do not know if the protective effects are caused by the antioxidants alone, or in combination with other nutrients (such as phytonutrients), or by some other nutrients in food that have not been investigated yet. Many nutrients work in **synergy,** enhancing chemical processes in the body.

Supplementation will not offset poor eating habits. Pills are no substitute for common sense. If you think your diet is not balanced, you first need to conduct a nutrient analysis (see Activity 5.1 on pages 143–144) to determine which nutrients you lack in sufficient amounts. Eat more of them, as well as foods that are high in antioxidants and phytonutrients. After you perform a nutrient assessment, a **registered dietitian** can help you decide what supplement(s), if any, might be necessary.

The American Heart Association does not recommend antioxidant supplements until more definite research is available. If you take supplements in pill form, look for products that meet the disintegration

---

KEY TERMS

Synergy A reaction in which the result is greater than the sum of its two parts.

Registered dietitian (RD) A person with a college degree in dietetics who meets all certification and continuing education requirements of the American Dietetic Association or Dietitians of Canada.

standards of the U.S. Pharmacopoeia (USP), as shown on the bottle. The USP symbol suggests that the supplement should completely dissolve in 45 minutes or less. Supplements that do not dissolve, of course, cannot get into the bloodstream.

CRITICAL THINKING

Do you take supplements? • If so, for what purposes are you taking them? • And do you think you could restructure your diet so you could do without them?

Probiotics

Yogurt is rated in the "super foods" category because, in addition to being a good source of calcium, riboflavin, and protein, it contains probiotics. These health-promoting microorganisms live in the intestines and help break down foods and prevent disease-causing organisms from settling in. Probiotics have been found to offer protection against gastrointestinal infections, to boost immune activity, and to even help fight certain types of cancer.

When selecting yogurt, look for products with L-acidophilus, Bifidus, and inulin, which is a prebiotic (a substance on which probiotics feed). A soluble fiber, inulin appears to enhance calcium absorption. Avoid yogurt with added fruit, jam, sugar, and candy.

Fish

The presence in fish of potential contaminants, in particular mercury, has created concern. Mercury, a naturally occurring trace mineral, can be released into the air from industrial pollution. As mercury falls into streams and oceans, it accumulates in the aquatic food chain. Large-size fish accumulate larger amounts of mercury because they eat medium- and small-size fish. Of particular concern are shark, swordfish, king mackerel, pike, bass, and tilefish that have higher levels.

The American Heart Association recommends consuming fish twice a week. The risk for adverse effects from eating fish is extremely low and primarily theoretical in nature.[9] For most people, eating two servings (up to 6 ounces) of fish per week poses no health threat. Pregnant and nursing women and young children, however, should avoid mercury in fish.

The best recommendation is to balance the risks against the benefits. If you are concerned, consume no more than 12 ounces per week of a variety of fish and shellfish that are lower in mercury, including canned light tuna, wild salmon, shrimp, pollock, catfish, and scallops. A review of over 200 studies on the effects of fish consumption on health concluded that the benefits exceed the potential risks, and seafood appears to be the single most important food a person can consume for good health.[10]

Eating Disorders

Eating disorders are medical illnesses that involve critical disturbances in eating behaviors, thought to stem from some combination of environmental pressures. These disorders are characterized by an intense fear of becoming fat, which does not disappear even after the individual has lost extreme amounts of weight. The two most common types of eating disorders are **anorexia nervosa** and **bulimia nervosa,** although **binge eating,** also known as

---

BEHAVIOR MODIFICATION PLANNING

Guidelines for a Healthy Diet

- Base your diet on a large variety of foods.
- Consume ample amounts of green, yellow, and orange fruits and vegetables.
- Eat foods high in complex carbohydrates, including at least three 1-ounce servings of whole-grain foods per day.
- Obtain most of your vitamins and minerals from food sources.
- Eat foods rich in vitamin D.
- Maintain adequate daily calcium intake and consider a bone supplement with vitamin D_3.
- Consume protein in moderation.
- Limit daily fat, trans fat, and saturated fat intake.
- Limit cholesterol consumption to less than 300 mg per day.
- Limit sodium intake to 2,400 mg per day.
- Limit sugar intake.
- If you drink alcohol, do so in moderation (one daily drink for women and two for men).
- Consider taking a daily multivitamin (preferably one that includes vitamin D_3).

Try It
Carefully analyze the above guidelines and note the areas where you can improve your diet. Work on one guideline each week until you are able to adhere to all of the above guidelines.

compulsive overeating, is recognized as an eating disorder as well.

Most people who have eating disorders are afflicted by significant family and social problems. They may lack fulfillment in many areas of their lives. The eating disorder then becomes the coping mechanism to avoid dealing with these problems. Taking control over their own body weight helps them feel that they are restoring some sense of control over their lives.

Anorexia nervosa and bulimia nervosa are common in industrialized nations where society encourages low-calorie diets and thinness. Although frequently seen in young women, the majority seeking treatment are between the ages of 25 and 50. Surveys, nonetheless, indicate that as many as 40 percent of college-age women are struggling with an eating disorder.

Eating disorders are not limited to women. Every 1 in 10 cases exists in men. But because the role of men in society and their body image are viewed differently, these cases often go unreported.

Individuals who have clinical depression and obsessive-compulsive behavior are more susceptible. About half of all people with eating disorders have some sort of chemical dependency (alcohol or drugs), and a majority of them come from families with alcohol- and drug-related problems. Of reported cases of eating disorders, a large number involve individuals who are or have been victims of sexual molestation.

Eating disorders develop in stages. Typically, individuals who are already dealing with significant issues in life start a diet. At first they feel in control and are happy about the weight loss even if they are not overweight. Encouraged by the prospect of weight loss and the control they can exert over their own weight, the individual takes dieting to an extreme and often combines it with exhaustive exercise and the overuse of laxatives and diuretics.

Although a genetic predisposition may contribute, most cases are environmentally related. The syndrome typically emerges following emotional issues or a stressful life event and the uncertainty about the ability to cope efficiently. Life experiences that can trigger the syndrome might be: gaining weight, starting the menstrual period, beginning college, losing a boyfriend, having poor self-esteem, being socially rejected, starting a professional career, or becoming a wife or a mother.

The eating disorder now takes on a life of its own and becomes the primary focus of attention every day for the individuals afflicted with it. Their self-worth revolves around what the scale reads, their relationship with food, and their perception of how they look.

Anorexia Nervosa

An estimated 1 percent of the population in the United States is anorexic. Anorexic individuals seem to fear weight gain more than death from starvation. Furthermore, they have a distorted image of their body and think of themselves as being fat, even when they are emaciated.

Anorexics commonly develop obsessive and compulsive behaviors and emphatically deny their condition. They are preoccupied with food, meal planning, and grocery shopping, and they have unusual eating habits. As they lose weight and their health begins to deteriorate, anorexics feel weak and tired. They might realize they have a problem, but they will not stop the starvation and refuse to consider the behavior abnormal.

Once they have lost a lot of weight and malnutrition sets in, physical changes become more visible. Typical changes are **amenorrhea** (stoppage of menstruation), digestive problems, extreme sensitivity to cold, hair and skin problems, fluid and electrolyte abnormalities (which may lead to an irregular heartbeat and sudden stopping of the heart), injuries to nerves and tendons, immune-function abnormalities, anemia, growth of fine body hair, mental confusion, inability to concentrate, lethargy, depression, dry skin, lower skin and body temperature, and osteoporosis.

Diagnostic criteria for anorexia nervosa are:[11]

- Refusal to maintain body weight over a minimal normal weight for age and height (weight loss leading to maintenance of body weight less than 85 percent of that expected or failure to make expected weight gain during periods of growth, leading to body weight less than 85 percent of that expected)

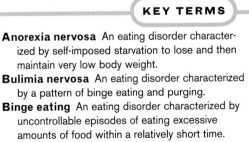

KEY TERMS

Anorexia nervosa An eating disorder characterized by self-imposed starvation to lose and then maintain very low body weight.

Bulimia nervosa An eating disorder characterized by a pattern of binge eating and purging.

Binge eating An eating disorder characterized by uncontrollable episodes of eating excessive amounts of food within a relatively short time.

Amenorrhea Cessation of regular menstrual flow.

- Intense fear of gaining weight or becoming fat, even though underweight
- Disturbance in the way in which one's body weight, size, or shape is perceived; undue influences of body weight or shape on self-evaluation; or denial of the seriousness of the current low body weight
- In postmenarcheal females, amenorrhea (absence of at least three consecutive menstrual cycles). (A woman is considered to have amenorrhea if her periods occur only following estrogen therapy.)

Many of the changes induced by anorexia nervosa can be reversed. Individuals with this condition can get better with professional therapy, but may also turn to bulimia nervosa, or may die. Twenty percent of anorexics die as a result of their condition. Anorexia nervosa has the highest mortality rate of all psychosomatic illnesses today. The disorder, however, is curable. But treatment almost always requires professional help, and the sooner it is started, the better the chances for reversibility and cure.

Therapy consists of a combination of medical and psychological techniques to restore proper nutrition, prevent medical complications, and modify the environment or events that triggered the syndrome.

Seldom can anorexics overcome the problem by themselves. They strongly deny their condition. They are able to hide it and deceive friends and relatives. Based on their behavior, many of them meet all of the characteristics of anorexia nervosa, but it goes undetected because both thinness and dieting are socially acceptable. Only a well-trained clinician is able to diagnose anorexia nervosa.

Bulimia Nervosa

Bulimia nervosa is more prevalent than anorexia nervosa. As many as one in every five women on college campuses may be bulimic, according to some estimates. Bulimia nervosa also is more prevalent than anorexia nervosa in males, although bulimia is still much more prevalent in females.

Bulimics usually are healthy-looking people, well educated, and near recommended body weight. They seem to enjoy food and often socialize around it. In actuality, they are emotionally insecure, rely on others, and lack self-confidence and self-esteem. Recommended weight and food are important to them.

The binge–purge cycle usually occurs in stages. As a result of stressful life events or the simple compulsion to eat, bulimics engage periodically in binge eating that may last an hour or longer.

With some apprehension, bulimics anticipate and plan the cycle. Next they feel an urgency to begin, followed by large and uncontrollable food consumption, during which they may eat several thousand calories (up to 10,000 calories in extreme cases). After a short period of relief and satisfaction, feelings of deep guilt, shame, and intense fear of gaining weight ensue. Purging seems to be an easy answer, as the bingeing cycle can continue without fear of gaining weight.

The diagnostic criteria for bulimia nervosa are:[12]

- Recurrent episodes of binge eating. An episode of binge eating is characterized by both of the following: (a) Eating in a discrete period of time (for example, within any two-hour period) an amount of food that is definitely more than most people would eat during a similar period and under similar circumstances. (b) A sense of lack of control over eating during the episode (a feeling that one cannot stop eating or control what or how much one is eating).
- Inappropriate compensatory behaviors recur to prevent weight gain, such as self-induced vomiting; misuse of laxatives, diuretics, enemas, or other medications; fasting; or excessive exercise.
- The binge eating and inappropriate compensatory behaviors both occur, on average, at least twice a week for three months.
- Self-evaluation is unduly influenced by body shape and weight.

The most typical form of purging is self-induced vomiting. Bulimics, too, frequently ingest strong laxatives and emetics. Near-fasting diets and strenuous bouts of exercise are common. Medical problems associated with bulimia nervosa include cardiac arrhythmias, amenorrhea, kidney and bladder damage, ulcers, colitis, tearing of the esophagus or stomach, tooth erosion, gum damage, and general muscular weakness.

Unlike anorexics, bulimics realize that their behavior is abnormal and feel great shame about it. Fearing social rejection, they pursue the binge–purge cycle in secrecy and at unusual hours of the day.

Bulimia nervosa can be treated successfully when the person realizes that this destructive behavior is not the solution to life's problems. A change in attitude can prevent permanent damage or death.

Binge-Eating Disorder

Binge-eating disorder is probably the most common of the three eating disorders. About 2 percent of American adults are afflicted with binge-eating disorder in a six-month period. Although most people think they overeat from time to time, eating more than one should now and then does not mean that the individual has a binge-eating disorder. The disorder is slightly more common in women than in men; three women for every two men have the disorder.

Binge-eating disorder is characterized by uncontrollable episodes of eating excessive amounts of food within a relatively short time. The causes of binge-eating disorder are unknown, although depression, anger, sadness, boredom, and worry can trigger an episode. Unlike bulimics, binge eaters do not purge; thus, most people with this disorder are either overweight or obese. Typical symptoms of binge-eating disorder include:

- Eating what most people think is an unusually large amount of food
- Eating until uncomfortably full
- Eating out of control
- Eating much faster than usual during binge episodes
- Eating alone because of embarrassment of how much food is being consumed
- Feeling disgusted, depressed, or guilty after overeating

Treatment

Treatment for eating disorders is available on most school campuses through the school's counseling center or the health center. Local hospitals also offer treatment for these conditions. Many communities have support groups, frequently led by professional personnel and often free of charge. All information and the identity of the individual are kept confidential so the person need not fear embarrassment or repercussion when seeking professional help.

2005 Dietary Guidelines for Americans

The 2005 Dietary Guidelines for Americans (see Figure 5.5) provide science-based advice to promote health and to reduce risk for major chronic diseases through diet and physical activity. The recommen-

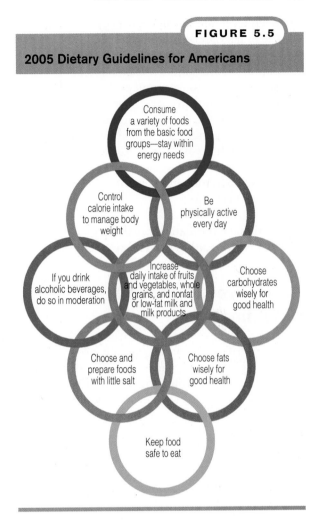

FIGURE 5.5

2005 Dietary Guidelines for Americans

dations are to the general public age 2 years and older and based on the preponderance of scientific and medical knowledge that is current at the time of publication of the committee's report. The extensive review of the evidence has led to the development of the following recommendations:[13]

1. Consume a variety of foods within and among the basic food groups while staying within energy needs.
2. Control calorie intake to manage body weight.
3. Be physically active every day.
4. Increase daily intake of fruits and vegetables, whole grains, and nonfat or low-fat milk and milk products.
5. Choose fats wisely for good health.
6. Choose carbohydrates wisely for good health.
7. Choose and prepare foods with little salt.
8. If you drink alcoholic beverages, do so in moderation.

9. Keep food safe to eat.
10. Clean hands, contact surfaces, and fruits and vegetables. (This does not apply to meat and poultry, which should not be washed.)
11. Separate raw, cooked, and ready-to-eat foods while shopping, preparing, or storing.
12. Cook foods to a safe temperature.
13. Chill (refrigerate) perishable foods promptly.
14. Avoid higher-risk foods (e.g., deli meats and frankfurters that have not been reheated to a safe temperature and may therefore contain *Listeria* bacteria).

Additional information on these guidelines are posted at www.health.gov/dietaryguidelines.

A Lifetime Commitment to Wellness

Proper nutrition, a sound exercise program, and quitting smoking (for those who smoke) are the three factors that do the most for health, longevity, and quality of life. Achieving and maintaining a balanced diet is not as difficult as most people would think. The difficult part for most people is retraining themselves to follow a lifetime healthy nutrition plan; that is, one that:

- Emphasizes fruits, vegetables, whole grains, and fat-free or low-fat milk and milk products
- Includes lean meats, poultry, fish, beans, eggs, and nuts (in moderation)
- Is low in saturated fats, trans fatty acids, cholesterol, salt (sodium), and added sugars

A well-balanced diet contains a variety of foods from all food groups, including wise selection of foods from animal sources. No single food can provide all the necessary nutrients and other beneficial substances in the amounts the body needs. For good nutrition, you should meet the recommended daily amounts of food from the different food groups in MyPyramid. Within each food group, choose a variety of foods. Food items vary, and each item provides different combinations of nutrients and other substances needed for good health.

In spite of ample scientific evidence linking poor dietary habits to early disease and mortality rates, many people are not willing to change their eating patterns. Even when faced with obesity, elevated blood lipids, hypertension, and other nutrition-related conditions, many people do not change. They remain in the precontemplation stage of change (see the discussion of behavior modification in Chapter 1).

The motivating factor to change one's eating habits seems to be a major health breakdown, such as a heart attack, a stroke, or cancer. An ounce of prevention is worth a pound of cure. The sooner you implement the dietary guidelines presented in this chapter, the better will be your chances of preventing chronic diseases and reaching a higher state of wellness.

CRITICAL THINKING

What factors in your life and the environment have contributed to your current dietary habits? • Do you need to make changes? • What may prevent you from doing so?

WWW WEB INTERACTIVE

The Mayo Clinic. This very informative website will show you how to balance your dietary intake with your physical activity to maintain healthy weight. To find your healthy weight, go to "Program & Tools" and click "Healthy Weight." You provide personal information regarding your age, gender, height, weight, and activity level, and the Mayo Clinic provides you with a healthy diet plan to meet your goals. It's fun and educational.
http://www.mayoclinic.com

The Nutrition Analysis Tools and System. This interactive website allows you to enter a variety of foods to receive a complete nutritional review of your diet based on the Recommended Dietary Allowances for your age and gender.
http://nat.crgq.com

ASSESS YOUR BEHAVIOR

Log on to *academic.cengage.com/login* *and take a wellness inventory to assess the behaviors that might benefit most from healthy change.*

1. Are whole grains, fruits, and vegetables the staple of your diet?

2. Are you meeting your personal MyPyramid recommendations for daily fruits, vegetables, grains, meat (or substitutes) and legumes, and milk?

3. Are there dietary changes that you need to implement to meet energy, nutrition, and disease risk-reduction guidelines and improve health and wellness? If so, list these changes and indicate what you will do to make it happen.

ASSESS YOUR KNOWLEDGE

Log on to *academic.cengage.com/login* *to assess your understanding of this chapter's topics by taking the chapter pre-test and exploring the modules recommended in your Personalized Study Plan.*

1. The science of nutrition studies the relationship of
   a. vitamins and minerals to health.
   b. foods to optimal health and performance.
   c. carbohydrates, fats, and proteins to the development and maintenance of good health.
   d. the macronutrients and micronutrients to physical performance.
   e. kilocalories to calories in food items.

2. Faulty nutrition often plays a crucial role in the development and progression of which disease?
   a. Cardiovascular disease
   b. Cancer
   c. Osteoporosis
   d. Diabetes
   e. All are correct choices.

3. According to MyPyramid, daily vegetable consumption is measured in
   a. servings.
   b. ounces.
   c. cups.
   d. calories.
   e. All of the above are correct.

4. The daily recommended amount of fiber intake for adults 50 years and younger is
   a. 10 grams per day for women and 12 grams for men.
   b. 21 grams per day for women and 30 grams for men.
   c. 28 grams per day for women and 35 grams for men.

   d. 25 grams per day for women and 38 grams for men.
   e. 45 grams per day for women and 50 grams for men.

5. Unhealthy fats include
   a. unsaturated fatty acids.
   b. monounsaturated fats.
   c. polyunsaturated fatty acids.
   d. saturated fats.
   e. alpha-linolenic acid.

6. The daily recommended carbohydrate intake is
   a. 45 to 65 percent of total calories.
   b. 10 to 35 percent of total calories.
   c. 20 to 35 percent of total calories.
   d. 60 to 75 percent of total calories.
   e. 35 to 50 percent of total calories.

7. The amount of a nutrient that is estimated to meet the nutrient requirement of half the healthy people in specific age and gender groups is known as the
   a. Estimated Average Requirement.
   b. Recommended Dietary Allowance.
   c. Daily Value.
   d. Adequate Intake.
   e. Dietary Reference Intake.

8. The percent fat intake for an individual who on a given day consumes 2,385 calories with 106 grams of fat is
   a. 44 percent of total calories.
   b. 17.7 percent of total calories.
   c. 40 percent of total calories.
   d. 31 percent of total calories.
   e. 22.5 percent of total calories.

CONTINUED

9. Treatment of anorexia nervosa
  a. almost always requires professional help.
  b. is often accomplished in the home.
  c. is most successful when friends take the initiative to help.
  d. requires that the individual be placed in the environment where the disorder started.
  e. is best done under the supervision of a physician.

10. Which of the following is *not* a goal of the 2005 Dietary Guidelines for Americans?
  a. Increase daily intake of fruits and vegetables, whole grains, and nonfat or low-fat milk and milk products.
  b. Be physically active each day.
  c. Choose carbohydrates wisely for good health.
  d. Control calorie intake to manage body weight.
  e. All are correct choices.

Correct answers can be found at the back of the book.

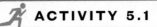

Nutrient Analysis

Name _____ Date _____

Course _____ Section _____

Age _____ Weight _____ Height _____ Gender M F   (Pregnant–P, Nursing–N)

Activity Rating for computer
software use (check one):
- ○ Sedentary
- ○ Lightly active
- ○ Moderately active
- ○ Very active
- ○ Extremely active

No.	Food	Amount	Calories*	Grains	Vegetables	Fruits	Milk	Meat and Beans	Oils
1									
2									
3									
4									
5									
6									
7									
8									
9									
10									
11									
12									
13									
14									
15									
16									
17									
18									
19									
20									
21									
22									
23									
24									
25									
26									
27									
28									
29									
30									
Totals									
Recommended amounts (obtain online at http://mypyramid.gov based on age, sex, and activity level)									
Deficiencies									

*See list of nutritive value of selected foods in Appendix E.

Name _____   Date _____

Course _____   Section _____

Age _____ Weight _____ Height _____   Gender M   F   (Pregnant–P, Nursing–N)

Activity Rating for computer   ◯ Sedentary
software use (check one):   ◯ Lightly active
                               ◯ Moderately active
                               ◯ Very active
                               ◯ Extremely active

No.	Food	Amount	Calories*	Grains	Vegetables	Fruits	Milk	Meat and Beans	Oils
1									
2									
3									
4									
5									
6									
7									
8									
9									
10									
11									
12									
13									
14									
15									
16									
17									
18									
19									
20									
21									
22									
23									
24									
25									
26									
27									
28									
29									
30									
Totals									
Recommended amounts (obtain online at http://mypyramid.gov based on age, sex, and activity level)									

Deficiencies _____

*See list of nutritive value of selected foods in Appendix E.

Weight Management

© Dylan Ellis/Corbis

OBJECTIVES

- Recognize myths and fallacies regarding weight management
- Understand the physiology of weight control
- Become familiar with the effects of diet and exercise on resting metabolic rate
- Recognize the role of a lifetime exercise program in a successful weight management program
- Learn to write and implement weight reduction and weight maintenance programs
- Identify behavior modification techniques that help a person adhere to a lifetime weight maintenance program

A good physical fitness program will include achieving and maintaining recommended body weight as a major objective. Two terms commonly used with reference to the condition of weighing more than recommended are **overweight** and **obesity.** Obesity levels are established at a point at which excess body fat can lead to significant health problems.

Obesity is a health hazard of epidemic proportions in most developed countries. According to the World Health Organization, an estimated 35 percent of the adult population in industrialized nations is obese. Obesity has been established at a body mass index (BMI) of 30 or higher.

The number of people who are overweight and obese in the United States has increased dramatically in the past decade and a half, a direct result of physical inactivity and poor dietary habits. More than 66 percent of U.S. adults ages 20 and older are overweight (have BMIs greater than 25), and 32 percent are obese.[1] More than 120 million people are overweight, and 30 million are obese. The prevalence of obesity is even higher in ethnic groups, especially African Americans and Hispanic Americans.

As illustrated in Figure 6.1, the U.S. obesity epidemic continues to escalate. In 1990, not a single state reported an obesity rate above 20 percent of the state's total population. By the year 2006, only four states had a rate of obesity of less than 20 percent, 22 states had a prevalence of 25 percent or greater, and two of these states had reached a rate above 30 percent.

Most of the blame for the alarming increase in obesity lies in the amount of food we eat and our lack of physical activity. According to the U.S. Department of Agriculture, the average daily caloric intake in the United States increased from 3,100 calories per person in the 1960s to 3,700 calories in the 1990s. Further, as the nation continues to evolve into a more mechanized and automated society (relying on escalators, elevators, remote controls, computers, electronic mail, cell phones, and automatic-sensor doors), the amount of required daily physical activity continues to decrease. We are being lulled into a high-risk, sedentary lifestyle.

About 44 percent of all women and 29 percent of all men are on a diet at any given moment. People spend about $40 billion yearly attempting to lose weight. More than $10 billion goes to memberships in weight reduction centers and another $30 billion to diet food sales. Furthermore, according to the National Institutes of Health, the total cost attributable to obesity-related disease is approximately $100 billion per year.

FIGURE 6.1

Incidence of obesity in the United States (based on BMI ≥30 or 30 pounds overweight), 1990, 2000, and 2006.

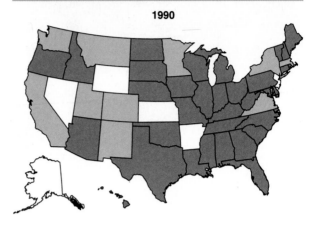

1990

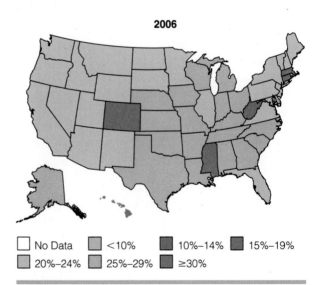

2000

2006

| | No Data | | <10% | | 10%–14% | | 15%–19% |
| | 20%–24% | | 25%–29% | | ≥30% |

SOURCE: *Obesity Trends Among U.S. Adults Between 1985 and 2006* (Atlanta: Centers for Disease Control and Prevention, 2007).

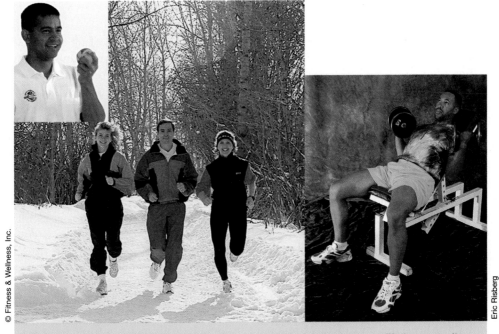

Achieving and maintaining a high physical fitness percent body fat requires a lifetime commitment to regular physical activity, exercise, and proper nutrition.

As the second leading cause of preventable death in the United States, excessive body weight and physical inactivity cause more than 112,000 deaths each year.[2] Obesity is presently more prevalent than smoking (19 percent), poverty (14 percent), and problem drinking (6 percent).[3] Obesity, cigarette smoking, and unhealthy lifestyle habits are the most critical public health problems that we face in the 21st century.

The American Heart Association has identified obesity as one of the six major risk factors for coronary heart disease. Obesity is associated with poor health status and is a risk factor for hypertension, congestive heart failure, high blood lipids, atherosclerosis, stroke, thromboembolitic disease, varicose veins, type 2 diabetes, osteoarthritis, gallbladder disease, sleep apnea, asthma, ruptured intervertebral disks, and arthritis. Estimates also indicate that 14 percent of all cancer deaths in men and 20 percent in women are related to current overweight and obesity patterns in the United States.[4] Furthermore, obesity is implicated in psychological maladjustment and a higher accidental death rate. Extremely obese people have worse mental health related to quality of life.

A primary objective of overall physical fitness and enhanced quality of life is to attain recommended body composition. Individuals at recommended body weight are able to participate in a wide variety of moderate to vigorous activities without functional limitations. These people have the freedom to enjoy most of life's recreational activities and reach their fullest potential. Excessive body weight does not afford an individual the fitness level to enjoy vigorous lifetime activities such as basketball, soccer, racquetball, surfing, mountain cycling, and mountain climbing. Maintaining high fitness and recommended body weight gives a person a degree of independence throughout life that the majority of people in developed nations no longer enjoy.

CRITICAL THINKING

Do you consider yourself overweight? • If so, how long have you had a weight problem, what attempts have you made to lose weight, and what has worked best for you?

KEY TERMS

Overweight Excess body weight when compared with a given standard such as height or recommended percent body fat.

Obesity A chronic disease characterized by an excessively high amount of body fat (about 20 percent above recommended weight or a BMI of 30 or above).

Tolerable Weight

Many people want to lose weight so they will look better. That's a noteworthy goal. The problem, however, is that they often have a distorted image of what they would really look like if they were to reduce to what they think is their ideal weight. Hereditary factors play a big role, and only a small fraction of the population has the genes for a "perfect body." **Tolerable weight** is a more realistic goal. This is a realistic standard that is not "ideal" but is "acceptable." It is likely to be closer to the health-fitness standard than the physical-fitness standard for many people.

The media have a great influence on people's perception of what constitutes ideal body weight. Most people rely on fashion, fitness, and beauty magazines to determine what they should look like. The "ideal" body shapes, physiques, and proportions shown in these magazines are rare and are achieved through airbrushing and medical reconstruction.[5] Many individuals, primarily young women, go to extremes in attempts to achieve these unrealistic body shapes. Failure to attain a "perfect body" often leads to eating disorders.

When people set their own target weight, they should be realistic. Attaining the "high physical fitness" percent body fat standard shown in Chapter 2, Table 2.12 (page 51) is extremely difficult for some. It is even more difficult to maintain, unless the person makes a commitment to a vigorous lifetime exercise program and permanent dietary changes. Few people are willing to do that. The "moderate" percent body fat category is more realistic for many people.

A question you should ask yourself is: Am I happy with my weight? Part of enjoying a higher quality of life is being happy with yourself. If you are not, you either need to do something about it or learn to live with it.

If your percent of body fat is higher than the health fitness standard shown in Table 2.12 (or a BMI above 25), you should try to reach and stay in this category, for health reasons. This is the category that seems to pose no detriment to health. If you have achieved the health fitness standard but would like to be more fit, ask yourself a second question: How badly do I want it? Enough to implement lifetime exercise and dietary changes? If you are not willing to change, you should stop worrying about your weight and deem the health fitness standard tolerable for you.

Fad Dieting

Only about 10 percent of all people who begin a traditional weight loss program (without exercise) are able to lose the desired weight. Worse, less than 5 percent of this group are able to keep the weight off for a significant time. Traditional diets have failed in helping people keep the weight off because few diet programs incorporate lifetime changes in food selection and overall increases in daily physical activity and exercise as the keys to successful weight loss and maintenance.

Fad diets continue to deceive people. Capitalizing on hopes that the latest diet to hit the market will really work this time, fad diets continue to appeal to people of all shapes and sizes. These diets may work for a while, but their success is usually short-lived. Most of these diets are low in calories and deprive the body of certain nutrients, generating a metabolic imbalance that can be detrimental to health. With many of these diets, a large amount

How to Recognize Fad Diets

Fad diets have characteristics in common. These diets typically

- are nutritionally unbalanced.
- rely primarily on a single food (for example, grapefruit).
- are based on testimonials.
- were developed according to "confidential research."
- are based on a "scientific breakthrough."
- promote rapid and "painless" weight loss.
- promise miraculous results.
- restrict food selection.
- are based on pseudo claims that excessive weight is related to a specific condition such as insulin resistance, combinations or timing of nutrient intake, food allergies, hormone imbalances, certain foods (fruits, for example).
- require the use of selected products.
- use liquid formulas instead of foods.
- misrepresent salespeople as individuals qualified to provide nutrition counseling.
- fail to provide information on risks associated with weight loss and of the diet use.
- do not involve physical activity.
- do not encourage healthy behavioral changes.
- are not supported by the scientific community or national health organizations.
- fail to provide information for weight maintenance upon completion of diet phase.

of weight loss is in the form of water and protein, not fat.

On a crash diet, close to half of the weight loss is in lean (protein) tissue (see Figure 6.2). When the body uses protein instead of a combination of fats and carbohydrates as a source of energy, the individual loses weight as much as 10 times faster. This is because a gram of protein produces less than half the amount of energy than fat does. In the case of muscle protein, one-fifth of protein is mixed with four-fifths of water. Each pound of muscle yields only one-tenth the amount of energy as a pound of fat. As a result, most of the weight loss is in the form of water, which on the scale, of course, looks good.

Among the popular diets on the market in recent years has been the low-carbohydrate/high-protein (LCHP) diet plans. Although variations exist among them, in general "low-carb" diets limit the intake of carbohydrate-rich foods. Examples of these diets are the Atkins Diet, The Zone, Protein Power, the Scarsdale Diet, The Carb Addict's Diet, and Sugar Busters.

Rapid weight loss occurs during LCHP diets because the low-carbohydrate intake forces the liver to produce glucose. The source for most of this glucose is body protein. As mentioned, protein is mostly water; thus, weight is lost rapidly. When a person terminates the diet, the body rebuilds some of the protein tissue and the person quickly regains some weight. Two studies in the *New England Journal of Medicine* indicated that individuals on an LCHP diet for six months lost about twice as much weight as those on a low-fat diet.[6] After a year, however, participants in the LCHP diet had regained more weight than those on the low-fat diet plan.

Are Low-Carb/High-Protein Diets More Effective?

A few studies suggest that, at least over the short term, low-carb/high-protein (LCHP) diets are more effective than carbohydrate-based diets in producing weight loss. These results are preliminary and controversial. In LCHP diets:

- much of the weight loss is water and muscle protein, not body fat. Some of this weight is regained quickly upon resuming regular dietary habits.
- few people are able to stay on the diet for more than a few weeks at a time. Most stop dieting before achieving their target weight.
- participants are rarely found on a national weight-loss registry of people who have lost 30 pounds and kept off the weight for a minimum of 6 years.
- food choices are severely restricted. With less variety available, individuals tend to eat less (800–1,200 calories/day) and thus lose more weight.
- the allowed foods may promote heart disease and cancer and increase the risk for osteoporosis.
- the allowed foods are fundamentally high in fat (about 60 percent fat calories).
- the food program carries high risks for people with diabetes, high blood pressure, heart disease, or kidney disease.
- participants are given no information about long-term healthy eating patterns.

Years of research will be required to determine the extent to which long-term adherence to LCHP diets increases the risk for heart disease, cancer, and kidney or bone damage. LCHP diets are contrary to the nutrition advice of most leading national health organizations (which recommend a diet low in animal fat and saturated fat and high in complex carbohydrates). Without fruits, vegetables, and whole grains, high-protein diets lack many vitamins, minerals, phytonutrients, and fiber—all dietary factors that protect against an array of ailments and diseases.

The major risk associated with long-term adherence to LCHP diets might be the increased risk for

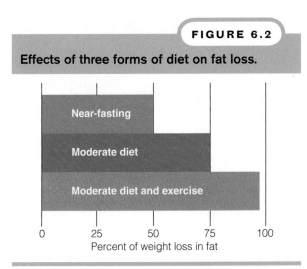

FIGURE 6.2

Effects of three forms of diet on fat loss.

Near-fasting

Moderate diet

Moderate diet and exercise

0   25   50   75   100
Percent of weight loss in fat

Adapted from *Alive Man: The Physiology of Physical Activity* by R. J. Shephard (Springfield, IL: Charles C. Thomas, 1975): 484–488.

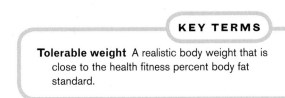

KEY TERMS

Tolerable weight A realistic body weight that is close to the health fitness percent body fat standard.

heart disease, because high-protein foods are also high in fat content. Low-carbohydrate intake also produces loss of vitamin B, calcium, and potassium. Side effects commonly associated with these diets are weakness, nausea, bad breath, constipation, irritability, lightheadedness, and fatigue. Potential bone loss can further accentuate the risk for osteoporosis. Long-term adherence to an LCHP diet also can increase the risk for cancer. If you choose to go on an LCHP diet for longer than a few weeks, let your physician know so that he or she may monitor your blood lipids, bone density, and kidney function.

Some diets allow only certain specialized foods. If people would realize that no "magic" foods provide all the necessary nutrients, that a person has to eat a variety of foods to be well nourished, the diet industry would not be as successful. Most of these diets create a nutritional deficiency, which can be detrimental to health. Some people eventually get tired of eating the same thing day in and day out and start eating less—which results in weight loss. If they achieve the lower weight without making permanent dietary changes, however, they gain back the weight quickly if they return to their old eating habits.

A few diets recommend exercise along with caloric restrictions—the best method for weight reduction, of course. People who adhere to these programs will succeed, so the diet has achieved its purpose. Unfortunately, if the people do not change their food selection and activity level permanently, they gain back the weight once they discontinue dieting and exercise.

Principles of Weight Management

Traditional concepts related to weight control have centered on three assumptions:

1. Balancing food intake against output allows a person to achieve recommended weight.
2. Fat people just eat too much.
3. The human body doesn't care how much (or little) fat is stored.

Although these statements contain some truth, they still are open to much debate and research. We now know that the causes of obesity are complex and combine genetic, behavior, and lifestyle factors.

Energy-Balancing Equation

In keeping with the **energy-balancing equation,** if caloric intake exceeds output, the person gains weight; when caloric output is more than intake, the individual loses weight. Each pound of fat equals 3,500 calories. Therefore, theoretically, to increase body fat (weight) by 1 pound, a person would have to consume an excess of 3,500 calories. Equally, to lose 1 pound, the individual would have to decrease caloric intake by 3,500 calories. This principle seems straightforward, but the human body is not quite that simple.

The genetic instinct to survive tells the body that fat storage is vital, and therefore the body's weight-regulating mechanism, or **setpoint,** sets an acceptable fat level for each person. This setpoint remains somewhat constant or may climb gradually because of poor lifestyle habits.

Diet and Metabolism

Under strict calorie reduction (fewer than 800 calories per day), the body makes compensatory metabolic adjustments in an effort to maintain its fat storage. The **basal metabolic rate (BMR)** may drop dramatically against a consistent negative caloric balance, and the person may be on a plateau for days or even weeks without losing much weight. When the dieter goes back to the normal or even below-normal caloric intake, at which the weight

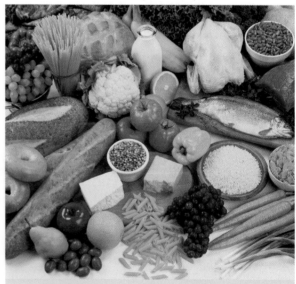

A wide variety of foods is required to maintain a well-nourished body.

may have been stable for a long time, he or she quickly regains the fat lost as the body strives to restore a comfortable fat level.

These findings were substantiated by research conducted at Rockefeller University in New York,[7] which showed that the body resists maintaining altered weight. Obese and lifetime nonobese individuals were used in the investigation. Following a 10 percent weight loss, in an attempt to regain the lost weight, the body compensated by burning up to 15 percent fewer calories than expected for the new reduced weight (after accounting for the 10 percent loss). The effects were similar in the obese and nonobese participants. These results imply that after a 10 percent weight loss, a person would have to eat less or exercise more to account for the estimated deficit of about 200 to 300 daily calories.

In this same study, when the participants were allowed to increase their weight to 10 percent above their "normal" body weight (pre–weight loss), the body burned 10 percent to 15 percent more calories than expected. This indicates an attempt by the body to waste energy and return to the preset weight. The study provides another indication that the body is highly resistant to weight changes unless the person incorporates additional lifestyle changes to ensure successful weight management. (Methods to manage weight will be discussed later in this chapter.)

This research shows why most dieters regain the weight they lose through dietary means alone. Let's use a practical illustration: Jim would like to lose some body fat, and assumes that he has reached a stable body weight at an average daily caloric intake of 2,500 calories (no weight gain or loss at this daily intake). In an attempt to lose weight rapidly, he now goes on a strict low-calorie diet (or, even worse, a near-fasting diet). Immediately the body activates its survival mechanism and readjusts its metabolism to a lower caloric balance.

After a few weeks of dieting at under 800 calories per day, the body now can maintain its normal functions at 2,000 calories per day. Having lost the desired weight, Jim terminates the diet but realizes that the original intake of 2,500 calories per day will have to be lower to maintain the new lower weight. To adjust to the new lower body weight, he restricts his intake to about 2,200 calories per day. Jim is surprised to find that even at this lower daily intake (300 fewer calories), his weight comes back at a rate of about 1 pound every two to three weeks. After the diet ends, this new lowered metabolic rate may take several months to kick back up to its normal level.

From this explanation, individuals clearly should not go on very low calorie diets. Doing so will decrease the resting metabolic rate and deprive the body of basic daily nutrients required for normal function. Very low calorie diets should be used only in conjunction with dietary supplements and under proper medical supervision.[8] Furthermore, research indicates that people who go on very low calorie diets are not as effective in keeping the weight off once they terminate the diet.

Under no circumstances should a person go on a diet that calls for below 1,200 and 1,500 calories, respectively, for women and men. Weight (fat) is gained over months and years, not overnight. Equally, weight loss should be gradual, not abrupt. A daily caloric intake of 1,200 to 1,500 calories provides the necessary nutrients if properly distributed over the various food groups (meeting the minimum daily required servings from each group). Of course, the individual has to learn which foods meet the requirements and yet are low in fat, sugar, and calories.

Furthermore, when a person tries to lose weight by dietary restrictions alone, **lean body mass** (muscle protein, along with vital organ protein) decreases. The amount of lean body mass lost depends entirely on the caloric limitation. When a person goes on a near-fasting diet, up to half of the weight lost can be lean body mass, and the other half actual fat loss. If the diet is combined with exercise, close to 100 percent of the weight loss is in the form of fat, and lean tissue actually may increase (see Figure 6.2). Loss of lean body mass is not good, because it weakens the organs and muscles and slows the metabolism.

Reduction in lean body mass is common in people on severely restricted diets. No diet with caloric intakes below 1,200 to 1,500 calories will prevent loss of lean body mass. Even at this intake level, some loss is inevitable unless the diet is combined

---

KEY TERMS

Energy-balancing equation A body weight formula stating that when caloric intake equals caloric output, weight remains unchanged.

Setpoint Body weight and body fat percentage unique to each person that are regulated by genetic and environmental factors.

Basal metabolic rate (BMR) Lowest level of caloric intake necessary to sustain life.

Lean body mass Nonfat component of the human body.

with exercise. Although many diets claim they do not alter the lean component, the simple truth is that regardless of what nutrients may be added to the diet, caloric restrictions always prompt a loss of lean tissue.

Too many people go on low-calorie diets again and again. Every time they do, the metabolic rate slows as more lean tissue is lost. People in their 40s and older who weigh the same as they did when they were 20 often think they are at recommended body weight. During this span of 20 years or more, however, they may have dieted too many times without exercising. Shortly after terminating each diet, they regain the weight, but much of that gain is in fat. Maybe at age 20 they weighed 150 pounds, of which only 15 percent was fat. Now, at age 40, even though they still weigh 150 pounds, they might be 30 percent fat (see Figure 6.3, and also Figure 2.2 in Chapter 2, page 44). At recommended body weight, they wonder why they are eating so little and still having trouble staying at that weight.

Further, data indicate that diets high in fat and refined carbohydrates, near-fasting diets, and perhaps even artificial sweeteners, keep people from losing weight and, in reality, contribute to fat gain. The only practical and sensible way to lose fat weight is to combine exercise and a sensible diet high in complex carbohydrates and low in fat and sugar.

Because of the effects of proper food management on body weight, most of the successful dieter's effort should be spent in retraining eating habits, increasing the intake of complex carbohydrates and high-fiber foods, and decreasing the consumption of refined carbohydrates (sugars) and fats. This change in eating habits will bring about a decrease in total daily caloric intake. One gram of carbohydrates provides only 4 calories, as contrasted with 9 calories per gram of fat. Thus, you could eat twice the volume of food (by weight) when substituting carbohydrates for fat. Some fat, however, is recommended in the diet—preferably polyunsaturated and monounsaturated fats. These so-called good fats do more than help protect the heart; they help delay hunger pangs.

A "diet" cannot be viewed as a temporary tool to aid in weight loss but, instead, as a permanent change in eating behaviors to ensure weight management and better health. The role of increased physical activity also must be considered because successful weight loss and recommended body composition seldom are attainable without a moderate reduction in caloric intake combined with a regular exercise program.

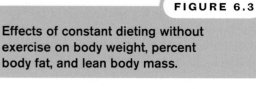

FIGURE 6.3

Effects of constant dieting without exercise on body weight, percent body fat, and lean body mass.

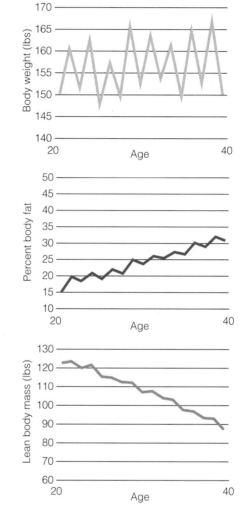

Exercise: The Key to Successful Weight Management

A more effective way to tilt the energy-balancing equation in your favor is by burning calories through physical activity. Exercise also seems to exert control over how much a person weighs. If, starting at age 25, a person only gains 1 pound of weight per year, this represents a simple energy surplus of under 10 calories per day ($10 \times 365 = 3,650$). In many cases, most of the additional weight accumulated in middle age comes from people becoming less physically active and not from increased caloric intake. Dr. Jack Wilmore, a leading exercise physiologist and expert weight management researcher, stated:[9]

> Physical inactivity is certainly a major, if not the primary, cause of obesity in the United States today. A certain minimal level of activity might be necessary for us to accurately balance our caloric intake to our caloric expenditure. With too little activity, we appear to lose the fine control we normally have to maintain this incredible balance. This fine balance amounts to less than 10 calories per day, or the equivalent of one potato chip.

Exercise enhances the rate of weight loss and is vital in maintaining the weight loss. Not only will exercise maintain lean tissue, but advocates of the setpoint theory say that exercise resets the fat thermostat to a new, lower level.

A few individuals can lose weight by participating in 30 minutes of exercise per day, but most people need 60 to 90 minutes of daily physical activity for proper weight management (the 30 minutes of exercise are included as part of the 60 to 90 minutes of physical activity).

Although 30 minutes of moderate-intensity activity per day provides substantial health benefits, the Institute of Medicine of the National Academy of Sciences recommends that people trying to manage their weight accumulate 60 minutes of moderate-intensity physical activity most days of the week.[10] The evidence shows that people who maintain recommended weight typically accumulate an hour or more of daily physical activity. As illustrated in Figure 6.4, greater weight loss can be achieved by combining a diet with an exercise program. Of even greater significance, however, only individuals who remain physically active for over 60 minutes per day are able to keep the weight off (see Figure 6.5).

Further, data from the National Weight Control Registry (http://www.nwcr.ws/) indicate that individuals who have lost at least 30 pounds and kept them off for a minimum of six years typically accumulate 90 minutes of daily activity. Those who are less active gradually regain the lost weight. Individuals who completely stop physical activity regain almost 100 percent of the weight within 18 months of discontinuing the weight loss program (see Figure 6.5). Thus, if weight management is *not* a consideration, 30 minutes of daily activity provides health benefits. To prevent weight gain, 60 minutes of daily

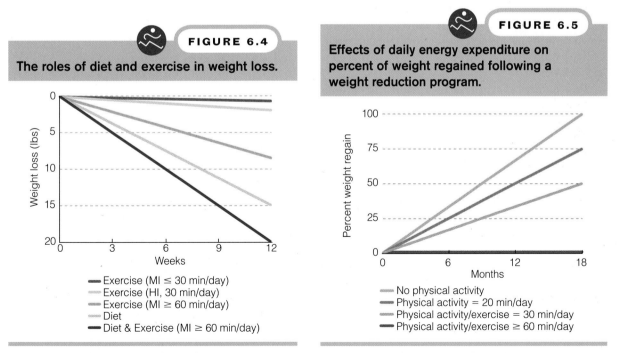

FIGURE 6.4

The roles of diet and exercise in weight loss.

- Exercise (MI ≤ 30 min/day)
- Exercise (HI, 30 min/day)
- Exercise (MI ≥ 60 min/day)
- Diet
- Diet & Exercise (MI ≥ 60 min/day)

American College of Sports Medicine, "Position Stand: Appropriate Intervention Strategies for Weight Loss and Prevention for Weight Regain for Adults," *Medicine and Science in Sports and Exercise* 33 (2001): 2145–2156.

FIGURE 6.5

Effects of daily energy expenditure on percent of weight regained following a weight reduction program.

- No physical activity
- Physical activity = 20 min/day
- Physical activity/exercise = 30 min/day
- Physical activity/exercise ≥ 60 min/day

American College of Sports Medicine, "Position Stand: Appropriate Intervention Strategies for Weight Loss and Prevention for Weight Regain for Adults," *Medicine and Science in Sports and Exercise* 33 (2001): 2145–2156.

activity is recommended; to maintain substantial weight loss, 90 minutes may be required.

A combination of aerobic and strength-training exercises works best in weight-loss programs. Aerobic exercise is the best to offset the setpoint, and the continuity and duration of these types of activities cause many calories to be burned in the process. Unfortunately, of those individuals who are attempting to lose weight, only 19 percent of women and 22 percent of men decrease their caloric intake and exercise above an average of 25 or more minutes per day.[11]

Strength training is critical in helping maintain lean body mass. Although the increase in BMR through increased muscle mass is presently being debated in the literature and merits further research, data indicate that each additional pound of muscle tissue raises the BMR in the range of 6 to 35 calories per day.[12] The latter figure is based on calculations that an increase of 3 to 3.5 pounds of lean tissue through strength training increased basal metabolic rate by about 105 to 120 calories per day.[13]

Most likely, the benefit of strength training goes beyond the new muscle tissue itself. Maybe a pound of muscle tissue requires only 6 calories per day to sustain itself, but as all muscles undergo strength training, they also undergo increased protein synthesis to build and repair themselves, resulting in increased energy expenditure of 1 to 1.5 calories per pound in all trained muscle tissue. Such an increase would explain the increase in BMR of 105 to 120 calories in some research studies.

To examine the effects of a small increase in BMR on long-term body weight, let's use a very conservative estimate of an additional 50 calories per day as a result of a regular strength-training program. An increase of 50 calories represent an additional 18,250 calories per year (50 × 365), or the equivalent of 5.2 pounds of fat (18,250 ÷ 3,500). This increase in BMR would more than offset the typical adult weight gain of 1 to 2 pounds per year.

This figure of 18,250 calories per year does not include the actual energy cost of the strength-training workout. An energy expenditure of only 150 calories per strength-training session, done twice per week, over a year's time would represent 15,600 calories (150 × 2 × 52) or the equivalent of another 4.5 pounds of fat (15,600 ÷ 3,500).

In addition, although the amounts seem small, the previous calculations do not account for the increase in metabolic rate following the strength-training workout (the time it takes the body to return to its pre-workout resting rate—about two hours). Depending on the intensity and length of training (see Chapter 7, page 174), this recovery energy expenditure ranges from 20 to 100 calories following each strength-training workout.[14] All these "apparently small" changes make a big difference in the long run.

Although size (inches) and percent body fat both decrease when sedentary individuals begin an exercise program, body weight often remains the same or might even increase during the first couple of weeks after beginning the program. Exercise helps to increase muscle tissue, connective tissue, blood volume (as much as 500 mL, or the equivalent of 1 pound, following the first week of aerobic exercise), enzymes and other structures within the cell, and glycogen (which binds water). All of these changes lead to a higher functional capacity of the human body. With exercise, most of the weight loss becomes apparent after a few weeks of training, when the lean component has stabilized.

The Myth of Spot-Reducing

Research has revealed the fallacy of spot-reducing, or losing cellulite, as some people call the fat deposits that bulge out in certain areas of the body. These deposits are simply enlarged fat cells from accumulated body fat. Merely doing several sets of sit-ups daily will not get rid of fat in the midsection of the body. When fat comes off, it does so throughout the entire body, not just in the exercised area. Although the greatest proportion of fat may come off the biggest fat deposits, the caloric output of a few sets of sit-ups has almost no effect on reducing total body fat. A person has to exercise regularly for extended periods of time to really see results.

Exercise Safety

Dieting never has been fun and never will be. People who are overweight and are serious about losing weight will have to make exercise a regular part of their daily life, along with proper food management and a sensible cut in caloric intake. Some precautions are in order, because excessive body fat is a risk factor for cardiovascular disease. Depending on the extent of the weight problem, a medical examination and possibly a stress ECG may be necessary before undertaking vigorous exercise. A physician should be consulted in this regard.

Significantly overweight individuals also may have to choose activities in which they will not have to

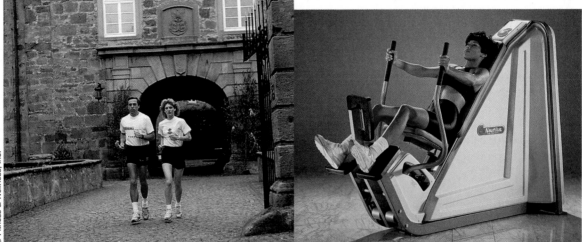

Regular participation in a combined lifetime aerobic and strength-training exercise program is the key to successful weight management.

support their own body weight but still will be effective in burning calories. Injuries to joints and muscles are common in overweight individuals who participate in weight-bearing exercises such as prolonged walking, jogging, and aerobics. Better alternatives for overweight people are riding a bicycle (either road or stationary), water aerobics, walking in a shallow pool, or running in place in deep water (treading water). The latter three modes of exercise are gaining quickly in popularity because little skill is required to participate. These activities seem to be just as effective as other forms of aerobic activity in helping individuals lose weight without the pain and the fear of injuries.

One final benefit of prolonged exercise for weight control is that it allows fat to be burned more efficiently. Both carbohydrates and fats are sources of energy. When the glucose levels begin to drop during prolonged exercise, more fat is used as energy substrate. Equally important is that fat-burning enzymes increase with aerobic training. Fat is lost primarily by burning it in muscle. Therefore, as the concentration of the enzymes increases, so does the ability to burn fat.

Low-Intensity Versus High-Intensity Exercise for Weight Loss

Some individuals promote low-intensity exercise over high-intensity exercise for the purpose of losing weight. Compared with high-intensity exercise, a greater proportion of calories burned during low-

BEHAVIOR MODIFICATION PLANNING

Weight-Maintenance Benefits of Lifetime Aerobic Exercise

The authors of this book have been jogging together a minimum of 15 miles per week (3 miles/5 times per week) for the past 30 years. Without considering the additional energy expenditure from their regular strength-training program and their many other sport and recreational activities, the energy cost of this regular jogging program over 30 years has been approximately 2,340,000 calories (15 miles × 100 calories/mile × 52 weeks × 30 years), or the equivalent of 668 pounds of fat (2,340,000 ÷ 3,500). In essence, without this 30-minute workout 5 times per week, the authors would weigh 810 and 784 pounds, respectively!

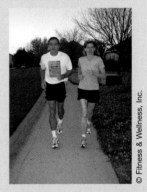

Try It
Ask yourself whether a regular aerobic exercise program is part of your long-term gratification and health enhancement program. If the answer is no, are you ready to change your behavior? Use the Behavior Change Planner to help you answer the question.

intensity exercise is derived from fat. The lower the intensity of exercise, the higher the percentage of fat utilization as a source of energy. In theory, if you are trying to lose fat, this principle makes sense, but in reality it is misleading. The bottom line when you are trying to lose weight is to burn more calories. When your daily caloric expenditure exceeds your intake, you lose weight. The more calories you burn, the more fat you lose.

During low-intensity exercise, up to 50 percent of the calories burned may be derived from fat (the other 50 percent from glucose [carbohydrates]). With intense exercise, only 30 to 40 percent of the caloric expenditure comes from fat. Overall, however, you can burn twice as many (or more) calories during high-intensity exercise, and subsequently more fat as well.

Let's look at a practical illustration. If you exercise for 30 minutes at a low intensity and burn 200 calories, about 100 of those calories (50 percent) would come from fat. If you exercise at high intensity during those same 30 minutes, you can burn 400 calories, with an even greater amount, 120 to 160 calories (30 to 40 percent), coming from fat as compared with only 100 during low-intensity exercise. Also, at the low-intensity pace, you would have to exercise twice as long to burn the same number of calories.

Moreover, high-intensity exercise by itself seems to trigger greater fat loss than low-intensity exercise. Research conducted at Laval University in Quebec, Canada, showed that subjects who performed a high-intensity, intermittent-training program lost more body fat than did a low- to moderate-intensity continuous aerobic endurance group.[15] Even more surprisingly, this finding occurred despite the fact that the high-intensity group burned fewer total calories per exercise session. The results support the notion that vigorous exercise is more conducive to weight loss than is low- to moderate-intensity exercise.

Before you start high-intensity exercise sessions, a word of caution is in order: Be sure that it is medically safe for you to participate in such activities and that you build up gradually to that level. If you are cleared to participate in high-intensity exercise, do not attempt to do too much too quickly, as you may suffer injuries and discouragement. You must allow your body a proper conditioning period of 8 to 12 weeks, or even longer for those with a moderate to serious weight problem. Also, high intensity does not mean high impact. High-impact activities are the most common cause of exercise-related injuries

(see the discussion on aerobics in Chapter 4, pages 102–103, and on acute sports injuries in Chapter 9, page 231).

The above information on high-intensity versus low-intensity exercise does not mean that low-intensity exercise is not effective. It provides substantial health benefits, and people who initiate exercise are more willing to participate and stay with low-intensity programs. Low-intensity exercise does promote weight loss, but it is not as effective as higher-intensity exercise. You will have to exercise longer to obtain the same results.

Designing Your Own Weight-Loss Program

In addition to exercise and food management, sensible adjustments in caloric intake are recommended. Most research finds that a negative caloric balance is required to lose weight. Perhaps the only exception is with people who are eating too few calories. A nutrient analysis often reveals that "faithful" dieters are not consuming enough calories. These people actually need to increase their daily caloric intake (combined with an exercise program) to get their metabolism to kick back up to a normal level.

Estimating Your Caloric Intake

With Activity 6.1 (pages 165–166) and Tables 6.1 and 6.2, you can estimate your daily energy (caloric) requirement. Because this is only an estimated value,

---

TABLE 6.1

Estimated Energy Requirement (EER) Based on Age, Body Weight, and Height (includes activities of independent living only and no moderate physical activity or exercise)

Men: EER = 662 − (9.53 × Age) + (15.91 × BW) + (539 × HT)

Women: EER = 354 − (6.91 × Age) + (9.36 × BW) + (726 × HT)

BW = body weight in kilograms (divide BW in pounds by 2.2046), HT = height in meters (multiply HT in inches by .0254).

SOURCE: National Academy of Sciences, Institute of Medicine, *Dietary Reference Intakes for Energy, Carbohydrates, Fiber, Fat, Protein and Amino Acids (Macronutrients)* (Washington, DC: National Academy Press, 2002).

TABLE 6.2

Caloric Expenditure of Selected Physical Activities

Activity*	Cal/lb/min	Activity*	Cal/lb/min	Activity*	Cal/lb/min
Aerobics		Gymnastics		Stationary Cycling	
Moderate	0.065	Light	0.030	Moderate	0.055
Vigorous	0.095	Heavy	0.056	Vigorous	0.070
Step Aerobics	0.070	Handball	0.064	Strength Training	0.050
Archery	0.030	Hiking	0.040	Swimming (crawl)	
Badminton		Judo/Karate	0.086	20 yds/min	0.031
Recreation	0.038	Racquetball	0.065	25 yds/min	0.040
Competition	0.065	Rope Jumping	0.060	45 yds/min	0.057
Baseball	0.031	Rowing (vigorous)	0.090	50 yds/min	0.070
Basketball		Running (on a level surface)		Table Tennis	0.030
Moderate	0.046	11.0 min/mile	0.070	Tennis	
Competition	0.063	8.5 min/mile	0.090	Moderate	0.045
Bowling	0.030	7.0 min/mile	0.102	Competition	0.064
Calisthenics	0.033	6.0 min/mile	0.114	Volleyball	0.030
Cycling (on a level surface)		Deep water**	0.100	Walking	
5.5 mph	0.033	Skating (moderate)	0.038	4.5 mph	0.045
10.0 mph	0.050	Skiing		Shallow pool	0.090
13.0 mph	0.071	Downhill	0.060	Water Aerobics	
Dance		Level (5 mph)	0.078	Moderate	0.050
Moderate	0.030	Soccer	0.059	Vigorous	0.070
Vigorous	0.055	Stairmaster		Wrestling	0.085
Golf	0.030	Moderate	0.070		
		Vigorous	0.090		

*Values are for actual time engaged in the activity.   ** Treading water

Adapted from:

P. E. Allsen, J. M. Harrison, and B. Vance, *Fitness for Life: An Individualized Approach* (Dubuque, IA: Wm. C. Brown, 1989).

C. A. Bucher and W. E. Prentice, *Fitness for College and Life* (St. Louis: Times Mirror/Mosby College Publishing, 1989).

C. F. Consolazio, R. E. Johnson, and L. J. Pecora, *Physiological Measurements of Metabolic Functions in Man* (New York: McGraw-Hill, 1963).

R. V. Hockey, *Physical Fitness: The Pathway to Healthful Living* (St. Louis: Times Mirror/Mosby College Publishing, 1989).

W. W. K. Hoeger et al., Research conducted at Boise State University, 1986–1993.

individual adjustments related to many of the factors discussed in this chapter may be necessary to establish a more precise value. Nevertheless, the estimated value does offer a beginning guideline for weight control or reduction.

The **estimated energy requirement (EER)** without additional planned activity and exercise is based on age, total body weight, and gender. Individuals who hold jobs that require a lot of walking or heavy manual labor burn more calories during the day than those who have sedentary jobs (such as working behind a desk). To estimate your EER, refer to Table 6.1. For example, the EER computation for a 20-year-old man, 71 inches tall, who weighs 160 pounds, would be as follows:

1. Body weight (BW) in kilograms = 72.6 kg (160 lbs ÷ 2.2046)
   Height in meters = 1.8 m (71 × 0.0254)

2. EER = 662 – (9.53 × Age) + (15.91 × BW) + (539 × Ht)
   EER = 662 – (9.53 × 20) + (15.91 × 72.6) + (539 × 1.8)
   EER = 662 – 190.6 + 1155 + 970
   EER = 2596

Thus, the EER to maintain body weight for this individual would be 2,596 calories per day.

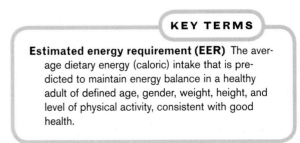

KEY TERMS

Estimated energy requirement (EER) The average dietary energy (caloric) intake that is predicted to maintain energy balance in a healthy adult of defined age, gender, weight, height, and level of physical activity, consistent with good health.

The second step is to determine the average number of calories this man burns daily as a result of exercise. To get this number, he must figure out the total number of minutes he exercises weekly and then figure the daily average exercise time. For instance, if he cycles at 10 miles per hour five times a week, 60 minutes each time, he exercises 300 minutes per week (5×60). The average daily exercise time is 42 minutes ($300 \div 7$, rounded off to the lowest unit).

Next, from Table 6.2, find the energy requirement for the activity (or activities) he has chosen for the exercise program. In the case of cycling (10 miles per hour), the requirement is .05 calories per pound of body weight per minute of activity (cal/lb/min). With a body weight of 160 pounds, this man would burn 8 calories each minute (body weight $\times$ .05, or $160 \times .05$). In 42 minutes, he burns approximately 336 calories (42×8).

The third step is to obtain the estimated total caloric requirement, with exercise, needed to maintain body weight. To do this, add the typical daily requirement (without exercise) and the average calories burned through exercise. In our example, it is 2,932 calories ($2,596 + 336$).

Therefore, this man has to consume fewer than 2,932 calories daily to lose weight. Because of the many factors that play a role in weight control, this is only an estimated daily requirement. Furthermore, to lose weight, we cannot predict that he will lose exactly 1 pound of fat in 1 week if he cuts his daily intake by 500 calories ($500 \times 7 = 3,500$ calories, or the equivalent of 1 pound of fat).

The daily energy requirement is only a target guideline for weight control. Periodic readjustments are necessary because individuals differ, and the estimated daily cost changes as you lose weight and modify your exercise habits.

To determine the target caloric intake to lose weight, multiply your current weight by 5 and subtract this amount from the total daily energy requirement (2,932 in our example) with exercise. For our moderately active male example, this would mean consuming only 2,366 calories per day to lose weight ($160 \times 5 = 800$ and $2,932 - 800 = 2,132$ calories).

This final caloric intake to lose weight should never be below 1,200 calories for women and 1,500 for men. If distributed properly over the various food groups, these figures are the lowest caloric intakes that provide the necessary nutrients the body needs. In terms of percentages of total calories, the daily distribution should be approximately 60 percent carbohydrates (mostly complex carbohydrates), less than 30 percent fat, and about 12 percent protein.

The time of day when food is consumed also may play a part in losing weight. When a person is attempting to lose weight, intake should consist of a minimum of 25 percent of the total daily calories for breakfast, 50 percent for lunch, and 25 percent or less at dinner. Breakfast, in particular, is a critical meal. Many people skip breakfast because it's the easiest meal to skip. Evidence, however, indicates that people who skip breakfast are hungrier later in the day and end up consuming more total daily calories than those who eat breakfast. Furthermore, regular breakfast eaters have less of a weight problem, lose weight more effectively, and have less difficulty maintaining lost weight.

If most of the daily calories are consumed during one meal (as in the typical evening meal) the body may perceive that something is wrong and will slow down the metabolism so it can store more calories in the form of fat. Also, eating most of the calories during one meal causes a person to go hungry the rest of the day, making it more difficult to adhere to the diet.

Monitoring Your Diet Through Daily Food Logs

To help you monitor and adhere to your diet plan, you may use the daily food intake record form in Activity 6.2, pages 167–170. First make a master copy so you can make copies as needed in the future. Guidelines are provided for 1,200-, 1,500-, 1,800-, and 2,000-calorie diet plans. These plans have been developed based on the MyPyramid food plan and the Dietary Guidelines for Americans to meet the Recommended Dietary Allowances. The objective is to meet (not exceed) the number of servings allowed for each diet plan. Each time you eat a serving of any food, record it in the appropriate box. Evidence indicates that people who monitor daily caloric intake are more successful at weight loss than those who don't self-monitor.

To lose weight, you should use the diet plan that most closely approximates your target caloric intake. The plan is based on the following caloric allowances for these food groups:

- Grains: 80 calories per serving.
- Fruits: 60 calories per serving.
- Vegetables: 25 calories per serving.
- Milk (use low-fat products): 120 calories per serving.

• Meat and beans: Use low-fat (300 calories per serving) frozen entrees or an equivalent amount if you prepare your own main dish (see the following discussion).

As you start your diet plan, pay particular attention to food serving sizes. Take care with cup and glass sizes. A standard cup is 8 ounces, but most glasses nowadays contain between 12 and 16 ounces. If you drink 12 ounces of fruit juice, in essence you are getting two servings of fruit because a standard serving is ¾ cup of juice.

Read food labels carefully to compare the caloric value of the serving listed on the label with the caloric guidelines provided above. Here are some examples:

• One slice of standard white bread has about 80 calories. A plain bagel may have 200 to 350 calories. Although it is low in fat, a 350-calorie bagel is equivalent to almost four servings in the bread, cereal, rice, and pasta group.
• The standard serving size listed on the food label for most cereals is 1 cup. As you read the nutrition information, however, you will find that for the same cup of cereal, one type of cereal has 120 calories and another cereal has 200 calories. Because a standard serving in the bread, cereal, rice, and pasta group is 80 calories, the first cereal would be 1½ servings and the second one 2½ servings.
• A medium-size fruit is usually considered to be 1 serving. A large fruit could provide as many as 2 or more servings.
• In the milk, yogurt, and cheese groups, 1 serving represents 120 calories. A cup of whole milk has about 160 calories, compared with a cup of skim milk, which contains 88 calories. A cup of whole milk, therefore, would provide 1⅓ servings in this food group.

Using Low-Fat Entrees

To be more accurate with caloric intake and to simplify meal preparation, use commercially prepared low-fat frozen entrees as the main dish for lunch and dinner meals (only one entree for the 1,200-calorie diet plan—see Activity 6.2, pages 167–170). Look for entrees that provide about 300 calories and no more than 6 grams of fat per entree. These two entrees can be used as the meat and beans group selections and will provide most of the daily protein requirement for the body. Along with each entree, supplement the meal with some of your servings from the other food groups.

This diet plan has been used successfully in weight loss research programs.[16] If you choose not to use these low-fat entrees, prepare a similar meal using 3 ounces (cooked) of lean meat, poultry, or fish with additional beans, vegetables, rice, or pasta that will provide 300 calories with fewer than 6 grams of fat per dish.

Analyze Your Intake

As you record your food choices, be sure to write the precise amount for each serving. If you choose to do so, you then can run a computerized nutrient analysis to verify your caloric intake and food distribution pattern (percent of total calories from carbohydrate, fat, and protein).

Behavior Modification and Adherence to a Lifetime Weight Management Program

Achieving and maintaining recommended body composition is by no means impossible, but it does require desire and commitment. If weight management is to become a priority in life, people must realize that they have to transform their behavior to some extent.

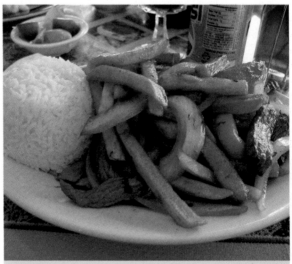

"Super-sized" portion sizes at restaurants in the United States contribute to the growing epidemic of obesity.

© Fitness & Wellness, Inc.

Weight Loss Strategies

1. *Make a commitment to change.* The first necessary ingredient is the desire to modify your behavior. You have to stop precontemplating or contemplating change and get going! You must accept that you have a problem and decide by yourself whether you really want to change. Sincere commitment increases your chances for success.

2. *Set realistic goals.* The weight problem developed over several years. Similarly, new lifetime eating and exercise habits take time to develop. A realistic long-term goal also will include short-term objectives that allow for regular evaluation and help maintain motivation and renewed commitment to attain the long-term goal.

3. *Incorporate exercise into the program.* Choosing enjoyable activities, places, times, equipment, and people to work out with will help you adhere to an exercise program. (See Chapters 6, 7, 8, and 9.)

4. *Differentiate hunger and appetite.* Hunger is the actual physical need for food. Appetite is a desire for food, usually triggered by factors such as stress, habit, boredom, depression, availability of food, or just the thought of food itself. Developing and sticking to a regular meal pattern will help control hunger.

5. *Eat less fat.* Each gram of fat provides 9 calories, and protein and carbohydrates provide only 4. In essence, you can eat more food on a low-fat diet because you consume fewer calories with each meal. Most of your fat intake should come from unsaturated sources.

6. *Pay attention to calories.* Just because food is labeled "low-fat" does not mean you can eat as much as you want. When reading food labels—and when eating—don't just look at the fat content. Pay attention to calories as well. Many low-fat foods are high in calories.

7. *Cut unnecessary items from your diet.* Substituting water for a daily can of soda would cut 51,100 (140 × 365) calories yearly from the diet—the equivalent of 14.6 (51,000 ÷ 3,500) pounds of fat.

8. *Maintain a daily intake of calcium-rich foods,* especially low-fat or nonfat dairy products.

9. *Add foods to your diet that reduce cravings,* such as eggs; small amounts of red meat, fish, poultry, tofu, oils, fats; and nonstarchy vegetables such as lettuce, green beans, peppers, asparagus, broccoli, mushrooms, and Brussels sprouts. Also increasing the intake of low-glycemic carbohydrates with your meals helps you go longer before you feel hungry again.

10. *Avoid automatic eating.* Many people associate certain daily activities with eating, for example, cooking, watching television, or reading. Most foods consumed in these situations lack nutritional value or are high in sugar and fat.

11. *Stay busy.* People tend to eat more when they sit around and do nothing. Occupying the mind and body with activities not associated with eating helps take away the desire to eat. Some options are walking; cycling; playing sports; gardening; sewing; or visiting a library, a museum, or a park. You also might develop other skills and interests not associated with food.

12. *Plan meals and shop sensibly.* Always shop on a full stomach, because hungry shoppers tend to buy unhealthy foods impulsively—and then snack on the way home. Always use a shopping list, which should include whole-grain breads and cereals, fruits and vegetables, low-fat milk and dairy products, lean meats, fish, and poultry.

13. *Cook wisely:*
    - Use less fat and fewer refined foods in food preparation.
    - Trim all visible fat from meats and remove skin from poultry before cooking.
    - Skim the fat off gravies and soups.
    - Bake, broil, boil, or steam instead of frying.
    - Sparingly use butter, cream, mayonnaise, and salad dressings.
    - Avoid coconut oil, palm oil, and cocoa butter.
    - Prepare plenty of foods that contain fiber.
    - Include whole-grain breads and cereals, vegetables, and legumes in most meals.
    - Eat fruits for dessert.
    - Stay away from soda pop, fruit juices, and fruit-flavored drinks.
    - Use less sugar, and cut down on other refined carbohydrates, such as corn syrup, malt sugar, dextrose, and fructose.
    - Drink plenty of water—at least six glasses a day.

14. Do not serve more food than you should eat. Measure the food in portions and keep serving dishes away from the table. Do not force yourself or anyone else to "clean the plate" after they are satisfied (including children after they already have had a healthy, nutritious serving).

15. Try "junior size" instead of "super size." People who are served larger portions eat more, whether they are hungry or not. Use smaller plates, bowls, cups, and glasses. Try eating half as much food as you commonly eat. Watch for portion sizes at restaurants as well: Supersized foods create supersized people.

16. Eat out infrequently. The more often people eat out, the more body fat they have. People who eat out six or more times per week consume an average of about 300 extra calories per day and 30 percent more fat than those who eat out less often.

17. Eat slowly and at the table only. Eating on the run promotes overeating because the body doesn't have enough time to "register" consumption and people overeat before the body perceives the fullness signal. Eating at the table encourages people to take time out to eat and deters snacking between meals. After eating, do not sit around the table but, rather, clean up and put away the food to avoid snacking.

18. Avoid social binges. Social gatherings tend to entice self-defeating behavior. Use visual imagery to plan ahead. Do not feel pressured to eat or drink and don't rationalize in these situations. Choose low-calorie foods and entertain yourself with other activities, such as dancing and talking.

19. Do not place unhealthy foods within easy reach. Ideally, avoid bringing high-calorie, high-sugar, or high-fat foods into the house. If they are there already, store them where they are hard to get to or see—perhaps the garage or basement.

20. Avoid evening food raids. Most people do really well during the day but then "lose it" at night. Take control. Stop and think. To avoid excessive nighttime snacking, stay busy after your evening meal. Go for a short walk; floss and brush your teeth, and get to bed earlier. Even better, close the kitchen after dinner and try not to eat anything 3 hours prior to going to sleep.

21. Practice stress management techniques (discussed in Chapter 7). Many people snack and increase their food consumption in stressful situations.

22. Get support. People who receive support from friends, relatives, and formal support groups are much more likely to lose and maintain weight loss than those without such support. The more support you receive, the better off you will be.

23. Monitor changes and reward accomplishments. Being able to exercise without interruption for 15, 20, 30, or 60 minutes; swimming a certain distance; running a mile—all these accomplishments deserve recognition. Create rewards that are not related to eating: new clothing, a tennis racquet, a bicycle, exercise shoes, or something else that is special and you would not have acquired otherwise.

24. Prepare for slip-ups. Most people will slip and occasionally splurge. Do not despair and give up. Reevaluate and continue with your efforts. An occasional slip won't make much difference in the long run.

25. Think positive. Avoid negative thoughts about how difficult changing past behaviors might be. Instead, think of the benefits you will reap, such as feeling, looking, and functioning better, plus enjoying better health and improving the quality of life. Avoid negative environments and unsupportive people.

Try It

In your Online Journal or class notebook, answer the following questions: How many of the above strategies do you use to help you maintain recommended body weight? Do you feel that any of these strategies specifically help you manage body weight more effectively? If so, explain why.

Modifying old habits and developing new, positive behaviors take time. Individuals who apply the management techniques provided in the Behavior Modification Planning box beginning on the previous page are more successful at changing detrimental behavior and adhering to a positive lifetime weight-control program. In developing a retraining program, people are not expected to use all of the strategies listed, but should pick the ones that apply to them.

CRITICAL THINKING

What behavioral strategies have you used to properly manage your body weight? • How do you think those strategies would work for others?

You Can Do It!

The challenge of taking off excessive body fat and keeping it off for good has no simple solution. Weight management is accomplished through lifetime commitment to physical activity and proper food selection. When taking part in a weight-reduction program, people have to decrease their caloric intake moderately and implement strategies to modify unhealthy eating behaviors.

Relapses into past negative behaviors are almost inevitable. Making mistakes is human and does not mean failure. Failure comes to those who give up and do not use previous experiences to build upon and, instead, develop skills that will prevent self-defeating behaviors in the future. Where there's a will, there's a way, and those who persist will reap the rewards.

www WEB INTERACTIVE

Aetna InteliHealth. This site provides articles on Healthful Lifestyles, including weight management. The Nutrition database offers tips on weight management, exercise and assessing your diet. Interactive tools include healthful recipe, food pyramid, and a body mass index calculator. **http://www.intelihealth.com**

*Log on to **academic.cengage.com/login** to track your progress in your exercise log and update your pedometer log if you are tracking your steps.*

1. Are you satisfied with your current body composition and quality of life? If not, are you willing to do something about it? If so, what do you plan to do to reach your goal?

2. Are physical activity, aerobic exercise, and strength training regular parts of your lifetime weight management program?

3. Do you weigh yourself regularly and make adjustments in energy intake and physical activity habits if your weight starts to slip upward?

4. Do you exercise portion control, watch your overall fat intake, and plan ahead before you eat out or attend social functions that entice overeating?

*Log on to **academic.cengage.com/login** to assess your understanding of this chapter's topics by taking the chapter pre-test and exploring the modules recommended in your Personalized Study Plan.*

1. Obesity is defined as a body mass index equal to or above
   a. 10.
   b. 25.
   c. 30.
   d. 45.
   e. 50.

2. The yearly estimated number of deaths attributed to excessive body weight and physical inactivity in the United States is
   a. 28,000.
   b. 55,000.
   c. 93,000.
   d. 112,000.
   e. 350,000.

3. Obesity increases the risk for
   a. hypertension.
   b. congestive heart failure.
   c. atherosclerosis.
   d. type 2 diabetes.
   e. all of the above.

4. Tolerable weight is a body weight
   a. that is not ideal but one that you can live with.
   b. that will tolerate the increased risk of chronic diseases.
   c. with a BMI range between 25 and 30.

d. that meets both ideal values for percent body weight and BMI.
   e. All are correct choices.

5. When the body uses protein instead of a combination of fats and carbohydrates as a source of energy,
   a. weight loss is very slow.
   b. a large amount of weight loss is in the form of water.
   c. muscle turns into fat.
   d. fat is lost very rapidly.
   e. fat cannot be lost.

6. One pound of fat represents
   a. 1,200 calories.
   b. 1,500 calories.
   c. 3,500 calories.
   d. 5,000 calories.
   e. None of the above.

7. The mechanism that seems to regulate how much a person weighs is known as
   a. setpoint.
   b. weight factor.
   c. basal metabolic rate.
   d. metabolism.
   e. energy-balancing equation.

8. The key to successful weight management is
   a. frequent dieting.
   b. very low calorie diets when "normal" dieting doesn't work.
   c. a lifetime physical activity program.
   d. regular low-carbohydrate/high-protein meals.
   e. All are correct choices.

CONTINUED

9. The daily amount of physical activity recommended for weight loss maintenance is
a. 15 to 20 minutes.
b. 20 to 30 minutes.
c. 30 to 60 minutes.
d. 60 to 90 minutes.
e. Any amount is sufficient as long as it is done daily.

10. A daily energy expenditure of 300 calories through physical activity is the equivalent of approximately _____ pounds of fat per year.
a. 12
b. 15
c. 22
d. 27
e. 31

Correct answers can be found at the back of the book.

Daily Food Intake Record: 1,200-Calorie Diet Plan

Name _____ Date _____

Course _____ Section _____

Instructions

The objective of the diet plan is to meet (not exceed) the number of servings allowed for the food groups listed. Each time you eat a particular food, record it in the space provided for each group along with the appropriate serving size. Be sure not to exceed the number of calories allowed per serving listed below. Instead of the meat and beans group, you are allowed to have a commercially available low-fat frozen entree for your meal (this entree should provide no more than 300 calories and less than 6 grams of fat). You can make additional copies of this form as needed.

Meat & Beans: 1 low-fat frozen entree
Milk: 2 servings
Fruits: 2 servings
Veggies: 3 servings
Grains: 6 servings

Bread, Cereal, Rice, Pasta Group (80 calories/serving): 6 servings

1 _____

2 _____

3 _____

4 _____

5 _____

6 _____

Vegetable Group (25 calories/serving): 3 servings

1 _____

2 _____

3 _____

Fruit Group (60 calories/serving): 2 servings

1 _____

2 _____

Milk Group (120 calories/serving, use low-fat milk and low-fat milk products): 2 servings

1 _____

2 _____

Low-fat Frozen Entrees (300 calories and less than 6 grams of fat): 1 serving

1 _____

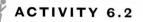
Daily Food Intake Record: 1,500-Calorie Diet Plan

Instructions

The objective of the diet plan is to meet (not exceed) the number of servings allowed for the food groups listed. Each time you eat a particular food, record it in the space provided for each group along with the appropriate serving size. Be sure not to exceed the number of calories allowed per serving listed below. Instead of the meat and beans group, you are allowed to have two commercially available low-fat frozen entree for your meal (this entree should provide no more than 300 calories and less than 6 grams of fat). You can make additional copies of this form as needed.

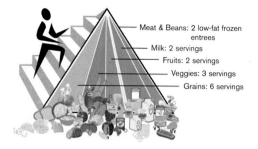

Meat & Beans: 2 low-fat frozen entrees
Milk: 2 servings
Fruits: 2 servings
Veggies: 3 servings
Grains: 6 servings

Bread, Cereal, Rice, Pasta Group (80 calories/serving): 6 servings

1 _____

2 _____

3 _____

4 _____

5 _____

6 _____

Vegetable Group (25 calories/serving): 3 servings

1 _____

2 _____

3 _____

Fruit Group (60 calories/serving): 2 servings

1 _____

2 _____

Milk Group (120 calories/serving, use low-fat milk and low-fat milk products): 2 servings

1 _____

2 _____

Low-fat Frozen Entrees (300 calories and less than 6 grams of fat): 2 servings

1 _____

2 _____

Daily Food Intake Record: 1,800-Calorie Diet Plan

Name _____   Date _____

Course _____   Section _____

Instructions

The objective of the diet plan is to meet (not exceed) the number of servings allowed for the food groups listed. Each time you eat a particular food, record it in the space provided for each group along with the appropriate serving size. Be sure not to exceed the number of calories allowed per serving listed below. Instead of the meat and beans group, you are allowed to have two commercially available low-fat frozen entrees for two of your meals (these entrees should provide no more than 300 calories and less than 6 grams of fat). You can make additional copies of this form as needed.

Meat & Beans: 2 low-fat frozen entrees
Milk: 2 servings
Fruits: 3 servings
Veggies: 5 servings
Grains: 8 servings

Bread, Cereal, Rice, Pasta Group (80 calories/serving): 8 servings

1 _____   5 _____

2 _____   6 _____

3 _____   7 _____

4 _____   8 _____

Vegetable Group (25 calories/serving): 5 servings

1 _____   4 _____

2 _____   5 _____

3 _____

Fruit Group (60 calories/serving): 3 servings

1 _____

2 _____

3 _____

Milk Group (120 calories/serving, use low-fat milk and low-fat milk products): 2 servings

1 _____

2 _____

Low-fat Frozen Entrees (300 calories and less than 6 grams of fat): 2 servings

1 _____

2 _____

Daily Food Intake Record: 2,000-Calorie Diet Plan

Instructions

The objective of the diet plan is to meet (not exceed) the number of servings allowed for the food groups listed. Each time you eat a particular food, record it in the space provided for each group along with the appropriate serving size. Be sure not to exceed the number of calories allowed per serving listed below. Instead of the meat and beans group, you are allowed to have two commercially available low-fat frozen entrees for two of your meals (these entrees should provide no more than 300 calories and less than 6 grams of fat). You can make additional copies of this form as needed.

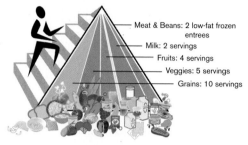

Meat & Beans: 2 low-fat frozen entrees
Milk: 2 servings
Fruits: 4 servings
Veggies: 5 servings
Grains: 10 servings

Bread, Cereal, Rice, Pasta Group (80 calories/serving): 10 servings

1 _____   6 _____

2 _____   7 _____

3 _____   8 _____

4 _____   9 _____

5 _____   10 _____

Vegetable Group (25 calories/serving): 5 servings

1 _____   4 _____

2 _____   5 _____

3 _____

Fruit Group (60 calories/serving): 4 servings

1 _____

2 _____

3 _____

4 _____

Milk Group (120 calories/serving, use low-fat milk and low-fat milk products): 2 servings

1 _____

2 _____

Low-fat Frozen Entrees (300 calories and less than 6 grams of fat): 2 servings

1 _____

2 _____

Stress Management

7

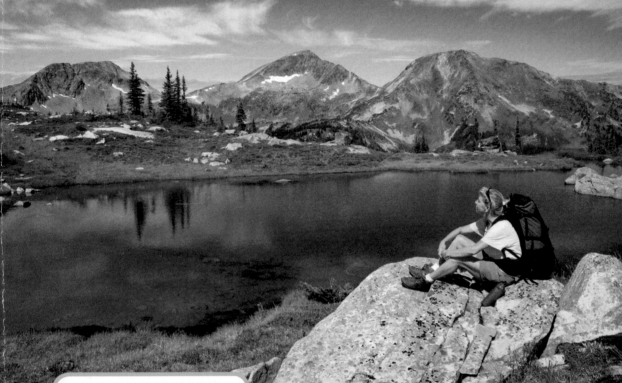

OBJECTIVES

- Define stress, eustress, and distress
- Explain how stress affects health and optimal performance
- Define the two major types of behavior patterns or personality types
- Learn whether you have a hostile personality
- Develop time-management skills
- Identify the major sources of stress in your life
- Define the role of physical exercise in reducing stress
- Learn to use various stress management techniques

© Frits Meyst/Adventure4ever.com/drr.net

Log on to **CengageNOW** at academic .cengage.com/login to find innovative study tools—including pre- and post-tests, personalized study plans, activities, labs, and the personal change planner.

Learning to live and get ahead today is not possible without stress. To succeed in an unpredictable world that changes with every new day, working under pressure has become the rule rather than the exception for most people. As a result, stress has become one of the most common problems we face. Current estimates indicate that the annual cost of stress and stress-related diseases in the United States exceeds $100 billion, a direct result of health care costs, lost productivity, and absenteeism.

The Mind/Body Connection

A growing body of evidence indicates that virtually every illness known to modern humanity—from arthritis to migraine headaches, from the common cold to cancer—is influenced for good or bad by our emotions. To a profound extent, emotions affect our susceptibility to disease and our immunity. The way we react to what comes along in life can determine in great measure how we will react to the disease-causing organisms that we face. The feelings we have and the ways we express them can either boost our immune system or weaken it.

Emotions cause physiological responses that can influence health. Certain parts of the brain are associated with specific emotions and specific hormone patterns. The release of certain hormones is associated with various emotional responses, and those hormones affect health. These responses may contribute to development of disease. Emotions have to be expressed somewhere, somehow. If they are suppressed repeatedly, as in stressful situations, and/or if a person feels conflict about controlling them, they often reveal themselves through physical symptoms. These physiological responses may weaken the immune system over time.

The immune system patrols and guards the body against attackers. This system consists of about a trillion cells called **lymphocytes** (the cells responsible for waging war against disease or infection) and about a hundred million trillion molecules called **antibodies.** The brain and the immune system are closely linked in a connection that allows the mind to influence both susceptibility and resistance to disease.

A fighting spirit also plays a major role in the recovery from illness. A fighting spirit involves the healthy expression of emotions, whether they are negative or positive. Many physicians believe that a patient's attitude, especially a fighting spirit, is the underlying factor in spontaneous remission from incurable illness. Fighters are not stronger or more capable than others—they simply do not give up easily. They enjoy better health and live longer, even when physicians and laboratory tests say they should not.

Stress

Every person has an optimal level of stress that is most conducive to adequate health and performance. When stress levels reach mental, emotional, and physiological limits, however, stress becomes distress and the person no longer functions effectively.

The body's response to stress has been the same ever since humans were first put on the earth. Stress prepares the organism to react to the stress-causing event, called the **stressor.** The difference is the way in which we react to stress. Many people thrive under stress. Others under similar circumstances are unable to handle it. An individual's reaction to a stress-causing agent determines whether stress is positive or negative.

Chronic negative reactions to stress raise the risk for many health disorders, including coronary heart disease, hypertension, eating disorders, ulcers, diabetes, asthma, depression, migraine headaches, sleep disorders, and chronic fatigue and may even play a role in the development of certain types of cancer. Crucial in maintaining emotional and physiologic stability is to recognize when stress has a negative effect and to overcome the stressful condition quickly and efficiently.

The good news is that stress can be self-controlled. Most people have accepted stress as a normal part of daily life, and even though everyone has to deal with it, few seem to understand it and know how to cope effectively. People should not try to avoid stress entirely, as a certain amount is necessary for optimum health, performance, and well-being. It is difficult to succeed and have fun in life without "hits, runs, and errors."

The Body's Reaction to Stress

Dr. Hans Selye, one of the foremost authorities on stress, defined it as "the nonspecific response of the human organism to any demand that is placed upon it."[1] "Nonspecific" indicates that the body reacts in a similar way regardless of the nature of the event that leads to the stress response. In simpler terms, stress is the body's mental, emotional, and physiological response to any situation that is new, threatening, frightening, or exciting.

The body responds to stress with a rapid-fire sequence of physical changes known as **fight or flight** (see Figure 7.1). The hypothalamus activates the sympathetic nervous system, and the pituitary gland triggers the release of catecholamines (hormones) from the adrenal glands. These hormonal changes increase heart rate, blood pressure, blood flow to active muscles and the brain, glucose levels, oxygen consumption, and strength—all necessary for the body to either fight or flee. In cases of both fight and flight, the body relaxes and stress dissipates. If the person is unable to take action, however, the muscles tense and tighten instead.

Stress isn't necessarily bad. Dr. Selye further defined stress as either **eustress** or **distress.** In both cases, the nonspecific response is almost the same. In eustress, health and performance continue to improve even as stress increases. With distress, health and performance begin to deteriorate.

CRITICAL THINKING

Can you identify sources of eustress and distress in your personal life during this past year? • Explain your emotional and physical response to each stressor and how the two differ.

Adaptation to Stress

Human physiology is such that the body continually strives to maintain a constant internal environment. This state of physiological balance, known as **homeostasis,** allows the body to function as effectively as possible. When a stressor triggers a nonspecific response, homeostasis is disrupted. This reaction to stressors, best explained by Dr. Selye through the **general adaptation syndrome (GAS),** is composed of three stages: alarm reaction, resistance, and exhaustion/recovery.

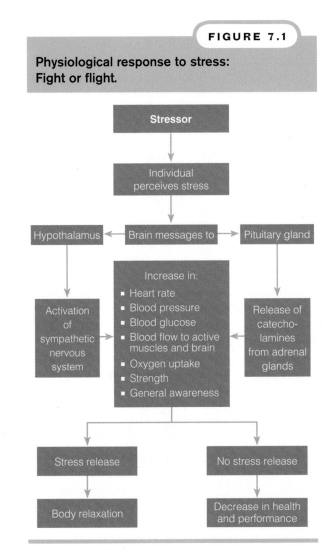

FIGURE 7.1

Physiological response to stress: Fight or flight.

SOURCE: *Lifetime Physical Fitness & Wellness,* by W. W. K. Hoeger and S. A. Hoeger (Belmont, CA: Wadsworth/Cengage Learning, 2009).

KEY TERMS

Stress The mental, emotional, and physiological response of the body to any situation that is new, threatening, frightening, or exciting.

Lymphocytes Immune system cells responsible for waging war against disease or infection.

Antibodies Substances produced by the white blood cells in response to an invading agent.

Stressor Stress-causing agent.

Fight or flight A series of physical responses activated automatically in response to environmental stressors.

Eustress Positive stress.

Distress Negative or harmful stress under which health and performance begin to deteriorate.

Homeostasis A natural state of equilibrium. The body attempts to maintain this equilibrium by constantly reacting to external forces that attempt to disrupt this fine balance.

General adaptation syndrome (GAS) A theoretical model that explains the body's adaptation to sustained stress which includes three stages: alarm reaction, resistance, and exhaustion/recovery.

Alarm Reaction

The alarm reaction is the immediate response to a stressor, whether positive or negative. During the alarm reaction, the body evokes an instant physiological reaction that involves the mobilization of systems and processes within the organism to minimize the threat to homeostasis (see "Coping with Stress," page 179). If the stressor subsides, the body recovers and returns to homeostasis.

Resistance

If the stressor persists, the body calls upon its limited reserves to build up resistance as it strives to maintain homeostasis. For a short while, the body copes effectively and meets the challenge of the stressor until it can be overcome (see Figure 7.2).

Exhaustion/Recovery

If stress becomes chronic and intolerable, the body spends its limited reserves and loses its ability to cope, entering the exhaustion/recovery stage. During this stage, the body functions at a diminished capacity while it recovers from stress. In due time, following an "adequate" recovery period, the body recuperates and is able to return to homeostasis. If chronic stress persists during the exhaustion stage, however, immune function is compromised, which can damage body systems and lead to disease.

An example of the stress response through the general adaptation syndrome can be illustrated in college test performance. As you prepare to take an exam, you experience an initial alarm reaction. If you understand the material, study for the exam, and do well (eustress), the body recovers and stress is dissipated. If, however, you are not adequately prepared and fail the exam, the resistance stage is triggered. You are now concerned about your grade, and you remain in the resistance stage until the next exam. If you prepare and do well, the body recovers. But if you fail once again and no longer can bring up your grade, exhaustion sets in, with possible physical and emotional breakdowns as a result. Exhaustion may be aggravated if you are struggling in other courses as well.

The exhaustion stage is often manifested in athletes and the most ardent fitness participants. Staleness is usually a consequence of overtraining. Peak performance can be sustained for only about two to three weeks at a time. Any attempts to continue intense training after peaking leads to exhaustion, diminished fitness, and mental and physical problems associated with overtraining. Thus, athletes and some fitness participants also need an active recovery phase following the attainment of peak fitness.

Behavior Patterns

Common life events are not the only source of stress in life. All too often, individuals bring on stress as a result of their characteristic behavior patterns. The

---

FIGURE 7.2

General adaptation syndrome: The body's response to stress.

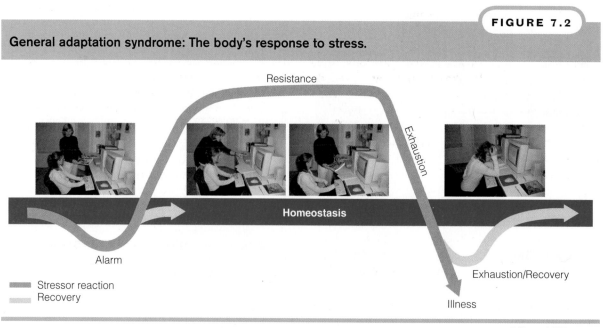

Resistance

Exhaustion

Homeostasis

Alarm

Exhaustion/Recovery

Illness

Stressor reaction
Recovery

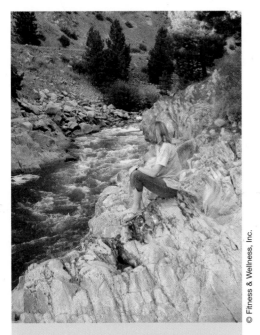

Taking time out during stressful life events is vital for good health and wellness.

© Fitness & Wellness, Inc.

two main types of behavior patterns are **Type A** and **Type B.** Each type is based on several characteristics that are used to classify people into one of these behavioral patterns.

Type A behavior characterizes a primarily hard driving, overly ambitious, aggressive, at times hostile and overly competitive person. Type A individuals often set their own goals, are self-motivated, try to accomplish many tasks at the same time, are excessively achievement oriented, and have a sense of time urgency. By contrast, Type B behavior is characteristic of calm, casual, relaxed, easygoing individuals. Type B people take one thing at a time, do not feel pressured or hurried, and seldom set their own deadlines.

Over the years, experts have indicated that individuals classified as Type A have a significantly higher incidence of disease, especially cardiovascular conditions.[2] Not all typical Type A people, however, are at higher risk for disease. Type A individuals who are chronically angry and hostile are at higher risk.[3] The questionnaire provided in Figure 7.3 can help you determine whether you have a hostile personality.

Some experts believe that emotional stress is far more likely than physical stress to trigger a heart attack. Especially vulnerable are people who are impatient and are readily annoyed when they have to wait for someone or something—an employee, a traffic light, in a restaurant line.

Research also is focusing on individuals who have anxiety, depression, and feelings of helplessness when they encounter setbacks and failures in life. People who lose control of their lives, those who give up on their dreams in life, knowing that they could and should be doing better, may be more

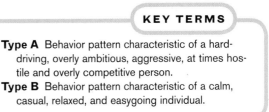

KEY TERMS

Type A Behavior pattern characteristic of a hard-driving, overly ambitious, aggressive, at times hostile and overly competitive person.

Type B Behavior pattern characteristic of a calm, casual, relaxed, and easygoing individual.

FIGURE 7.3

Hostility and heart disease risk scale.

HOSTILITY COULD HARM YOUR HEART

Experts now conclude that feelings of hostility increase your risk of heart disease. Dr. Redford Williams, Duke University Medical Center, has designed a questionnaire to help you determine whether you have a hostile personality. Circle the answer that most closely fits how you would respond to the given situation:

1. A teenager drives by my yard blasting the car stereo:
   A. I begin to understand why teenagers can't hear.
   B. I can feel my blood pressure starting to rise.

2. A boyfriend/girlfriend calls at the last minute "too tired to go out tonight." I'm stuck with two $15 tickets:
   A. I find someone else to go with.
   B. I tell my friend how inconsiderate he/she is.

3. Waiting in the express checkout line at the supermarket where a sign says "No More Than 10 Items Please":
   A. I pick up a magazine and pass the time.
   B. I glance to see if anyone has more than 10 items.

4. Most homeless people in large cities:
   A. Are down and out because they lack ambition.
   B. Are victims of illness or some other misfortune.

5. At times when I've been very angry with someone:
   A. I was able to stop short of hitting him/her.
   B. I have, on occasion, hit or shoved him/her.

6. When I am stuck in a traffic jam:
   A. I am usually not particularly upset.
   B. I quickly start to feel irritated and annoyed.

7. When there's a really important job to be done:
   A. I prefer to do it myself.
   B. I am apt to call on my friends to help.

8. The cars ahead of me start to slow and stop as they approach a curve:
   A. I assume there is a construction site ahead.
   B. I assume someone ahead had a fender-bender.

9. An elevator stops too long above where I'm waiting:
   A. I soon start to feel irritated and annoyed.
   B. I start planning the rest of my day.

10. When a friend or coworker disagrees with me:
    A. I try to explain my position more clearly.
    B. I am apt to get into an argument with him or her.

11. At times when I was really angry in the past:
    A. I have never thrown things or slammed a door.
    B. I've sometimes thrown things or slammed a door.

12. Someone bumps into me in a store:
    A. I pass it off as an accident.
    B. I feel irritated at their clumsiness.

13. When my spouse (significant other) is fixing a meal:
    A. I keep an eye out to make sure nothing burns.
    B. I talk about my day or read the paper.

14. Someone is hogging the conversation at a party:
    A. I look for an opportunity to put him/her down.
    B. I soon move to another group.

15. In most arguments:
    A. I am the angrier one.
    B. The other person is angrier than I am.

Score one point for each of these answers: 1. B, 2. B, 3. B, 4. A, 5. B, 6. B, 7. A, 8. B, 9. A, 10. B, 11. B, 12. B, 13. A, 14. A, 15. A. If you scored 4 or more points you may be hostile. Questions 1, 6, 9, 12, and 15 reflect anger. Questions 2, 5, 10, 11, and 14 reflect aggression. Questions 3, 4, 7, 8, and 13 reflect cynicism. If you scored 2 points in any category, you should work on that area of your personality.

SOURCE: *Anger Kills*, by Redford B. Williams and Virginia Williams. Copyright © 1993 by Redford B. Williams, M.D., and Virginia Williams, Ph.D. Reprinted by permission of Random House, Inc.

likely to have heart attacks than hard-driving people who enjoy their work.

Many of the Type A characteristics are learned behaviors. Consequently, if people can learn to identify the sources of stress, they can change their behavioral responses. The main assessment tool to determine behavioral type is the structured interview, in which the interviewee is asked to reply to several questions that describe Type A and Type B behavior patterns. The interviewer notes the responses to the questions and also mental, emotional, and physical behaviors the individual exhibits as he or she replies to each question. Based on the answers and the associated behaviors, the interviewer rates the person along a continuum ranging from Type A to Type B.

Changing a Type A Personality

- Make a contract with yourself to slow down and take it easy. Put it in writing. Post it in a conspicuous spot, then stick to the terms you set up. Be specific. Abstracts ("I'm going to be less uptight") don't work.
- Work on only one or two things at a time. Wait until you change one habit before you tackle the next one.
- Eat more slowly and eat only when you are relaxed and sitting down.
- If you smoke, quit.
- Cut down on your caffeine intake, because it increases the tendency to become irritated and agitated.
- Take regular breaks throughout the day, even as brief as 5 or 10 minutes, when you totally change what you're doing. Get up, stretch, get a drink of cool water, walk around for a few minutes.
- Work on fighting your impatience. If you're standing in line at the grocery store, study the interesting things people have in their carts instead of getting upset.
- Work on controlling hostility. Keep a written log. When do you flare up? What causes it? How do you feel at the time? What preceded it? Look for patterns and figure out what sets you off. Then do something about it. Either avoid the situations that cause you hostility or practice reacting to them in different ways.
- Plan some activities just for the fun of it. Load a picnic basket in the car and drive to the country with a friend. After a stressful physics class, stop at a theater and see a good comedy.
- Choose a role model, someone you know and admire who does not have a Type A personality. Observe the person carefully, then try out some techniques the person demonstrates.
- Simplify your life so you can learn to relax a little bit. Figure out which activities or commitments you can eliminate right now, then get rid of them.
- If morning is a problem time for you and you get too hurried, set your alarm clock half an hour earlier.

- Take time out during even the most hectic day to do something truly relaxing. Because you won't be used to it, you may have to work at it at first. Begin by listing things you'd really enjoy that would calm you. Include some things that take only a few minutes: Watch a sunset, lie out on the lawn at night and look at the stars, call an old friend and catch up on news, take a nap, sauté a pan of mushrooms and savor them slowly.
- If you're under a deadline, take short breaks. Stop and talk to someone for 5 minutes, take a short walk, or lie down with a cool cloth over your eyes for 10 minutes.
- Pay attention to what your own body clock is saying. You've probably noticed that every 90 minutes or so, you lose the ability to concentrate, get a little sleepy, and have a tendency to daydream. Instead of fighting the urge, put down your work and let your mind wander for a few minutes. Use the time to imagine and let your creativity run wild.
- Learn to treasure unplanned surprises: a friend dropping by unannounced, a hummingbird outside your window, a child's tightly clutched bouquet of wildflowers.
- Savor your relationships. Think about the people in your life. Relax with them and give yourself to them. Give up trying to control others and resist the urge to end relationships that don't always go as you'd like them to.

From *Wellness: Guidelines for a Healthy Lifestyle,* by W. W. K. Hoeger, L. Turner, and B. Q. Hafen (3d ed.) (Belmont, CA: Thomson Wadsworth, 2007).

Try It

If Type A describes your personality, pick three of the above strategies and apply them in your life this week. At the end of each day determine how well you have done that day and evaluate how you can improve the next day.

Vulnerability to Stress

Researchers have identified a number of factors that can affect the way in which people handle stress. How people deal with these factors actually can increase or decrease vulnerability to stress. The questionnaire provided in Figure 7.4 lists these factors so you can determine your vulnerability rating. Many of the items on this questionnaire are related to health, social support, self-worth, and nurturance (sense of being needed). All of the factors are crucial for a person's physical, social, mental, and emotional well-being. The questionnaire will help you identify specific areas in which you can make improvements to help you cope more efficiently.

The benefits of physical fitness are discussed extensively in this book. In addition, social support, self-worth, and nurturance are essential to cope effectively with stressful life events. These factors play a supportive and protective role in people's lives. The more integrated people are in society, the less vulnerable they are to stress and illness.

Positive correlations have been found between social support and health outcomes. People can draw upon social support to weather crises. Knowing that someone else cares, that people are there to lean on, that support is out there, is valuable for survival (or growth) in times of need.[4]

As you complete the questionnaire, you will notice that many of the items describe situations and

FIGURE 7.4

Stress vulnerability questionnaire.

Item	Strongly Agree	Mildly Agree	Mildly Disagree	Strongly Disagree
1. I try to incorporate as much physical activity* as possible in my daily schedule.	(1)	2	3	4
2. I exercise aerobically 20 minutes or more at least three times per week.	(1)	2	3	4
3. I regularly sleep 7 to 8 hours per night.	1	2	(3)	4
4. I take my time eating at least one hot, balanced meal a day.	1	(2)	3	4
5. I drink fewer than two cups of coffee (or equivalent) per day.	(1)	2	3	4
6. I am at recommended body weight.	(1)	2	3	4
7. I enjoy good health.	(1)	2	3	4
8. I do not use tobacco in any form.	(1)	2	3	4
9. I limit my alcohol intake to no more than one drink per day.	(1)	2	3	4
10. I do not use hard drugs (chemical dependency).	(1)	2	3	4
11. I have someone I love, trust, and can rely on for help if I have a problem or need to make an essential decision.	(1)	2	3	4
12. There is love in my family.	(1)	2	3	4
13. I routinely give and receive affection.	(1)	2	3	4
14. I have close personal relationships with other people who provide me with a sense of emotional security.	(1)	2	3	4
15. There are people close by whom I can turn to for guidance in time of stress.	(1)	2	3	4
16. I can speak openly about feelings, emotions, and problems with people I trust.	(1)	2	3	4
17. Other people rely on me for help.	(1)	2	3	4
18. I am able to keep my feelings of anger and hostility under control.	1	(2)	3	4
19. I have a network of friends who enjoy the same social activities I do.	(1)	2	3	4
20. I take time to do something fun at least once a week.	(1)	2	3	4
21. My religious beliefs provide guidance and strength to my life.	1	2	(3)	4
22. I often provide service to others.	(1)	2	3	4
23. I enjoy my job (major or school).	(1)	2	3	4
24. I am a competent worker.	(1)	2	3	4
25. I get along well with coworkers (or students).	(1)	2	3	4
26. My income is sufficient for my needs.	(1)	2	3	4
27. I manage time adequately.	(1)	2	3	4
28. I have learned to say "no" to additional commitments when I am already pressed for time.	1	2	(3)	4
29. I take daily quiet time for myself.	(1)	2	3	4
30. I practice stress management as needed.	(1)	2	3	4

Total Points: [   ]

Scoring:

0–30 points	Excellent (great resistance to stress)
31–40 points	Good (little vulnerability to stress)
41–50 points	Average (somewhat vulnerable to stress)
51–60 points	Fair (vulnerable to stress)
≥61 points	Poor (highly vulnerable to stress)

*Walk instead of driving, avoid escalators and elevators, or walk to neighboring offices, homes, and stores.

SOURCE: *Lifetime Physical Fitness & Wellness,* by W. W. K. Hoeger and S. A. Hoeger (Belmont, CA: Wadsworth/Cengage Learning, 2009).

behaviors that are within your own control. To make yourself less vulnerable to stress, you will want to improve certain behaviors. You should start by modifying the behaviors that are easiest to change before undertaking some of the most difficult ones.

Sources of Stress

Before addressing techniques that you can use to cope more effectively with stress, attempt to identify your current life stressors using the stress test provided in Figure 7.5. This test will help you determine stressors that you have encountered recently in your life. Think back over this past year and circle the "stress points" listed for each event that you experienced during this time. Then total the points and determine the amount of stress in your life during the past year.

Now, to help you cope more effectively, use the stress analysis form provided in Activity 7.1, pages 191–192. On this form, record the results of your stress questionnaires and list the stressors that affect you the most in your daily life. For each stressor, explain, in the box provided, the situation(s) under which it occurs, your response to it, the impact it is having in your life, and how you presently are handling the stressor. Based on what you have learned already, also indicate what you can do to either avoid the stressor or cope more effectively with it in the future. Common stressors in the lives of college students are depicted in Figure 7.6.

After completing the exercise in Activity 7.1, proceed to the discussion of relaxation techniques, pages 183–189. Once you have learned and mastered some of these techniques, return to your stress analysis and reevaluate your approach to cope with each stressor.

Coping with Stress

The ways in which people perceive and cope with stress seem to be more important in the development of disease than the amount and type of stress itself. If individuals perceive stress as a definite problem in their lives, when it interferes with optimal levels of health and performance, several techniques can help in coping more effectively.

First, of course, the person must recognize that a problem is present. Many people either do not want to believe they are under too much stress or they fail to recognize some of the typical symptoms of dis-

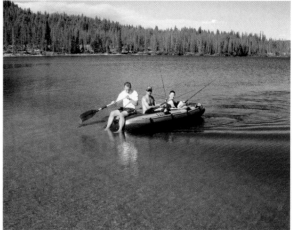

Regular leisure-time physical activity helps prevent psychological burnout.

tress. Noting some of the stress-related symptoms will help a person respond more objectively and initiate an adequate coping response.

When people have stress-related symptoms, they first should try to identify and remove the stressor or stress-causing agent. This is not as simple as it may seem, because in some situations, eliminating the stressor is not possible or a person may not even know what has caused it. If the cause is unknown, keeping a log of the time and days when the symptoms arise, as well as the events preceding and following the onset of symptoms, might be helpful.

For instance, a couple noted that every afternoon around 6 o'clock, the wife became nauseated and had abdominal pain. After seeking professional help, both were instructed to keep a log of daily events. It soon became clear that the symptoms did not appear on weekends but always started just before the husband came home from work during the week. Following some personal interviews with the couple, it was determined that the wife felt a lack of attention from her husband and responded subconsciously by becoming ill to the point at which she required personal attention and affection from her husband. Once the stressor was identified, they initiated appropriate behavior changes to correct the situation.

In many instances, however, the stressor cannot be removed. Examples of situations in which little or nothing can be done to eliminate the stress-causing agent are the death of a close family member, first year on the job, an intolerable boss, and a change in work responsibility. Nevertheless, stress

FIGURE 7.5

Stress test.

Take the Stress Test

To get a feel for the possible health impact of the various recent changes in your life, think back over the past year and circle the "stress points" listed for each of the events that you experienced during that time. Then add up your points. A total score of anywhere from about 250 to 500 or so would be considered a moderate amount of stress. If you score higher than that, you may face an increased risk of illness; if you score lower than that, consider yourself fortunate.

Health

An injury or illness which:

kept you in bed a week or more, or sent you to the hospital	74
was less serious than that	44
Major dental work	26
Major change in eating habits	27
Major change in sleeping habits	26
Major change in your usual type or amount of recreation	28

Work

Change to a new type of work	51
Change in your work hours or conditions	35

Change in your responsibilities at work:

more responsibilities	29
fewer responsibilities	21
promotion	31
demotion	42
transfer	32

Troubles at work:

with your boss	29
with coworkers	35
with persons under your supervision	35
other work troubles	28
Major business adjustment	60
Retirement	52

Loss of job:

laid off from work	68
fired from work	79
Correspondence course to help you in your work	18

Home and Family

Major change in living conditions	42

Change in residence:

move within the same town or city	25
move to a different town, city, or state	47
Change in family get-togethers	25
Major change in health or behavior of family member	55
Marriage	50
Pregnancy	67
Miscarriage or abortion	85

Gain of a new family member:

birth of a child	66
adoption of a child	65
a relative moving in with you	59
Spouse beginning or ending work	46

Child leaving home:

to attend college	41
due to marriage	41
for other reasons	45
Change in arguments with spouse	50
In-law problems	38

Change in the marital status of your parents:

divorce	59
remarriage	50

Separation from spouse:

due to work	53
due to marital problems	76
Divorce	96
Birth of grandchild	43
Death of spouse	119

Death of other family member:

child	123
brother or sister	102
parent	100

Personal and social

Change in personal habits	26
Beginning or ending school or college	38
Change of school or college	35
Change in political beliefs	24
Change in religious beliefs	29
Change in social activities	27
Vacation trip	24
New, close, personal relationship	37
Engagement to marry	45
Girlfriend or boyfriend problems	39
Sexual difficulties	44
"Falling out" of a close personal relationship	47
An accident	48
Minor violation of the law	20
Being held in jail	75
Death of a close friend	70
Major decision about your immediate future	51
Major personal achievement	36

Financial

Major change in finances:

increased income	38
decreased income	60
investment or credit difficulties	56
Loss or damage of personal property	43
Moderate purchase	20
Major purchase	37
Foreclosure on a mortgage or loan	58

Total Score: _____

Reprinted from *Journal of Psychosomatic Research,* Vol. 43, Miller and Rahe, "Life Changes Scaling for the 1990's," 1997, with permission from Elsevier Science.

FIGURE 7.6

Stressors in the lives of college students.

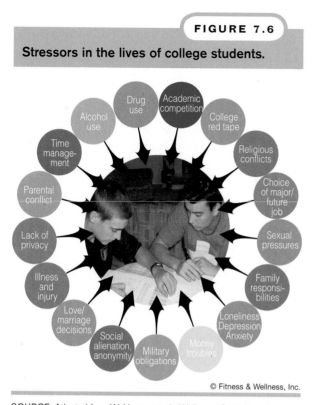

© Fitness & Wellness, Inc.

SOURCE: Adapted from W. Hoeger et al., *Wellness: Guidelines for a Healthy Lifestyle* (Belmont, CA: Thomson Wadsworth, 2007).

BEHAVIOR MODIFICATION PLANNING

Common Symptoms of Stress

- headaches
- muscular aches (mainly in neck, shoulders, and back)
- grinding teeth
- nervous tic, finger-tapping, toe-tapping
- increased sweating
- increase in or loss of appetite
- insomnia
- nightmares
- fatigue
- dry mouth
- stuttering
- high blood pressure
- tightness or pain in the chest
- impotence
- hives
- dizziness
- depression
- irritation
- anger
- hostility
- fear, panic, anxiety
- stomach pain, flutters
- nausea
- cold, clammy hands
- poor concentration
- pacing
- restlessness
- rapid heart rate
- low-grade infection
- loss of sex drive
- rash or acne

Try It

If you regularly experience some of the above symptoms, use your Online Journal or class notebook to keep a log of when these symptoms occur and under what circumstances. You may find out that a pattern emerges when experiencing distress in life.

can be managed through time management and relaxation techniques.

Time Management

According to Benjamin Franklin, "Time is the stuff life is made of." The current "hurry-up" style of life is not conducive to wellness. The hassles involved in getting through a typical day often lead to stress-related illnesses. People who do not manage their time properly may experience chronic stress, fatigue, despair, discouragement, and illness.

Based on various national surveys, almost 80 percent of Americans report that time moves too fast for them and more than 50 percent think they have to get everything done. The younger the respondents, the more they struggled with lack of time. Almost half wished they had more time for exercise and recreation, hobbies, and family.

Healthy and successful people are good time managers, able to maintain a pace of life within their comfort zone. In a survey of 1954 Harvard graduates from the school of business, only 27 percent had reached the goals they'd established in

college. All had rated themselves as superior time managers, and only 8 percent of the remaining graduates perceived themselves as superior time managers. The successful graduates attributed their success to "smart work," not necessarily "hard work."

Trying to achieve one or more goals in a limited time can create a tremendous amount of stress. Many people just don't seem to have enough hours in the day to accomplish their tasks. The greatest demands on our time, nonetheless, frequently are self-imposed—trying to do too much, too fast, too soon.

Although some time killers, such as eating, sleeping, and recreation, are necessary for health and wellness, in excess they will cause stress. To make better use of your time:

1. Find the time killers. Many people do not know how they spend each part of the day. Keep a 4- to 7-day log, and record your activities at half-hour intervals. As you go through your typical day, record the activities so you will remember all of them. At the end of each day, decide when you wasted time. You might be shocked by the amount of time you spent on the phone, sleeping (more than eight hours per night), or watching television.

2. Set long-range and short-range goals. Setting goals requires some in-depth thinking and helps put your life and daily tasks in perspective. Write down three goals that you want to accomplish: (a) in life, (b) 10 years from now, (c) this year, (d) this month, and (e) this week. You may want to file this form and review it in years to come.

3. Identify your immediate goals and prioritize them for today and this week. Each day, sit down and determine what you need to accomplish that day and that week. Rank your "today" and "this week" tasks in three categories: (a) top priority, (b) medium priority, and (c) trash. Top-priority tasks are clearly the most important ones. If you were to reap most of your productivity from 30 percent of your activities, which would they be? Medium-priority activities must be done but can wait a day or two. Trash activities are those that are not worth your time (for example, cruising the hallways).

4. Use a daily planner to help you organize and simplify your day. In this way you can access your priority list, appointments, notes, references, names, places, phone numbers, and addresses conveniently from your coat pocket or purse. Many individuals think that planning daily and weekly activities is a waste of time. A few minutes to schedule your time each day, however, will pay off in hours saved.

5. As you plan your day, be realistic and find your comfort zone. Determine what is the best way to organize your day. Which is the most productive time for work, study, errands? Are you a morning person, or are you getting most of your work done when other people are quitting for the day? Pick your best hours for top-priority activities. Be sure to schedule enough time for exercise and relaxation. Recreation is not necessarily wasted time. You need to take care of your physical and emotional well-being. Otherwise your life will be seriously imbalanced.

6. Take 10 minutes each night to figure out how well you accomplished your goals that day. Successful time managers evaluate themselves daily. This simple task will help you see the entire picture. Cross off the goals you accomplished, and carry over to the next day those you did not get done. You also may realize that some goals can be moved down to low priority or be trashed.

In addition to the above steps, the following general suggestions can help you make better use of your time:

- *Delegate.* When possible, delegate activities that someone else can do for you. Having another person type your paper while you prepare for an exam might be well worth the expense and your time.
- *Say "no."* Learn to say no to activities that keep you from getting your top priorities done. You

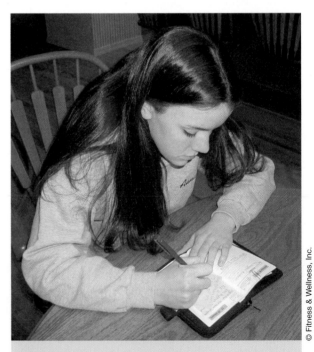

Planning and prioritizing your daily activities simplifies your days.

© Fitness & Wellness, Inc.

Common Time Killers

- watching television
- listening to radio/music
- sleeping
- eating
- daydreaming
- shopping
- socializing/parties
- recreation
- talking on the telephone
- worrying
- procrastinating
- drop-in visitors
- confusion (unclear goals)
- indecision (what to do next)
- interruptions
- perfectionism (every detail must be done)

in a park might distract you and become time killers.

- *Set aside "overtimes."* Regularly schedule time you did not think you would need as overtime to complete unfinished projects. Most people underschedule rather than overschedule time. The result is usually late-night burnout! If you schedule overtimes and get your tasks done, enjoy some leisure time, get ahead on another project, or work on some of your trash priorities. Plan time for *you.*
- *Set aside special time for yourself daily.* Life is not meant to be all work. Use your time to walk, read, or listen to your favorite music.
- *Reward yourself.* As with any other healthy behavior, positive change or a job well done deserves a reward. We often overlook the value of rewards, even if they are self-given. People practice behaviors that are rewarded and discontinue those that are not.

Relaxation Techniques

Stress management skills are essential to cope effectively and move forward in today's fast-paced world. Although you may reap benefits immediately after engaging in any of the several relaxation techniques described in this chapter, several months of regular practice may be necessary for total mastery. The relaxation exercises that follow should not be considered cure-alls or panaceas. If they do not prove to be effective, more specialized resources and professional help are indicated. In some instances a person's symptoms may not be caused by stress but, rather, may be related to an undiagnosed medical disorder.

Physical Activity

Physical exercise is one of the simplest tools to control stress. Exercise and fitness are thought to reduce the intensity of stress and recovery from a stressful event. The value of exercise in reducing stress is related to several factors, the main one being less muscular tension.

Imagine you are distressed after a miserable day at work. The job requires eight hours of work with an intolerable boss. To make matters worse, it is late, and on the way home the car in front of you is going much slower than the speed limit. The body's fight-or-flight mechanism is activated. Your heart rate and blood pressure shoot up, your breathing quickens

can do only so much in a single day. Nobody has enough time to do everything he or she would like to get done. Don't overload either. Many people are afraid to say no because they feel guilty if they do. Think ahead, and think of the consequences. Are you doing it to please others? What will it do to your well-being? Can you handle one more task? At some point you have to balance your activities and look at life and time realistically.

- *Protect against boredom.* Doing nothing can be a source of stress. People need to feel that they are contributing and that they are productive members of society. It also is good for self-esteem and self-worth. Set realistic goals, and work toward them each day.
- *Plan ahead for disruptions.* Even a careful plan of action can be disrupted. An unexpected phone call or visitor can ruin your schedule. Planning your response ahead of time will help you deal with these saboteurs.
- *Get it done.* Select only one task at a time, concentrate on it, and see it through. Many people do a little here, a little there, then do something else. In the end, nothing gets done. An exception to working on just one task at a time is when you are doing a difficult task. Rather than "killing yourself," interchange with another activity that is not as hard.
- *Eliminate distractions.* If you have trouble adhering to a set plan, remove distractions and trash activities from your eyesight. Television, radio, computers, magazines, open doors, or studying

and deepens, your muscles tense, and all systems say "go." Under the circumstances, you can take no action, and the stress will not be dissipated because you simply cannot hit your boss or the car in front of you. Instead, you could take action by "hitting" the tennis ball, the weights, the swimming pool, or the jogging trail. By engaging in physical activity, you are able to reduce the muscular tension and eliminate the physiological changes that triggered the fight-or-flight mechanism.

Physical exercise gives people an overall boost by:

- Lessening feelings of anxiety, depression, frustration, aggression, anger, and hostility
- Alleviating insomnia
- Providing an opportunity to meet social needs and develop new friendships
- Allowing people to share common interests and problems
- Developing self-discipline
- Providing the opportunity to do something enjoyable and constructive that will lead to better health and total well-being

Although exercise has enhanced the health and quality of life of millions of people, exercise, for a few, can become an obsessive behavior with potentially addictive qualities. Compulsive exercisers often express feelings of guilt and discomfort when they miss a day's workout. These individuals sometimes continue to exercise even when they are injured or ill and should get proper rest for adequate recovery. Under these circumstances, exercise becomes a biological stressor that will compromise performance and health. As a biological stressor, compulsive exercise or overtraining produces both physiological and psychological symptoms. Many physical activities (for example, jogging, basketball, aerobics) performed at high intensity levels or for unusually long periods (overtraining) can be detrimental to a person's physical and emotional well-being.

Psychological symptoms of overtraining include lower motivation, depression, sleep disturbances, increased irritability, and lack of confidence. Physiological symptoms include musculoskeletal injuries, lower performance, slower recovery time, chronic fatigue, decreased appetite, loss of weight and lean tissue, fat gain, increased muscle tension, higher resting heart rate and blood pressure, and even ECG abnormalities. If you experience any of these symptoms, you need to reevaluate your exercise program and make adjustments accordingly. People

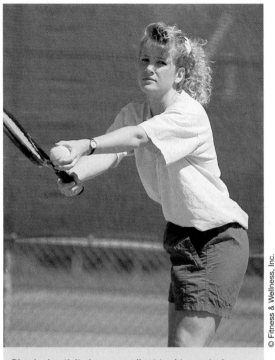

Physical activity is an excellent tool to control stress.

© Fitness & Wellness, Inc.

who exceed the recommended guidelines for fitness development and maintenance (see Chapters 3 and 4) are exercising for reasons other than health, and some actually may be aggravating an already stressful situation.

Progressive Muscle Relaxation

One of the most popular methods used to dissipate stress is **progressive muscle relaxation,** which enables individuals to relearn the sensation of deep relaxation. Acute awareness of how it feels to progressively tighten and relax the muscles releases muscle tension and teaches the body to relax at will. Feeling the tension during the exercises also helps the person to be more alert to signs of distress because this tension is similar to that experienced in stressful situations. In everyday life, these feelings then can cue the person to do relaxation exercises.

Relaxation exercises should be done in a quiet, warm, well-ventilated room. The exercises should encompass all muscle groups of the body. Most important is to pay attention to the sensation you feel each time you tense and relax your muscles.

The instructions can be read to the person, or memorized, or tape-recorded. You should set aside at least 20 minutes to complete the entire sequence.

Doing the exercises any faster will defeat their purpose. Ideally, you should complete the sequence twice a day.

First, stretch out comfortably on the floor, face up, with a pillow under your knees, and assume a passive attitude, allowing your body to relax as much as possible. Then contract each muscle group in sequence, taking care to avoid any strain. Tighten each muscle to only about 70 percent of the total possible tension to avoid cramping or some type of injury to the muscle itself.

To produce the relaxation effects, pay attention to the sensation of tensing and relaxing. Hold each contraction about 5 seconds, then allow the muscles to go totally limp. Take enough time to contract and relax each muscle group before going on to the next. An example of a complete progressive muscle relaxation sequence is as follows:

1. Point your feet, curling your toes downward. Study the tension in the arches and tops of your feet. Hold, and continue to note the tension, then relax. Repeat once again.
2. Flex the feet upward toward your face, and note the tension in your feet and calves. Hold, and relax. Repeat once more.
3. Push your heels down against the floor as if burying them in the sand. Hold, and note the tension at the back of the thigh. Relax. Repeat once more.
4. Contract your right thigh by straightening your leg, gently raising your leg off the floor. Hold, and study the tension. Relax. Repeat with the left leg. Hold and relax. Repeat each leg again.
5. Tense your buttocks by raising your hips ever so slightly off the floor. Hold, and note the tension. Relax. Repeat once again.
6. Contract your abdominal muscles. Hold them tight and note the tension. Relax. Repeat one more time.
7. Suck in your stomach. Try to make it reach your spine. Flatten your lower back to the floor. Hold, and feel the tension in the stomach and lower back. Relax. Repeat once more.
8. Take a deep breath and hold it, then exhale. Repeat. Note your breathing becoming slower and more relaxed.
9. Place your arms at the side of your body and clench both fists. Hold, study the tension, and relax. Repeat a second time.
10. Flex the elbow by bringing both hands to your shoulders. Hold tight and study the tension in the biceps. Relax. Repeat one more time.
11. Place your arms flat on the floor, palms up, and push the forearms hard against the floor. Note the tension on the triceps. Hold, and relax. Repeat once more.
12. Shrug your shoulders, raising them as high as possible. Hold, and note the tension. Relax. Repeat once again.

BEHAVIOR MODIFICATION PLANNING

Characteristics of Good Stress Managers

Good stress managers
- are physically active, eat a healthy diet, and get adequate rest every day.
- believe they have control over events in their life (have an internal locus of control, see pages 16–18).
- understand their own feelings and accept their limitations.
- recognize, anticipate, monitor, and regulate stressors within their capabilities.
- control emotional and physical responses when distressed.
- use appropriate stress management techniques when confronted with stressors.
- recognize warning signs and symptoms of excessive stress.
- schedule daily time to unwind, relax, and evaluate the day's activities.
- control stress when called upon to perform.
- enjoy life despite occasional disappointments and frustrations.
- look success and failure squarely in the face and keep moving along a predetermined course.
- move ahead with optimism and energy and do not spend time and talent worrying about failure.
- learn from previous mistakes and use them as building blocks to prevent similar setbacks in the future.
- give of themselves freely to others.
- find deep meaning in life.

Try It
Change for many people is threatening, but often required. Pick three of the above strategies and apply them in your life. After several days, determine the usefulness of these strategies in your physical, mental, social, and emotional well-being.

KEY TERMS

Progressive muscle relaxation A relaxation technique that involves contracting, then relaxing muscle groups in the body in succession.

13. Gently push your head backward. Note the tension in the back of the neck. Hold, then relax. Repeat one more time.

14. Gently bring the head against the chest, push forward, hold, and note the tension in the neck. Relax. Repeat a second time.

15. Press your tongue toward the roof of your mouth. Hold, study the tension, and relax. Repeat once more.

16. Press your teeth together. Hold, and study the tension. Relax. Repeat one more time.

17. Close your eyes tightly. Hold them closed and note the tension. Relax, leaving your eyes closed. Do this one more time.

18. Wrinkle your forehead and note the tension. Hold, and relax. Repeat one more time.

When time is a factor during the daily routine and you are not able to go through the entire sequence, you may do only the exercises specific to the area that feels most tense. Performing a partial sequence is better than not doing the exercises at all. Completing the entire sequence, of course, yields the best results.

Breathing Techniques

Breathing exercises, too, can be an antidote to stress. These exercises have been used for centuries in Asian countries to improve mental, physical, and emotional stamina. In breathing exercises, the person concentrates on "breathing away" the tension and inhaling fresh air to the entire body. Breathing exercises can be learned in only a few minutes and require considerably less time than the progressive muscle relaxation exercises.

As with any other relaxation technique, these exercises should be done in a quiet, pleasant, well-ventilated room. Any of the three examples of breathing exercises presented here will help relieve tension induced by stress.

Deep Breathing

Lie with your back flat against the floor, and place a pillow under your knees, feet slightly separated, with your toes pointing outward. (This exercise also may be done while sitting up in a chair or standing straight up.) Place one hand on your abdomen and the other hand on your chest. Breathe in and out slowly so the hand on your abdomen rises when you inhale and falls as you exhale. The hand on your chest should not move much at all. Repeat the exercise about 10 times. Then scan your body for ten-

sion, and compare your present tension with the tension you felt at the beginning of the exercise. Repeat the entire process once or twice more.

Sighing

Using the abdominal breathing technique, breathe in through your nose to a specific count (such as 4, 5, or 6). Now exhale through pursed lips to double the intake count (such as 8, 10, or 12). Repeat the exercise 8 to 10 times whenever you feel tense.

Complete Natural Breathing

Sit in an upright position or stand straight up. Breathing through your nose, fill your lungs gradually from the bottom up. Hold your breath for several seconds. Now exhale slowly by allowing your chest and abdomen to relax completely. Repeat the exercise 8 to 10 times.

Meditation

Hundreds of scientific studies have verified that **meditation** induces relaxation and alleviates the harmful physiological effects of stress. Meditation is a mental exercise that can bring about psychological and physical benefits. Regular meditation has been shown to decrease blood pressure, stress, anger, anxiety, fear, negative feelings, and chronic pain and to increase activity in the brain's left frontal region—an area associated with positive emotions.[5] The objective of meditation is to gain control over one's attention by clearing the mind and blocking out the stressor(s) responsible for the higher tension.

This technique can be learned rather quickly and can be used frequently during times of increased stress. Initially, choose a room that is comfortable, quiet, and free of all disturbances (including telephones). After learning the technique, you will be able to meditate just about anywhere. A time block of approximately 15 minutes, twice a day, is suggested for meditation.

1. Sit in a chair or in a quiet place in an upright position with your hands resting either in your lap or on the arms of the chair. Close your eyes and focus on your breathing. Allow your body to relax as much as possible. Do not consciously try to relax, because trying means work. Rather, assume a passive attitude and concentrate on your breathing.

2. Allow your body to breathe regularly, at its own rhythm, and repeat in your mind the word

"one" every time you inhale, and the word "two" every time you exhale. Paying attention to these two words keeps distressing thoughts from entering into your mind.

3. Continue to breathe in this way about 15 minutes. Because the objective of meditation is to bring about a hypometabolic (slower metabolism) state leading to body relaxation, do not use an alarm clock to remind you that the 15 minutes have expired. The alarm will only trigger the stress response again, defeating the purpose of the exercise. Opening your eyes once in a while to keep track of the time is fine, but do not rush or anticipate the end of the 15 minutes. This time has been set aside for meditation, and you need to relax, take your time, and enjoy the exercise.

CRITICAL THINKING

List the most significant stressor that you face as a college student. • What technique(s) have you used to manage this situation, and in what way has it helped you cope?

Yoga

Yoga is an excellent stress-coping technique. **Yoga** is a school of thought in the Hindu religion that seeks to help the individual attain a higher level of spirituality and peace of mind. Although its philosophical roots can be considered spiritual, yoga is based on principles of self-care.

Yoga practitioners adhere to a specific code of ethics and a system of mental and physical exercises that promote control of the mind and the body. In Western countries, many people are mainly familiar with the exercise portion of yoga. This system of exercises (postures) can be used as a relaxation technique for stress management. The exercises include a combination of postures, diaphragmatic breathing, muscle relaxation, and meditation that help buffer the biological effects of stress.

Western interest in yoga exercises gradually developed over the last century, particularly since the 1970s. People pursue yoga exercises for their potential to dispel stress by raising self-esteem, clearing the mind, slowing respiration, promoting neuromuscular relaxation, and increasing body awareness. In addition, the exercises help control involuntary body functions, including heart rate, blood pressure, oxygen consumption, and metabolic rate.

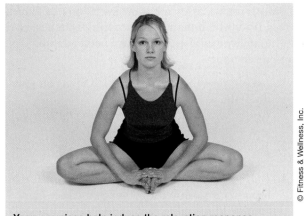

Yoga exercises help induce the relaxation response.

© Fitness & Wellness, Inc.

Doing yoga exercises can increase muscular flexibility, muscular strength and endurance, balance, and a better aligned musculoskeletal system.[6] Yoga is also used in many hospital-based programs for cardiac patients to help manage stress and decrease blood pressure.

Further, yoga exercises have been used to help treat chemical dependency and insomnia and to prevent injury. Research on patients with coronary heart disease who practiced yoga (among other lifestyle changes) has shown that it slows or even reverses atherosclerosis.[7] These patients were compared with others who did not use yoga as one of the lifestyle changes.

There are many different styles of yoga. Classes vary according to their emphasis. Some styles of yoga are athletic, and others are passive in nature. The most popular variety in the Western world is **hatha yoga,** which incorporates a series of static-stretching postures performed in specific sequences (also known as "asanas") that help induce the relaxation response. Participants hold the postures for several seconds while concentrating on breathing patterns, meditation, and body awareness.

KEY TERMS

Meditation A mental exercise in which the objective is to gain control over one's attention, clearing the mind and blocking out stressors.

Yoga A school of thought in the Hindu religion that seeks to help the individual attain a higher level of spirituality and peace of mind.

Hatha yoga A yoga style that incorporates a series of static-stretching postures performed in specific sequences.

Most yoga classes are now variations of hatha yoga, from which many of the typical stretches used in flexibility exercises today have been adapted. Examples include:

1. *Integral yoga* and *viny yoga,* which focus on gentle/static stretches
2. *Iyengar yoga,* which promotes muscular strength and endurance
3. *Yogalates,* incorporating Pilates exercises to increase muscular strength
4. *Power yoga* or *yogarobics,* a high-energy form that links many postures together in a dance-like routine to promote cardiorespiratory fitness.

As with flexibility exercises, the stretches in hatha yoga should not be performed to the point of discomfort. Instructors should not push participants beyond their physical limitations. Similar to other stress management techniques, yoga exercises are best performed in a quiet place for about 15 to 60 minutes per session. Many yoga participants like to perform the exercises daily.

To appreciate yoga exercise, a person has to experience it. We are only introducing yoga here. Although participants can practice yoga exercises with the instruction of a book or video, most participants take classes. Many of the postures are difficult and complex, and few individuals can master the entire sequence in the first few weeks.

Individuals who are interested in yoga exercise should initially pursue it under qualified instruction. Many universities offer yoga courses, and you also can check the phone book for a listing of yoga instructors or classes. Yoga courses are offered at many health clubs and recreation centers. Because instructors and yoga styles vary, you may want to observe a class before enrolling. You should look for an instructor whose views on wellness parallel your own. There are no national certification standards for instructors. If you are new to yoga, you are encouraged to compare a couple of instructors before you select a class.

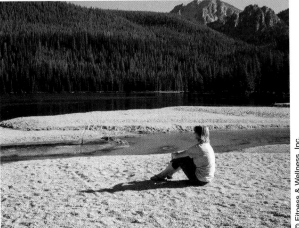

Visual imagery is an effective technique for coping with stress.

Visual Imagery

Visual or mental **imagery** has been used as a healing technique for centuries in various cultures around the world. In Western medicine, the practice of imagery is relatively new and not widely accepted among health care professionals. Imagery induces a state of relaxation that rids the body of the stress that leads to illness. It improves circulation and increases the delivery of healing antibodies and white blood cells to the site of illness.[8]

Visual imagery involves the creation of relaxing visual images and scenes in times of stress to elicit body and mind relaxation. Imagery works by offsetting the stressor with the visualization of relaxing scenes such as a sunny beach, a beautiful meadow, a quiet mountaintop, or some other peaceful setting. If you are ill, you can also visualize your white blood cells attacking an infection or a tumor. Imagery is also used in conjunction with breathing exercises, meditation, and yoga.

As with other stress management techniques, imagery should be performed in a quiet and comfortable environment. You can either sit or lie down for the exercise. If you lie down, use a soft surface and place a pillow under your knees. Be sure that your clothes are loose and that you are as comfortable as you can be.

Close your eyes and visualize one of your favorite scenes in nature. Place yourself into the scene and visualize yourself moving about and experiencing nature to its fullest. Enjoy the people, the animals, the colors, the sounds, the smells, and even the tem-

---

KEY TERMS

Imagery Mental visualization of relaxing images and scenes to induce body relaxation in times of stress or as an aid in the treatment of certain medical conditions, such as cancer, hypertension, asthma, chronic pain, and obesity.

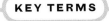

perature in your scene. After 10 to 20 minutes of visualization, open your eyes and compare the tension in your body and mind at this point with how you felt prior to the exercise. You can repeat this exercise as often as you deem necessary when you are feeling tension or stress.

Which Technique Is Best?

Each person reacts to stress differently. Therefore, the best strategy to alleviate stress depends mostly on the individual. Which technique you use does not matter as long as it works. You may want to experiment with all of them to find out which works best for you. Many people choose a combination of two or more.

All of the strategies discussed in this chapter help to block out stressors and promote mental and physical relaxation by diverting the attention to a different, nonthreatening action. Some of the techniques are easier to learn and take less time per session. Regardless of which technique you select, the time you spend doing stress management exercises (several times a day, as needed) is well worth the effort when stress becomes a significant problem in your life.

People need to learn to relax and take time for themselves. What makes people ill is not stress itself but, instead, the way they react to the stress-causing agent. Individuals who are diligent and start taking control of themselves find that they can enjoy a better, happier, and healthier life.

w w w WEB INTERACTIVE

Stress Assess. This is a three-part online educational tool developed by the National Wellness Institute at the University of Wisconsin–Stevens Point. This questionnaire is designed to increase your knowledge about stress and features separate evaluations for stress sources, distress symptoms, and stress-balancing strategies. Based on these results, you will learn healthy strategies to better manage your specific stressors.
http://wellness.uwsp.edu/Other/stress/

Are You Under Stress? Take the Discovery Health stress questionnaire to find out your level. The site offers 17 tips for dealing with stress and online stress resources.
http://health.discovery.com/centers/stress/ stress.html

ASSESS YOUR BEHAVIOR

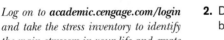

Log on to academic.cengage.com/login and take the stress inventory to identify the main stressors in your life and create a plan for dealing more effectively with them.

1. Are you able to channel your emotions and feelings to exert a positive effect on your mind, health, and wellness?

2. Do you use time management strategies on a regular basis?

3. Do you use stress management techniques, and do they allow you to be in control over the daily stresses of life?

*Log on to **academic.cengage.com/login** to assess your understanding of this chapter's topics by taking the chapter pre-test and exploring the modules recommended in your Personalized Study Plan.*

1. Positive stress is also referred to as
   a. eustress.
   b. poststress.
   c. functional stress.
   d. distress.
   e. physiostress.

2. Which of the following is *not* a stage of the general adaptation syndrome?
   a. Alarm reaction
   b. Resistance
   c. Compliance
   d. Exhaustion/recovery
   e. All are stages of the general adaptation syndrome.

3. Which of the following behaviors seems to have the greatest impact in increasing the risk for illness among Type A individuals?
   a. Hard-driven
   b. Overly ambitious
   c. Chronic hostility
   d. Overly competitive
   e. All increase the risk equally.

4. Effective time managers
   a. delegate.
   b. learn to say "no."
   c. protect against boredom.
   d. set aside "overtimes."
   e. do all of the above.

5. Hormonal changes that occur during a stress response
   a. decrease heart rate.
   b. increase blood pressure.
   c. diminish blood flow to the muscles.
   d. induce relaxation.
   e. sap the body's strength.

6. Exercise decreases stress levels by
   a. deliberately diverting stress to various body systems.
   b. metabolizing excess catecholamines.
   c. diminishing muscular tension.
   d. stimulating alpha-wave activity in the brain.
   e. doing all of the above.

7. Which of the following exercises is/are included in the progressive muscle relaxation technique?
   a. Pointing the feet
   b. Wrinkling the forehead
   c. Contracting the abdominal muscles
   d. Pressing the teeth together
   e. All of the above exercises are used.

8. The technique in which a person breathes in through the nose to a specific count and then exhales through pursed lips to double the intake count is known as
   a. sighing.
   b. deep breathing.
   c. meditation.
   d. autonomic ventilation.
   e. release management.

9. Meditation
   a. induces relaxation.
   b. alleviates the harmful physiologic effects of stress.
   c. can be performed just about anywhere.
   d. incorporates breathing exercises.
   e. includes all of the above.

10. Yoga exercises have been used successfully to
   a. stimulate ventilation.
   b. increase metabolism during stress.
   c. slow down atherosclerosis.
   d. decrease body awareness.
   e. accomplish all of the above.

Correct answers can be found at the back of the book.

A Healthy Lifestyle Approach

© Bloomimage/Corbis

OBJECTIVES

- Understand the importance of implementing a healthy lifestyle program
- Recognize the relationship between spirituality and wellness
- Identify the major risk factors for coronary heart disease

- Be able to differentiate physiological age and chronological age
- Become acquainted with cancer-prevention guidelines
- Learn the health consequences of chemical abuse and irresponsible sex

CENGAGENOW Log on to **CengageNOW** at academic
.cengage.com/login to find innovative
study tools—including pre- and post-tests,
personalized study plans, activities, labs, and the personal change planner.

Improving our health—the quality, and most likely the length, of our lives—is a matter of personal choice. The wellness approach—the combination of a fitness program and a healthy lifestyle program—can help accomplish these goals.

A Wellness Lifestyle

Wellness is the constant and deliberate effort to stay healthy and achieve the highest potential for well-being. Ten simple lifestyle habits can increase longevity significantly:

1. Be physically active (including exercise).
2. Do not use tobacco.
3. Eat a healthy diet.
4. Avoid snacking between meals.
5. Maintain recommended body weight.
6. Sleep 7 to 8 hours each night.
7. Decrease stress levels.
8. Drink alcohol moderately or not at all.
9. Surround yourself with healthy relationships.
10. Be informed about the environment and avoid environmental risk factors.
11. Increase education (more-educated people live longer).
12. Take personal safety measures.

Spiritual Well-Being

To enjoy a wellness lifestyle, a person has to practice behaviors that will lead to positive outcomes in the seven dimensions of wellness: physical, emotional, intellectual, social, environmental, occupational, and spiritual. These dimensions are interrelated; one dimension frequently affects the others. For example, a person who is emotionally down often has no desire to exercise, study, socialize with friends, or attend church and may be more susceptible to illness and disease. Because spirituality plays an important role and has not been discussed thus far, it merits some attention.

The definition of **spirituality** by the National Interfaith Coalition on Aging encompasses Christians and non-Christians alike. It assumes that all people are spiritual in nature. Spiritual health provides a unifying power that integrates the other dimensions of wellness (see Figure 8.1). Basic characteristics of spiritual people include a sense of meaning and direction in life, a relationship to a higher being, freedom, prayer, faith, love, closeness to others, peace, joy, fulfillment, and altruism.

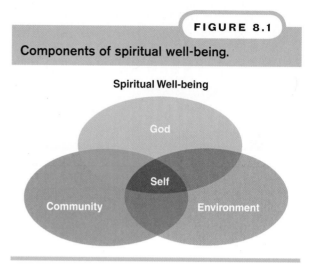

FIGURE 8.1

Components of spiritual well-being.

Religion has been a major part of cultures since the beginning of time. Although not everyone claims an affiliation with a certain religion or denomination, various surveys indicate that more than 90 percent of the U.S. population believes in God or a universal spirit functioning as God. People, furthermore, believe to a varying extent that (a) a relationship with God is meaningful; (b) God can grant help, guidance, and assistance in daily living; and (c) mortal existence has a purpose. If we accept any or all of these statements, attaining spirituality will have a definite effect on our happiness and well-being. Although the reasons why religious affiliation enhances wellness are difficult to determine, possible reasons include the promotion of healthy lifestyle behaviors, social support, assistance in times of crisis and need, and counseling to overcome one's weaknesses.

Altruism—a key attribute of spiritual people—seems to enhance health and longevity. Altruism has been the focus of several studies. Researchers believe that doing good for others is good for oneself, especially for the immune system. In a classic study of more than 2,700 people in Michigan,[1] the investigators found that people who did regular volunteer work lived longer. People who did not volunteer regularly (at least once a week) had a 250 percent greater mortality risk during the course of the study. In this same study, the authors found that the health benefits of altruism could be so powerful that even just watching films of altruistic endeavors enhances the formation of an immune system chemical that helps fight disease.

The relationship between spirituality and wellness, therefore, is meaningful in our quest for a better quality of life. As with other parameters of wellness, optimum spirituality requires development of the spiritual nature to its fullest potential.

Causes of Death

Of all deaths in the United States, approximately 59 percent are caused by cardiovascular disease and cancer.[2] Close to 80 percent of these deaths could be prevented by following a healthy lifestyle. The third and fourth leading causes of death—chronic lower respiratory disease (CLRD) and accidents—also are preventable, primarily by abstaining from tobacco and other drugs, wearing seat belts, and using common sense. Eight of the nine underlying causes of death in the United States (see Figure 8.2) are related to lifestyle and lack of common sense. The "big three"—tobacco use, poor diet and inactivity, and alcohol abuse—are responsible for more than 632,000 deaths annually.

Diseases of the Cardiovascular System

The most prevalent degenerative conditions in the United States are **cardiovascular diseases.** Based on 2004 vital statistics, almost 36 percent of

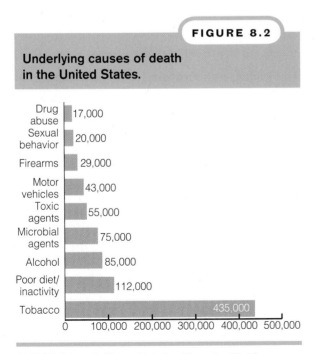

FIGURE 8.2

Underlying causes of death in the United States.

- Drug abuse — 17,000
- Sexual behavior — 20,000
- Firearms — 29,000
- Motor vehicles — 43,000
- Toxic agents — 55,000
- Microbial agents — 75,000
- Alcohol — 85,000
- Poor diet/inactivity — 112,000
- Tobacco — 435,000

(0 100,000 200,000 300,000 400,000 500,000)

SOURCE: Centers for Disease Control and Prevention, Atlanta.

TABLE 8.1

Estimated Prevalence and Yearly Number of Deaths from Cardiovascular Disease

	Prevalence	Deaths
All forms of cardiovascular diseases*	79,400,000	871,500
Coronary heart disease	15,800,000	**
Heart attack	7,900,000	452,300
Stroke	5,700,000	150,100
High blood pressure	72,000,000	54,200***

*Includes people with one or more forms of cardiovascular disease.

**Number of deaths included under heart attack.

***Mortality figures appear to be low because many heart attacks and stroke deaths are caused by high blood pressure.

SOURCE: American Heart Association, *Heart Disease and Stroke Statistics–2007: Update At-a-Glance* (Dallas: AHA).

all deaths in the United States were attributable to diseases of the heart and blood vessels.[3] More than 850,000 people die of cardiovascular diseases in the United States each year.

Types of Cardiovascular Disease and Their Prevalence

Examples of cardiovascular diseases are coronary heart disease, heart attack, peripheral vascular disease, congenital heart disease, rheumatic heart disease, atherosclerosis, strokes, high blood pressure, and congestive heart failure. According to estimates from the Centers for Disease Control and Prevention, if all deaths from the major cardiovascular diseases were eliminated, life expectancy in the United States would increase by about seven years. Table 8.1 provides the estimated prevalence and annual number of deaths caused by the major types of cardiovascular disease.

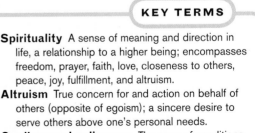

KEY TERMS

Spirituality A sense of meaning and direction in life, a relationship to a higher being; encompasses freedom, prayer, faith, love, closeness to others, peace, joy, fulfillment, and altruism.

Altruism True concern for and action on behalf of others (opposite of egoism); a sincere desire to serve others above one's personal needs.

Cardiovascular diseases The array of conditions that affect the heart and blood vessels.

The American Heart Association (AHA) estimated that the cost of heart and blood vessel disease in the United States exceeded $431.8 billion in 2007.[4] About 7.9 million people have heart attacks each year, and about a half a million of these people die as a result. More than half of these deaths occur within an hour of the onset of symptoms, before the person reaches the hospital.

Although heart and blood vessel disease is still the number-one health problem in the United States, the incidence declined by 28 percent between 1960 and 2000 (see Figure 8.3). The main reason for this dramatic decrease is health education. More people now are aware of the risk factors for cardiovascular disease and are changing their lifestyle to lower their potential risk for these diseases.

The heart and the coronary arteries are illustrated in Figure 8.4. The major form of cardiovascular disease is **coronary heart disease (CHD).** In CHD the arteries that supply the heart muscle with oxygen and nutrients are narrowed by fatty deposits such as cholesterol and triglycerides. Narrowing of the coronary arteries diminishes the blood supply to the heart muscle, which can precipitate a heart attack.

CHD is the single leading cause of death in the United States, accounting for approximately 20 percent of all deaths and about half of all cardiovascular deaths. More than half of the people who died suddenly from CHD had no previous symptoms of

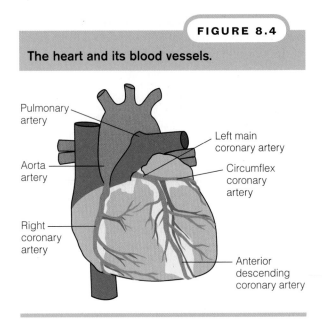

FIGURE 8.4

The heart and its blood vessels.

the disease. Further, the risk for death is greater in the least-educated segment of the population.

CRITICAL THINKING

What are your feelings about your own risk for diseases of the cardiovascular system? • Is this something that you need to concern yourself with at this point in your life? • Why or why not?

Risk Factors for CHD

The leading **risk factors** for the development of CHD are:

- Physical inactivity
- High blood pressure
- Excessive body fat
- Low HDL cholesterol
- Elevated LDL cholesterol
- Elevated triglycerides
- Elevated homocysteine
- Inflammation
- Diabetes
- Abnormal electrocardiograms
- Tobacco use
- Stress
- Personal and family history of cardiovascular disease
- Age
- Gender

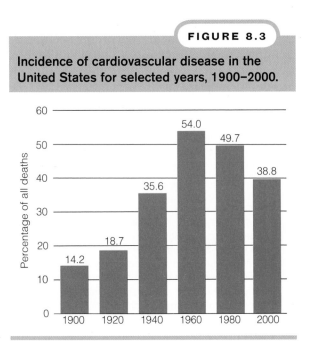

FIGURE 8.3

Incidence of cardiovascular disease in the United States for selected years, 1900–2000.

Warning Signals of a Heart Attack and Stroke

Any or all of the following signs may occur during a heart attack or a stroke. If you experience any of these and they last longer than a few minutes, call 911 and seek medical attention immediately. Failure to do so may cause irreparable damage and even result in death.

Warning Signs of a Heart Attack

Chest pain, discomfort, pressure, or squeezing that lasts for several minutes. These feelings may go away and return later.

Pain that radiates to the shoulders, neck, or arms.

Chest discomfort with shortness of breath, lightheadedness, sweating, nausea, or fainting.

Warning Signs of Stroke

Sudden weakness or numbness of the face, arm, or leg—particularly on one side of the body.

Sudden severe headache.

Sudden confusion, dizziness, or difficulty in speech and understanding.

Sudden difficulty walking, loss of balance or coordination.

Sudden visual difficulty.

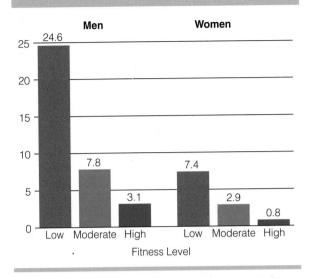

FIGURE 8.5

Relationship between fitness levels and cardiovascular mortality.

S. N. Blair, H. W. Kohl III, R. S. Paffenbarger, Jr., D. G. Clark, K. H. Cooper, and L. W. Gibbons, "Physical Fitness and All-Cause Mortality: A Prospective Study of Healthy Men and Women," *Journal of the American Medical Association* 262 (1989): 2395–2401.

An important concept in CHD risk management is that many of the risk factors are preventable and reversible. Approximately 90 percent of CHD can be prevented if people practice healthy lifestyle habits. The above risk factors are discussed in the following pages.

Physical Inactivity

Improving cardiorespiratory endurance through aerobic exercise has perhaps the greatest impact in reducing the overall risk for cardiovascular disease. In this day and age of mechanized societies, we cannot afford *not* to be physically active. Research data on the benefits of aerobic exercise in reducing cardiovascular disease are too impressive to be ignored.

Guidelines for implementing an aerobic exercise program are discussed thoroughly in Chapters 3 and 4. Following these guidelines will promote cardiorespiratory fitness, enhance health, and extend the lifespan. Even moderate amounts of aerobic exercise can reduce cardiovascular risk considerably. As shown in Figure 8.5, pioneer research conducted at the Aerobics Research Institute in Dallas showed a much higher incidence of cardiovascular deaths in low-fitness people compared with moderate- and high-fitness people.[5]

A regular aerobic exercise program helps to control most of the major risk factors that lead to heart and blood vessel disease. Aerobic exercise will:

- Increase cardiorespiratory endurance
- Decrease and control blood pressure
- Reduce body fat
- Lower blood lipids (cholesterol and triglycerides)
- Improve high-density lipoprotein cholesterol (see "Abnormal Cholesterol Profile" on page 199)
- Decrease low-grade (hidden) inflammation in the body
- Help control or decrease the risk for diabetes
- Increase and maintain good heart function, sometimes improving certain electrocardiographic abnormalities

KEY TERMS

Coronary heart disease (CHD) Condition in which the arteries that supply the heart muscle with oxygen and nutrients are narrowed by fatty deposits such as cholesterol and triglycerides.

Risk factors Lifestyle and genetic variables that may lead to disease.

- Encourage smoking cessation
- Alleviate stress
- Counteract a personal history of heart disease

High Blood Pressure (Hypertension)

Blood pressure should be checked regularly, regardless of whether it is elevated or not. **Blood pressure** is measured in milliliters of mercury (mm Hg) and usually expressed in two numbers. The higher number reflects the **systolic blood pressure,** the pressure exerted during the forceful contraction of the heart. The lower value, **diastolic blood pressure,** is taken during the heart's relaxation phase, when no blood is being ejected.

Ideally, blood pressure is 120/80 or below (see Table 8.2). Most major health organizations consider all blood pressures above 140/90 as **hypertension.** High blood pressure can be controlled with different types of medications, along with the lifestyle changes described below for people with mild hypertension. Because people respond differently to these medications, a physician may try several different medications to find out which produces the best results with the fewest side effects.

Recommended treatment for people with mild hypertension includes regular aerobic exercise, weight control, a low-salt/low-fat and high-potassium/high-calcium diet, lower alcohol and caffeine intake, smoking cessation, and stress management. People with high blood pressure should follow their physicians' advice and stay on any prescribed medication.

Adequate potassium intake seems to regulate water retention and lower blood pressure slightly. According to the Institute of Medicine of the National Academy of Sciences, we need to consume at least 4,700 mg of potassium per day. Most Americans get only half that amount. Food items high in potassium include vegetables (especially leafy green), citrus fruit, dairy products, fish, beans, and nuts.

In terms of salt (sodium) intake, a 2004 government report indicates that to either prevent or postpone the onset of hypertension, and to help some hypertensives control their blood pressure, we should consume less sodium than previously recommended.[6] Less than 1,500 mg of sodium is now recommended for people between 19 and 50 years of age. The current upper limit (UL) has been set at 2,300 mg per day. Among Americans and Canadians, about 95 percent of men and 75 percent of women exceed this limit.

Comprehensive reviews on the effects of aerobic exercise on blood pressure found that, in general, an individual can expect exercise-induced reductions of approximately 4 to 5 mm Hg in resting systolic blood pressure and 3 to 4 mm Hg in resting diastolic blood pressure.[7] Although these reductions do not seem large, a decrease of about 5 mm Hg in resting diastolic blood pressure has been associated with a 40 percent decrease in the risk for stroke and a 15 percent reduction in the risk for coronary heart disease.[8]

Even in the absence of any decrease in resting blood pressure, hypertensive individuals who exercise have a lower risk for all-cause mortality compared with hypertensive/sedentary individuals.[9] Exercise, not weight loss, is the major contributor to the lower blood pressure of exercisers. If the hypertensive/sedentary individuals discontinue aerobic exercise, they do not maintain these changes.

Aerobic exercise programs for hypertensive patients should be of moderate intensity. Training at 40 to 60 percent intensity seems to have the same effect in lowering blood pressure as training at 70 percent. High-intensity training (above 70 percent) in hypertensive patients may not lower the blood pressure as much as moderate-intensity exercise.

Another extensive review of research studies on the effects of at least four weeks of strength training on resting blood pressure yielded similar results.[10] Both systolic and diastolic blood pressures decreased by an average of 3 mm Hg. The participants in these studies, however, were primarily individuals with normal blood pressure. Of greater significance, the results showed that strength training did not cause an increase in resting blood pressure. More research remains to be done on hypertensive subjects.

Excessive Body Fat

As defined in Chapter 2, body composition refers to the fat and nonfat components of the human body. If a person has too much fat weight, he or she is overweight or obese. Obesity long has been recog-

TABLE 8.2

Blood Pressure Guidelines (expressed in mm Hg)

Rating	Systolic	Diastolic
Normal	≤120	≤80
Prehypertension	121–139	81–89
Hypertension	≥140	≥90

SOURCE: National Heart, Lung and Blood Institute.

nized as a factor contributing to coronary heart disease. The AHA lists obesity as one of the six major risk factors for this disease. The other five risk factors are tobacco smoke, high blood lipids, physical inactivity, high blood pressure, and diabetes mellitus.

Maintaining recommended body weight is essential in any cardiovascular risk-reduction program. For individuals with excessive body fat, even a modest weight reduction of 5 to 10 percent can reduce high blood pressure and total cholesterol levels.

The causes of obesity are complex, including an individual's combination of genetics, behavior, and lifestyle factors. Guidelines for a comprehensive weight management program are given in Chapter 6.

Abnormal Cholesterol Profile

The term **blood lipids** is used mainly with reference to cholesterol and triglycerides. Because these substances cannot float around freely in the water-based medium of the blood, they are packaged and transported in the blood by complex molecules called **lipoproteins.** If you have never had a blood lipid test, it is highly recommended. The blood test includes total **cholesterol, high-density lipoprotein (HDL)** cholesterol, **low-density lipoprotein (LDL)** cholesterol, and triglycerides. A significant elevation in blood lipids has been linked to heart and blood vessel disease.

A poor blood lipid profile is one of the most important predisposing factors in the development of CHD, accounting for almost half of all cases. The general recommendation by the National Cholesterol Education Program (NCEP) is to keep total cholesterol levels below 200 mg/dL (see Table 8.3). The risk for heart attack increases 2 percent for every 1 percent increase in total cholesterol.[11] Cholesterol levels between 200 and 239 mg/dL are borderline-high, and levels of 240 mg/dL and above indicate high risk for disease. Approximately 105 million American adults have total cholesterol values at or above 200 mg/dL.[12]

Although the average adult in the United States consumes between 400 and 600 mg of cholesterol daily, the body actually manufactures more than that. Saturated fats raise cholesterol levels more than anything else in the diet. The average saturated fat intake in the American diet produces approximately 1,000 mg of cholesterol per day.[13] Because of individual differences, some people can have a higher than normal intake of saturated fats and still maintain normal levels. Others, who have a lower intake, can have abnormally high levels.

TABLE 8.3

Standards for Blood Lipids

	Amount	Rating
Total Cholesterol	<200 mg/dL	Desirable
	200–239 mg/dL	Borderline high
	≥240 mg/dL	High risk
LDL Cholesterol	<100 mg/dL	Optimal
	100–129 mg/dL	Near or above optimal
	130–159 mg/dL	Borderline high
	160–189 mg/dL	High
	≥190 mg/dL	Very high
HDL Cholesterol	<40 mg/dL	Low (high risk)
	≥60 mg/dL	High (low risk)
Triglycerides	≤150 mg/dL	Desirable
	150–199 mg/dL	Borderline high
	200–499 mg/dL	High
	≥500 mg/dL	High risk

SOURCE: National Cholesterol Education Program.

As important as it is, total cholesterol is not the most accurate predictor of cardiovascular risk. Many heart attacks occur in people who have only slightly elevated total cholesterol. More significant is the

KEY TERMS

Blood pressure A measure of the force exerted against the walls of the vessels by the blood flowing through them.

Systolic blood pressure Pressure exerted by the blood against the walls of the arteries during the forceful contraction (systole) of the heart.

Diastolic blood pressure Pressure exerted by the blood against the walls of the arteries during the relaxation phase (diastole) of the heart.

Hypertension Chronically elevated blood pressure.

Blood lipids Cholesterol and triglycerides.

Lipoproteins Complex molecules that transport cholesterol in the bloodstream.

Cholesterol A waxy substance, technically a steroid alcohol, found only in animal fats and oil; used in making cell membranes, as a building block for some hormones, in the fatty sheath around nerve fibers, and in other necessary substances.

High-density lipoprotein (HDL) Cholesterol-transporting molecules in the blood (good cholesterol).

Low-density lipoprotein (LDL) Cholesterol-transporting molecules in the blood (bad cholesterol).

way in which cholesterol is carried in the bloodstream. Cholesterol is transported primarily in the form of HDL and LDL cholesterol.

In a process known as reverse cholesterol transport, HDLs act as scavengers, removing cholesterol from the body and preventing plaque from forming in the arteries. The strength of HDL is in the protein molecules found in their coatings. When HDL comes in contact with cholesterol-filled cells, these protein molecules attach to the cells and take their cholesterol. LDL cholesterol, on the other hand, tends to release cholesterol, which then may penetrate the lining of the arteries and speed up the process of **atherosclerosis.**

Saturated fats are found mostly in meats and dairy products and seldom in foods of plant origin. Poultry and fish contain less saturated fat than beef does but should be eaten in moderation (about 3 to 6 ounces per day). Unsaturated fats are mainly of plant origin and cannot be converted to cholesterol.

The NCEP guidelines provided in Table 8.3 state that an LDL cholesterol value below 100 mg/dL is optimal. Values above 160 mg/dL present high risk for cardiovascular disease. A genetic variation of LDL cholesterol, known as Lp(a), is noteworthy because a high level of these particles leads to earlier development of atherosclerosis. Certain substances in the arterial wall are thought to interact with Lp(a), leading to premature formation of plaque.

The more HDL cholesterol, the better. HDL cholesterol, the "good cholesterol," offers some protection against heart disease. Actually, low levels of HDL cholesterol could be the best predictor of CHD and may be more significant than the total cholesterol value. A low level of HDL cholesterol has the strongest relationship to CHD at all levels of total cholesterol, including levels below 200 mg/dL.

The recommended HDL cholesterol values to minimize the risk for CHD are a minimum of 40 mg/dL. HDL cholesterol levels above 60 mg/dL actually may reduce the risk for CHD. For the most part, HDL cholesterol is determined genetically. Generally, women have higher levels than men. The female sex hormone estrogen tends to raise HDL, so premenopausal women have a much lower incidence of heart disease. African American children and adult men have higher HDL values than whites. HDL cholesterol also decreases with age.

Increasing HDL Cholesterol. Increasing HDL cholesterol improves the cholesterol profile and lessens the risk for CHD. Habitual aerobic exercise,

weight loss, niacin, and quitting smoking help raise HDL cholesterol. Drug therapy also may promote higher HDL cholesterol levels.

There is a clear relation between HDL cholesterol and a regular vigorous aerobic exercise program (an intensity above 6 METs [metabolic equivalents], for at least 20 minutes three times per week—see Chapters 3 and 4). Individual responses to aerobic exercise differ, but generally, the more you exercise, the higher your HDL cholesterol level.

Lowering LDL Cholesterol. When more LDL cholesterol is present than the cells can use, cholesterol seems not to cause a problem until it is oxidized by **free radicals.** When oxidized, white blood cells invade the arterial wall, take up the cholesterol, and clog the arteries. If LDL cholesterol is higher than ideal, it can be lowered by losing body fat, manipulating the diet, taking medication, and participating in a regular aerobic exercise program.

The antioxidant effect of vitamins C and E can reduce the risk for CHD. A single unstable free radical (an oxygen compound produced during metabolism) can damage LDL particles. Vitamin C seems to inactivate free radicals and slow the oxidation of LDL cholesterol. Vitamin E may protect LDL from oxidation, preventing heart disease, but studies suggest that it does not seem to be helpful in reversing damage once it has taken place.[14]

To decrease LDL cholesterol, the diet should be low in saturated fat, cholesterol, and trans fatty acids. It should also be high in fiber. Saturated fat should be replaced by monounsaturated and polyunsaturated fats because the latter tend to decrease LDL cholesterol. Exercise is important, as dietary manipulation by itself is not as effective in lowering LDL cholesterol as a combination of diet plus aerobic exercise.

Foods that contain trans fatty acids, hydrogenated fat, or partially hydrogenated vegetable oil should be avoided. Studies indicate that these foods elevate cholesterol as much as saturated fats do. Hydrogen is frequently added to monounsaturated and polyunsaturated fats to increase shelf life and to solidify them so they are more spreadable. Margarine and spreads, commercially produced crackers and cookies, dairy products, meats, and fast foods often contain trans fatty acids. The labels "partially hydrogenated" and "trans fat" indicate that the product carries a health risk just as high as that of saturated fat.

In 2006, the AHA became the first major health organization to issue dietary guidelines for trans fat intake. In the 2006 revision of its *Diet and Lifestyle Recommendations,* the AHA limits trans fat intake to less than 1 percent of the total daily caloric intake.[15] This amount represents about 2 grams of trans fats a day for a 2,000 calorie diet or 1.5 grams for 1,500 calories and 3 grams for 3,000 calories. Because the U.S. Food and Drug Administration (FDA) now requires that all food labels list the trans fat content, you can keep better track of your daily trans fat intake by paying attention to food labels. Additional information on trans fats is found under the "Trans Fatty Acids" section in Chapter 5 (see page 123).

The FDA allows food manufacturers to label any product that has less than half a gram of trans fat per serving as zero. Be aware that if you eat three or four servings of a particular food near a half a gram of trans fat, you may be getting your maximum daily allowance (1 gram per 1,000 calories of daily caloric intake). Thus, you are encouraged to look at the list of ingredients and search for the words "partially hydrogenated" as an indicator of hidden trans fats.

Now that trans fats are listed on food labels, companies are looking to reformulate their products to reduce or eliminate these fats. Some products which once had a high trans fat content now have none. As a consumer, you are encouraged to check food labels often to obtain current information.

To have a significant effect in lowering LDL cholesterol, total daily fiber intake must be in the range of 25 to 38 grams per day (see the discussion of fiber in Chapter 5), and total fat consumption can be in the range of 30 percent of total daily caloric intake, as long as most of the fat is unsaturated fat and the average cholesterol consumption is lower than 200 mg per day.

The fiber intake of most people in the United States averages less than 15 grams per day. Fiber, in particular the soluble type, has been shown to lower cholesterol. Soluble fiber dissolves in water and forms a gel-like substance that encloses food particles. This property helps bind and excrete fats from the body. Soluble fibers are found primarily in oats, fruits, barley, legumes, and psyllium.

Psyllium, a grain that is added to some multigrain breakfast cereals, also helps lower LDL cholesterol. As little as 3 daily grams of psyllium can lower LDL cholesterol by 20 percent. Commercially available fiber supplements that contain psyllium (such as Metamucil) can be used to increase soluble fiber intake. Three daily tablespoons will add about 10 grams of soluble fiber to the diet.

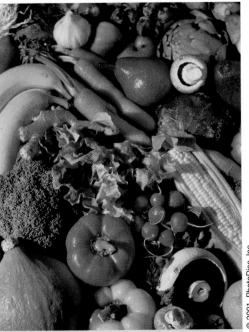

© 2001, PhotoDisc, Inc.

Phytonutrients found in abundance in fruits and vegetables seem to have a powerful effect in decreasing risk for cancer.

The incidence of heart disease is low in populations in which daily fiber intake exceeds 30 grams per day. Further, a 1996 Harvard University Medical School study on 43,000 middle-aged men who were followed for more than six years showed that increasing fiber intake to 30 daily grams resulted in a 41 percent reduction in heart attacks.[16]

Research on the effects of a 30 percent fat diet has shown that it has little or no effect in lowering cholesterol and that CHD actually continues to progress in people who have the disease. Thus, some practitioners recommend a 10 percent or less fat-calorie diet combined with aerobic exercise program while trying to lower cholesterol.

One drawback of very low fat (less than 25 percent) diets is that they tend to lower HDL cholesterol and increase triglycerides. If HDL cholesterol is

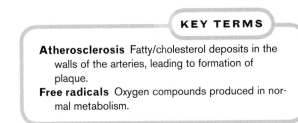

KEY TERMS

Atherosclerosis Fatty/cholesterol deposits in the walls of the arteries, leading to formation of plaque.
Free radicals Oxygen compounds produced in normal metabolism.

already low, monounsaturated and polyunsaturated fats should be added to the diet. Olive, canola, corn, soybean oils, and nuts are sample food items that are high in monounsaturated fats and polyunsaturated fats. A specialized nutrition book or online software can be consulted to determine food items that are high in monounsaturated and polyunsaturated fats.

Margarines and salad dressings now are available on the market that contain stanol ester, a plant derived compound that lowers cholesterol. Over time, about 3 grams of margarine or 6 tablespoons of salad dressing containing stanol ester lowers LDL cholesterol by 14 percent.

To lower LDL cholesterol levels, the following general dietary guidelines are recommended:

- Consume between 25 and 38 grams of fiber daily, including a minimum of 10 grams of soluble fiber (good sources are oats, fruits, barley, legumes, and psyllium).
- Increase consumption of vegetables, fruits, whole grains, and beans.
- Do not consume more than 200 mg of dietary cholesterol a day.
- Consume red meats (3 ounces per serving) fewer than three times per week and no organ meats (such as liver and kidneys).
- Do not eat commercially baked foods.
- Avoid foods that contain trans fats, hydrogenated fat, or partially hydrogenated vegetable oil.
- Increase intake of omega-3 fatty acids by eating two or three omega-3-rich fish meals per week.
- Consume 25 grams of soy protein a day.
- Drink low-fat milk (1 percent or less fat, preferably) and use low-fat dairy products.
- Do not use coconut oil, palm oil, or cocoa butter.
- Limit egg consumption to fewer than three eggs per week (this is for people with high cholesterol only; others may consume eggs in moderation).
- Use margarines and salad dressings that contain stanol ester instead of butter and regular margarine.
- Bake, broil, grill, poach, or steam food instead of frying.
- Refrigerate cooked meat before adding to other dishes. Remove fat hardened in the refrigerator before mixing the meat with other foods.
- Avoid fatty sauces made with butter, cream, or cheese.
- Maintain recommended body weight.

Elevated Triglycerides

Triglycerides, also known as free fatty acids, make up most of the fat in our diet and most of the fat that circulates in the blood. In combination with cholesterol, triglycerides speed up formation of plaque in the arteries. Triglycerides are carried in the bloodstream primarily by very low density lipoproteins (VLDLs) and **chylomicrons.**

Although these fatty acids are found in poultry skin, lunch meats, and shellfish, they are manufactured mainly in the liver from refined sugars, starches, and alcohol. High intake of alcohol and sugars (honey included) significantly raises triglyceride levels. The level can be lowered by cutting down on the previously mentioned foods along with pastries, candies, soft drinks, fruit juices, white bread, pasta, and alcohol. In addition, cutting down on overall fat consumption, quitting smoking, reducing weight (if overweight), and doing aerobic exercise are helpful. A desirable blood triglyceride level is less than 150 mg/dL (see Table 8.3).

Blood Lipid–Lowering Medications. Effective medications are available to treat elevated cholesterol and triglycerides. Most notable among them are the statins group (Lipitor, Mevacor, Pravachol, Lescol, and Zocor), which can lower cholesterol by up to 60 percent in two to three months. Statins slow down cholesterol production and increase the liver's ability to remove blood cholesterol. They also decrease triglycerides and produce a small increase in HDL levels.

Other drugs effective in reducing LDL cholesterol are bile acid sequestrants that bind cholesterol found in bile acids. Cholesterol subsequently is excreted in the stools. These drugs are often used in combination with statin drugs.

High doses (1.5 to 3 grams per day) of nicotinic acid or niacin (a B vitamin) also help lower LDL cholesterol and triglycerides and increase HDL cholesterol. (A fourth group of drugs, known as fibrates, is primarily used to lower triglycerides.)

It is better to lower LDL cholesterol without medication, because drugs can often cause undesirable side effects. People with heart disease often must take cholesterol-lowering medication, but it is best if medication is combined with lifestyle changes to augment the cholesterol-lowering effect.

Elevated Homocysteine

Clinical data indicating that many heart attack victims have normal cholesterol levels have led researchers to look for other risk factors that may contribute to atherosclerosis. Although it is not a blood lipid, a high concentration of **homocyste-ine** in the blood is thought to enhance the formation of plaque and subsequently lead to blockage of the arteries. The body uses homocysteine to help build proteins and carry out cellular metabolism. Homocysteine forms during an intermediate step in the creation of another amino acid. This process requires the presence of folate and vitamins B_6 and B_{12}.

Typically, homocysteine is metabolized rapidly, so it does not accumulate in the blood or damage the arteries. Many people, however, have high blood levels of homocysteine. This might be attributable to either a genetic inability to metabolize homocysteine or a deficiency in the vitamins required for its conversion.

Homocysteine is typically measured in micromoles per liter (μmol/L). A level below 9.0 μmol/L is desirable, while above 13.0 μmol/L is viewed as elevated. A 10-year follow-up study of people with high homocysteine levels showed that those individuals with a level above 14.25 μmol/L had almost twice the risk for stroke compared with individuals whose level was below 9.25 μmol/L.[17] Homocysteine accumulation is theorized to be toxic because it may:

1. Damage the inner lining of the arteries (the initial step in the process of atherosclerosis)
2. Stimulate the proliferation of cells that contribute to plaque formation
3. Encourage clotting that may completely obstruct an artery

Keeping homocysteine from accumulating in the blood seems to be as simple as eating the recommended daily servings of vegetables, fruits, grains, and some meat and legumes. Increasing evidence that folate can prevent heart attacks has led to the recommendation that people consume 400 mcg per day of folate.

Unfortunately, estimates indicate that most Americans do not get 400 daily mcg of folate. Five daily servings of fruits and vegetables can provide sufficient levels of folate and vitamin B_6 to remove and clear homocysteine from the blood. People who consume these five servings are unlikely to derive extra benefits from a vitamin B-complex supplement. Vitamin B_{12} is found primarily in animal flesh and animal products. Vitamin B_{12} deficiency is rarely a problem, as 1 cup of milk or an egg provides the daily requirement. The body also recycles most of this vitamin; therefore, it takes years to develop a deficiency.

Inflammation

For years it has been known that inflammation plays a role in CHD and that inflammation hidden deep in the body is a common trigger of heart attacks, even when cholesterol levels are normal or low and arterial plaque is minimal. Low-grade inflammation can occur in a variety of places throughout the body.

To evaluate ongoing inflammation, physicians have turned to **C-reactive protein (CRP),** whose level in the blood increases with inflammation. People with elevated CRP are more prone to cardiovascular events. The evidence shows that CRP blood levels elevate years before a first heart attack or stroke and that individuals with elevated CRP have twice the risk for a heart attack. The risk for a heart attack is even higher in people with both elevated CRP and cholesterol, resulting in an almost ninefold increase in risk (see Figure 8.6).

Because high CRP levels might be a better predictor of future heart attacks than high cholesterol alone, a test known as *high-sensitivity CRP* (hs-CRP) is used to measure inflammation in the blood vessels. The term "high-sensitivity" was derived from the test's capability to detect small amounts of CRP in the blood.

Hs-CRP test results provide a good measure of the probability of plaque rupturing within the arterial wall. The two main types of plaque are soft and hard. Soft plaque is the most likely to rupture. Ruptured plaque releases clots into the bloodstream that can lead to a heart attack or a stroke. Other evidence has linked high CRP levels to high blood pressure and colon cancer. Guidelines for hs-CRP levels are given in Table 8.4.

CRP is increased by several factors, including obesity, excessive alcohol intake, and high-protein

---

KEY TERMS

Triglycerides Fats formed by glycerol and three fatty acids.

Chylomicrons Molecules that transport triglycerides in the blood.

Homocysteine Intermediate amino acid in the interconversion of two other amino acids: methionine and cysteine.

C-reactive protein (CPR) A protein whose level in the blood increases with inflammation (which may be hidden deep in the body); elevation of this protein is an indicator of potential cardiovascular events.

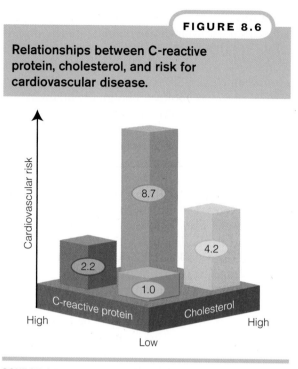

SOURCE: Adapted from P. Libby, P. M. Ridker, and A. Maseri, "Inflammation and Atherosclerosis," *Circulation* 105 (2002): 1135–1143.

FIGURE 8.6

Relationships between C-reactive protein, cholesterol, and risk for cardiovascular disease.

Cardiovascular risk

8.7

2.2

1.0

4.2

C-reactive protein

Cholesterol

High

Low

High

diets. Recent evidence further indicates that high-fat, fast-food meals increase CRP levels for several hours following the meals.[18] Cooking meat and poultry at high temperatures creates damaged proteins (advanced glycosylation end-products [AGEs]) that trigger inflammation.

CRP levels decrease with statin drugs, which also lower cholesterol and reduce inflammation. Exercise, proper nutrition, and aspirin are also helpful. With weight loss, CRP levels decrease proportional to the amount of fat lost. Omega-3 fatty acids (found in salmon, tuna, and mackerel fish) inhibit proteins that cause inflammation, and aspirin therapy also helps by controlling inflammation.

TABLE 8.4

High-Sensitivity CRP Guidelines

Amount	Rating
<1 mg/L	Low risk
1–3 mg/L	Average risk
>3 mg/L	High risk

Source: T. A. Pearson, et. al. "Markers of Inflammation and Cardiovascular Disease." *Circulation* 107 (2003): 499–511.

Diabetes

In people who have **diabetes mellitus,** the pancreas totally stops producing insulin (or does not produce enough to meet the body's needs) or the cells become resistant to the effects of insulin. The role of insulin is to "unlock" the cells and escort glucose into the cell. Diabetes affects about 20 million people in the United States, and about 1 million new cases are diagnosed each year. Between 1980 and 2003, the prevalence of diabetes more than doubled.

The incidence of cardiovascular disease and death in the diabetic population is quite high. More than 75 percent of people with diabetes mellitus die from cardiovascular disease. People with chronically elevated blood glucose levels may have problems metabolizing fats, which can make them more susceptible to atherosclerosis, coronary disease, heart attacks, high blood pressure, and strokes. Diabetics also tend to have lower HDL cholesterol and higher triglyceride levels.

Chronic high blood sugar can also lead to nerve damage, vision loss, kidney damage, and lower immune function (making the individual more susceptible to infections). Diabetics are four times more likely to become blind and 20 times more likely than nondiabetics to develop kidney failure. Nerve damage in the lower extremities makes the person less aware of injury and infection. A small untreated sore can lead to severe infection, gangrene, and even lead to an amputation.

An eight-hour fasting blood glucose level of 126 mg/dL or higher on two separate tests confirms a diagnosis of diabetes. A level of 126 or higher should be brought to the attention of a physician. This guideline has changed from previous years, in which a level above 140 had been used to diagnose diabetes.

Types of Diabetes. Diabetes is of two types: type 1, or **insulin-dependent diabetes mellitus (IDDM),** and type 2, or **non-insulin-dependent diabetes mellitus (NIDDM).** Type 1 has also been known as "juvenile diabetes," because it is found mainly in young people. With type 1, the pancreas produces little or no insulin. With type 2, the pancreas either does not produce sufficient insulin or it produces adequate amounts but the cells become insulin-resistant, thereby keeping glucose from entering the cell. Type 2 accounts for 90 to 95 percent of all diabetes cases.

Although diabetes has a genetic predisposition, adult-onset (type 2) diabetes is related closely to overeating, obesity, and lack of physical activity.

More than 80 percent of type 2 diabetics are overweight or have a history of excessive weight. In most cases, this condition can be corrected through a special diet, a weight loss program, and a regular exercise program.

A diet high in complex carbohydrates (unrefined whole grains) and water-soluble fibers (found in fruits, vegetables, oats, and beans), low in saturated fat, and low in sugar is helpful in treating diabetes. Several research reports have shown that a habitual aerobic exercise program (walking, cycling, or swimming four or five times per week) increases the body's receptivity to insulin.

Aerobic exercise helps prevent type 2 diabetes in the first place. The protective effect is even greater in those who have risk factors such as obesity, high blood pressure, and family propensity. The preventive effect is attributed to less body fat and better sugar and fat metabolism resulting from the regular exercise program. Evidence also suggests that consumption of low-fat dairy products lowers the risk for type 2 diabetes. Individuals who consume the most dairy products have a 23 percent lower incidence of the disease.

Both moderate-intensity and vigorous physical activity have been associated with increased insulin sensitivity and decreased risk for diabetes. The key to increase and maintain proper insulin sensitivity is regularity of the exercise program. Failure to maintain habitual physical activity voids the benefits.

Aggressive weight loss, especially if combined with increased activity, often allows type 2 diabetic patients to normalize their blood sugar level without the use of medication. Individuals who have high blood glucose levels should consult a physician to decide on the best treatment.

Metabolic Syndrome. As the cells resist the action of insulin, the pancreas releases even more insulin in an attempt to keep the blood glucose level from rising. A chronic rise in insulin seems to trigger a series of abnormalities referred to as **metabolic syndrome.** These abnormal conditions include low HDL cholesterol, high triglycerides, and an increased blood-clotting mechanism. Many individuals with metabolic syndrome also have high blood pressure. All of these conditions increase the risk for CHD and other diabetic-related conditions (blindness, infection, nerve damage, and kidney failure). Approximately 70 million Americans are afflicted by metabolic syndrome.

People with metabolic syndrome have an abnormal insulin response to carbohydrates, in particular those that are absorbed rapidly (high-glycemic foods). Metabolic syndrome research indicates that a low-fat/high-carbohydrate dietary plan may not be the best for prevention of CHD and actually could increase the risk for this disease in people with high insulin resistance and glucose intolerance. It might be best for these people to distribute their daily caloric intake so they derive 45 percent of their calories from carbohydrates (primarily low-glycemic), 40 percent from fat, and 15 percent from protein.[19] Of the 40 percent fat calories, 30 to 35 percent should come from mono- and polyunsaturated fats and only 5 to 10 percent should be provided by saturated fat.

Individuals with metabolic syndrome also benefit from weight loss (if overweight), exercise, and smoking cessation. Insulin resistance drops by about 40 percent in overweight people who lose 20 pounds. Forty-five minutes of daily aerobic exercise enhances insulin efficiency by 25 percent. Smoking, on the other hand, increases insulin resistance.

Abnormal Electrocardiograms

An **electrocardiogram (ECG or EKG)** is taken at rest, during the stress of exercise, and during recovery. An exercise or stress ECG also is known as a graded exercise stress test or a maximal exercise tolerance test. Similar to a high-speed road test on a car, a stress ECG reveals the heart's tolerance

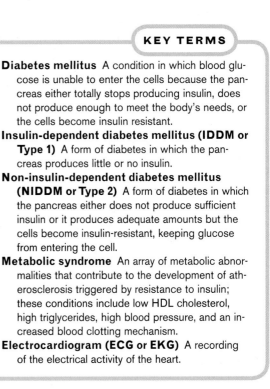

KEY TERMS

Diabetes mellitus A condition in which blood glucose is unable to enter the cells because the pancreas either totally stops producing insulin, does not produce enough to meet the body's needs, or the cells become insulin resistant.

Insulin-dependent diabetes mellitus (IDDM or Type 1) A form of diabetes in which the pancreas produces little or no insulin.

Non-insulin-dependent diabetes mellitus (NIDDM or Type 2) A form of diabetes in which the pancreas either does not produce sufficient insulin or it produces adequate amounts but the cells become insulin-resistant, keeping glucose from entering the cell.

Metabolic syndrome An array of metabolic abnormalities that contribute to the development of atherosclerosis triggered by resistance to insulin; these conditions include low HDL cholesterol, high triglycerides, high blood pressure, and an increased blood clotting mechanism.

Electrocardiogram (ECG or EKG) A recording of the electrical activity of the heart.

2006 American Heart Association Diet and Lifestyle Recommendations for Cardiovascular Disease Risk Reduction

- Balance caloric intake and physical activity to achieve or maintain a healthy body weight.
- Consume a diet rich in vegetables and fruits.
- Consume whole-grain, high-fiber foods.
- Consume fish, especially oily fish, at least twice a week.
- Limit your intake of saturated fat to less than 7 percent and trans fat to less than 1 percent of total daily caloric intake.
- Limit cholesterol intake to less than 300 mg per day.
- Minimize your intake of beverages and foods with added sugars.
- Choose and prepare foods with little or no salt.
- If you consume alcohol, do so in moderation.
- When you eat food that is prepared outside of the home, follow the above recommendations.
- Avoid use of and exposure to tobacco products.
- Be physically active.
- Aim for recommended levels of LDL cholesterol, HDL cholesterol, and triglycerides.
- Aim for a normal blood pressure.
- Aim for normal blood glucose levels.

Try It

In your Online Journal or class notebook, record which of the above recommendations you fall short on and propose at least one thing you could do to improve.

3. Hypertensive and diabetic individuals
4. Cigarette smokers
5. Individuals with a family history of CHD, syncope, or sudden death before age 60
6. People with an abnormal resting ECG
7. All individuals with symptoms of chest discomfort, dysrhythmias, syncope, or **chronotropic incompetence**

Tobacco Use

More than 46 million adults and 3.5 million adolescents in the United States smoke cigarettes. Each day, an additional 3,000 people under the age of 18 become smokers. Cigarette smoking is the single largest preventable cause of illness and premature death in the United States. If we include all related deaths, tobacco is responsible for more than 440,000 unnecessary deaths per year. Smoking has been linked to cardiovascular disease, cancer, bronchitis, emphysema, and peptic ulcers.

About 53,000 of those yearly deaths are of nonsmokers who were exposed to secondhand smoke in their daily life. Both fatal and nonfatal cardiac events increase greatly in people who are exposed to passive smoking. Some 37,000 yearly deaths from heart disease are attributed to secondhand smoke. Even in regular smokers, adaptations to the harmful effects of smoking are slight, so the adverse effects are much greater to nonsmokers.

Secondhand smoke is ranked behind active smoking and alcohol as the third leading preventable cause of death in the United States. Passive smoking

to high-intensity exercise. Based on the findings, ECGs may be interpreted as normal, equivocal, or abnormal.

A **stress electrocardiogram (stress ECG)** frequently is used to diagnose coronary heart disease. It also is administered to determine cardiorespiratory fitness levels, to screen individuals for preventive and cardiac rehabilitation programs, to detect abnormal blood pressure response during exercise, and to establish actual or functional maximal heart rate for purposes of participation in exercise.

Not every adult who wishes to start or continue in an exercise program needs a stress ECG. Those most indicative for this type of test are:

1. Men over age 45 and women over age 55
2. People with a total cholesterol level above 200 mg/dL, or an HDL cholesterol level below 35 mg/dL

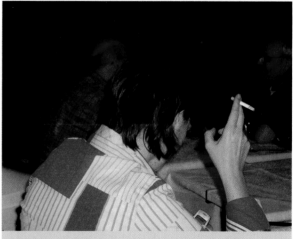

© Fitness & Wellness, Inc.

Cigarette smoking is the single largest preventable cause of illness and premature death in the United States.

is a significant risk factor for heart disease in children and adults alike. Between 150,000 and 300,000 children under the age of 18 months suffer from respiratory tract infections due to secondhand smoke exposure.

In relation to coronary disease, smoking speeds up the process of atherosclerosis and also produces a threefold increase in the risk for sudden death following a **myocardial infarction.** Smoking increases heart rate and blood pressure and irritates the heart, which can trigger fatal cardiac **arrhythmias.** As far as the extra load on the heart is concerned, smoking one pack of cigarettes per day is the equivalent of carrying between 50 and 75 pounds of excess body fat! Another harmful effect is a decrease in HDL cholesterol, the "good" type that helps control blood lipids.

The risk for cardiovascular disease starts to decrease the moment a person quits smoking. After cessation, the risk approaches that of a lifetime non-smoker. Pipe and cigar smoking and chewing tobacco also increase the risk for heart disease. Even if no smoke is inhaled, toxic substances are absorbed through the membranes of the mouth and end up in the bloodstream.

Quitting tobacco use is not easy. The addictive properties of nicotine make quitting difficult, and physical and psychological withdrawal symptoms set in. A six-step plan to help people stop smoking is contained in Figure 8.7.

The most important factor in quitting cigarette smoking is a sincere desire to do so. More than 95 percent of successful ex-smokers have been able to quit on their own, either by quitting cold turkey or by using self-help kits available from organizations such as the American Cancer Society (ACS), the AHA, and the American Lung Association. Only 3 percent of ex-smokers quit as a result of formal cessation programs.

Stress

Stress has become a part of life. People have to deal daily with goals, deadlines, responsibilities, and pressures. The **stressor** itself is not what creates the health hazard but, rather, the individual's response to it.

The human body responds to stress by producing more catecholamines to prepare the body for **fight or flight.** If the person fights or flees, the body metabolizes the higher levels of catecholamines and is able to return to a normal state. If, however, a person is under constant stress and is unable to take action (as in the death of a close relative or friend, loss of a job, trouble at work, or financial insecurity), the catecholamines remain elevated in the bloodstream.

People who are not able to relax place a constant low-level strain on the cardiovascular system that could manifest itself in heart disease. In addition, when a person is in a stressful situation, the coronary arteries that feed the heart muscle constrict, reducing the oxygen supply to the heart. If the blood vessels are largely blocked by atherosclerosis, abnormal heart rhythms or even a heart attack may follow.

As outlined in Chapter 7, individuals who are under a lot of stress and do not cope well with it need to take measures to counteract the effects of stress in their lives. Identifying and learning how to cope with the sources of stress will improve health and quality of life.

Physical activity is one of the best ways to relieve stress. When a person takes part in physical activity, the body metabolizes excess catecholamines and is

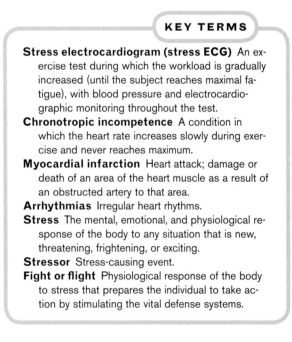

FIGURE 8.7

Six-step smoking cessation approach.

The following six-step plan has been developed as a guide to help you quit smoking. The total program should be completed in 4 weeks or less. Steps one through four should take no longer than 2 weeks. A maximum of 2 additional weeks are allowed for the rest of the program.

Step One. Decide positively that you want to quit. Now prepare a list of the reasons why you smoke and why you want to quit.

Step Two. Initiate a personal diet and exercise program. Exercise and decreased body weight cause a greater awareness of healthy living and increase motivation for giving up cigarettes.

Step Three. Decide on the approach you will use to stop smoking. You may quit cold turkey or gradually decrease the number of cigarettes smoked daily. Many people have found that quitting cold turkey is the easiest way to do it. Although it may not work the first time, after several attempts, all of a sudden smokers are able to overcome the habit without too much difficulty. Tapering off cigarettes can be done in several ways. You may start by eliminating cigarettes that you do not necessarily need, you can switch to a brand lower in nicotine or tar every couple of days, you can smoke less of each cigarette, or you can simply decrease the total number of cigarettes smoked each day.

Step Four. Set the target date for quitting. In setting the target date, choosing a special date may add a little extra incentive. An upcoming birthday, anniversary, vacation, graduation, family reunion—all are examples of good dates to free yourself from smoking.

Step Five. Stock up on low-calorie foods—carrots, broccoli, cauliflower, celery, popcorn (butter- and salt-free), fruits, sunflower seeds (in the shell), sugarless gum, and plenty of water. Keep such food handy on the day you stop and the first few days following cessation. Replace it for cigarettes when you want one.

Step Six. This is the day that you will quit smoking. On this day and the first few days thereafter, do not keep cigarettes handy. Stay away from friends and events that trigger your desire to smoke. Drink large amounts of water and fruit juices and eat low-calorie foods. Replace the old behavior with new behavior. You will need to replace smoking time with new positive substitutes that will make smoking difficult or impossible. When you desire a cigarette, take a few deep breaths and then occupy yourself by doing a number of things such as talking to someone else, washing your hands, brushing your teeth, eating a healthy snack, chewing on a straw, doing dishes, playing sports, going for a walk or bike ride, going swimming, and so on.

If you have been successful and stopped smoking, a lot of events still can trigger your urge to smoke. When confronted with such events, people rationalize and think, "One won't hurt." It will not work! Before you know it, you will be back to the regular nasty habit. Be prepared to take action in those situations. Find adequate substitutes for smoking. Remind yourself of how difficult it has been and how long it has taken you to get to this point. As time goes on, it will only get easier rather than worse.

---

able to return to a normal state. Exercise also steps up muscular activity, which contributes to muscular relaxation.

Personal and Family History

Individuals who have a family history of, or already have experienced, cardiovascular problems are at higher risk than those who never have had a problem. People with this history should be encouraged strongly to keep the other risk factors as low as possible. Because most risk factors are reversible, the risk for future problems will decrease significantly.

Age and Gender

Age becomes a risk factor for men over age 45 and women over age 55. The greater incidence of heart disease may stem in part from lifestyle changes as we get older (less physical activity, poor nutrition, obesity, and so on). Earlier in life, men are at greater risk for cardiovascular disease than women are. Following menopause, the risk for women increases. Based on final mortality statistics for 2002, more women (461,100) than men (410,400) died from cardiovascular disease.[20]

Young people should not think they are immune from heart disease. The process begins early in life.

Autopsies conducted in people who have died in their 20s reveal that many of them already exhibit early stages of atherosclerosis. Other studies have found elevated blood cholesterol levels in children as young as 10 years old.

Even though the aging process cannot be stopped, it certainly can be slowed. The concept of **chronological age** versus **physiological age** is important in longevity. Some individuals in their 60s or older have the body of a 35 year old. And 35 year olds often are in such poor condition and health that they almost seem to have the body of a 60 year old. Managing risk factors and developing positive lifestyle habits are the best ways to slow natural aging.

Cancer

Cell growth is controlled by **deoxyribonucleic acid (DNA)** and **ribonucleic acid (RNA).** When nuclei lose their ability to regulate and control cell growth, cell division is disrupted and mutant cells may develop. Some of these cells may grow uncontrollably and abnormally, forming a mass of tissue called a tumor, which can be either **benign** or **malignant.** Although benign tumors can interfere with normal bodily functions, they rarely cause death.

About 23 percent of all deaths in the United States come from **cancer.** Each year, over 1.4 million new cases are reported and more than half a million people die from cancer.[21] Over 100 types of cancer can develop in the body. Cancer cells grow for no reason and multiply, destroying normal tissue. If the spread of cells is not controlled, death ensues. A cell may duplicate as many as 100 times.

Normally, the DNA molecule is duplicated perfectly during cell division. In a few cases the DNA molecule is not replicated exactly but specialized enzymes repair it quickly. Occasionally, cells with defective DNA keep dividing and ultimately form a small tumor. As more mutations occur, the altered cells continue to divide and can become malignant. A decade or more can pass between carcinogenic exposure or mutations and the time cancer is diagnosed. A critical turning point in the development of cancer is when a tumor reaches about 1 million cells. At this stage it is referred to as **carcinoma in situ,** when it has not spread. Such an undetected tumor may go for months or years without any significant growth.

While encapsulated, a tumor does not pose a serious threat to human health. To grow, the tumor requires more oxygen and nutrients. In time, a few of the cancer cells start producing chemicals that enhance **angiogenesis.** Cells break away from a malignant tumor and, through the new blood vessels, migrate to other parts of the body, in a process called **metastasis,** where they can cause new cancer.

Although the immune system and the blood turbulence destroy most cancer cells, only one abnormal cell lodging elsewhere can start a new cancer. These cells also will grow and multiply uncontrollably, destroying normal tissue. Once cancer cells metastasize, treatment becomes more difficult. Therapy can kill most cancer cells, but a few cells may become resistant to treatment. These cells then can grow into a new tumor that will not respond to the same treatment.

As with cardiovascular disease, cancer is largely preventable. As much as 80 percent of all human cancer is related to lifestyle or environmental factors (including diet, tobacco use, excessive use of alcohol, sexual and reproductive activity, and exposure to environmental hazards). Equally important is that more than 9.8 million Americans with a history of cancer were alive in 2005. Currently, 6 in 10 people diagnosed with cancer are expected to be alive five years from the initial diagnosis.

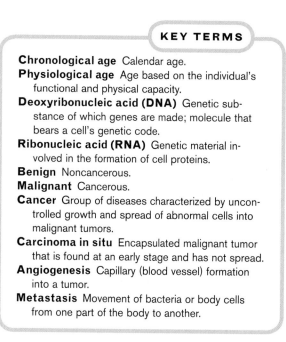

KEY TERMS

Chronological age Calendar age.

Physiological age Age based on the individual's functional and physical capacity.

Deoxyribonucleic acid (DNA) Genetic substance of which genes are made; molecule that bears a cell's genetic code.

Ribonucleic acid (RNA) Genetic material involved in the formation of cell proteins.

Benign Noncancerous.

Malignant Cancerous.

Cancer Group of diseases characterized by uncontrolled growth and spread of abnormal cells into malignant tumors.

Carcinoma in situ Encapsulated malignant tumor that is found at an early stage and has not spread.

Angiogenesis Capillary (blood vessel) formation into a tumor.

Metastasis Movement of bacteria or body cells from one part of the body to another.

Guidelines for Preventing Cancer

The biggest factor in fighting cancer today is health education. People need to be informed about the risk factors for cancer and the guidelines for early detection. The most effective way to protect against cancer is to change negative lifestyle habits and behaviors. Activity 8.1, pages 223–224, is a questionnaire regarding the risk factors and preventive measures discussed below.

Making Dietary Changes

The ACS estimates that one-third of all cancers in the United States are related to nutrition. A healthy diet, therefore, is crucial to decrease the risk for cancer. The diet should be predominantly vegetarian—high in fiber and low in fat (particularly from animal sources). **Cruciferous vegetables** (cauliflower, broccoli, cabbage, Brussels sprouts, and kohlrabi), tea, vitamin D, calcium, and omega-3 fats are encouraged. If alcohol is consumed, it should be used in moderation. Obesity should be avoided.

Brightly colored fruits and vegetables are also encouraged. These fruits and vegetables contain **carotenoids** and vitamin C. Lycopene, one of the many carotenoids (a phytonutrient—see discussion below), has been linked to lowered risk for cancers of the prostate, colon, and cervix. Lycopene is especially abundant in cooked tomato products.

The evidence for vitamin D in protecting against cancer continues to mount each day. Vitamin D is the most powerful regulator of cell growth and keeps cells from becoming malignant. The protective effect of vitamin D appears to be strongest against breast, colon, and prostate cancers and possibly lung and digestive cancers. You should strive for "safe sun" exposure, that is, up 15 minutes of unprotected sun exposure, on most days of the week between the hours of 10:00 a.m. and 4:00 p.m. For people living in the northern United States and Canada, with limited sun exposure during the winter months, a vitamin D_3 supplement of up to 2,000 IU per day is strongly recommended.

Researchers also believe that the antioxidant effect of vitamins and the mineral selenium helps protect the body from free radicals. Antioxidants are thought to absorb free radicals before they can cause damage, and they also interrupt the sequence of reactions once damage has begun.

Many studies have linked low intake of fiber to increased risk for colon cancer. Fiber binds to bile acids in the intestine for excretion from the body in the stools. The interaction of bile acids with intestinal bacteria releases cancer-causing byproducts. Bile-acid production increases with increased fat content in the small intestine.

Grains are high in fiber and contain vitamins and minerals—folate, selenium, and calcium—that seem to decrease the risk for colon cancer. Selenium also protects against prostate cancer and possibly lung cancer. Calcium may protect against colon cancer by preventing rapid growth of cells in the colon, especially in people with colon polyps.

Phytonutrients. A promising horizon in cancer prevention is the discovery of **phytonutrients.** These compounds, found in abundance in fruits and vegetables, seem to exert a powerful effect in preventing cancer by blocking the formation of cancerous tumors and disrupting the process at almost every step of the way. Experts recommend that to obtain the highest possible protection, produce should be consumed several times during the day (instead of in one meal) to maintain effective phytonutrient levels throughout the day. Phytonutrient blood levels drop within three hours of consuming the produce.

Polyphenols (a phytonutrient) are cancer-fighting antioxidants found in tea. They are known to block the formation of **nitrosamines** and quell the activation of carcinogens. Polyphenols also are thought to fight cancer by shutting off the formation of cancer cells, turning up the body's natural detoxification defenses, and thereby suppressing progression of the disease. Different types of tea contain different mixtures of polyphenols. White tea appears to have the highest amount, followed by green and black tea. Herbal teas do not provide the same benefits as regular tea.

Observational data on tea-drinking habits in China showed that people who regularly drank green tea had about half the risk for chronic gastritis and stomach cancer and the risk decreased further as the number of years of drinking green tea increased. In Japan, where people drink green tea regularly but smoke twice as much as people in the United States, the incidence of lung cancer is half that of the United States.

The antioxidant effect of one of the polyphenols in green tea—epigallocatechin gallate, or EGCG—is at least 25 times more effective than vitamin E and 100 times more effective than vitamin C at protecting cells and the DNA from damage believed to cause cancer, heart disease, and other diseases associated with free radicals.[22] EGCG is also twice as strong as the red wine antioxidant resveratrol, which helps prevent heart disease.

Other Dietary Factors. High fat intake may promote cancer and excessive weight. Some experts recommend that in a cancer prevention diet, total fat intake should be limited to less than 20 percent of total daily calories. Fat intake should consist of primarily monounsaturated and omega-3 fats. Omega-3 fats, found in many types of fish, flaxseeds, and flaxseed oil, seem to offer protection against colorectal, pancreatic, breast, oral, esophageal, and stomach cancers. Omega-3 fats block the synthesis of prostaglandins, bodily compounds that promote growth of tumors.

Foods high in vitamin C may deter some cancers. Salt-cured, smoked, and nitrite-cured foods have been associated with cancers of the esophagus and stomach. Processed meats should be consumed sparingly and always with orange juice or other foods rich in vitamin C. Vitamin C seems to discourage the formation of nitrosamines.

Cooking protein at high temperature should be avoided or done so only occasionally. The data suggest that grilling, broiling, or frying meat, poultry, or fish at high temperatures to "medium well" or "well done" leads to the formation of carcinogenic substances known as heterocyclic amines (HCAs) and polycyclic aromatic hydrocarbons (PAHs). Individuals who prefer their meat medium well or well done have a much higher risk for colorectal and stomach cancers.

Cooking proteins at high temperatures changes amino acids into HCAs that collect on the surface of meats. Charring meat increases their formation to an even greater extent. PAHs are formed when fat drips onto the rocks or coals of the grill. The subsequent fire flare-up releases smoke that coats the food with PAHs.

An electric contact grill such as a George Foreman grill is preferable when cooking meats because cooking temperatures are easily controlled. When cooking on an outdoor grill, line the grill with foil to keep the drippings off the rocks or coals. Microwaving the meat for a couple of minutes before barbecuing also decreases the risk, as long as the fluid released by the meat is discarded. Most of the potential **carcinogens** collect in this solution. For an occasional outdoor barbecue, trim off excess fat to avoid flare-ups and turn meats over frequently to decrease HCA formation. Removing the skin before serving and cooking at lower heat to "medium" also lowers the risk.

Mixing soy protein in powder form with meats also seems to decrease the formation of carcinogens when cooking meats. Soy foods may help because soy contains isoflavones (phytonutrients) that prevent cancer. Presently, it is not known if the health benefits of soy are related to isoflavones by themselves or in combination with other nutrients found in soy. Experts caution women with breast cancer or a history of this disease to limit soy intake because it may stimulate cancer cells by closely imitating the actions of estrogen.

Based on the traditional diets of people in China and Japan, including children, who regularly consume soy foods, there doesn't seem to be an unsafe level of consumption. Soy protein powder supplementation, however, may not be safe, because this may elevate soy protein intake to an unnaturally high level.

People who consume alcohol should do so in moderation, because too much alcohol raises the risk for developing certain cancers, especially when it is combined with tobacco smoking or smokeless tobacco. In combination, these substances significantly increase the risk for cancers of the mouth, larynx, throat, esophagus, and liver. The combined action of heavy use of alcohol and tobacco can increase cancer of the oral cavity fifteenfold.

Maintaining recommended body weight also is encouraged. Obesity may be associated with cancers of the colon, rectum, breast, prostate, endometrium, and kidney.

Abstaining from Tobacco

Cigarette smoking by itself is a major health hazard. As stated earlier in this chapter, if we include all related deaths, smoking is responsible for more

---

KEY TERMS

Cruciferous vegetables Plants that produce cross-shaped leaves (cauliflower, broccoli, cabbage, Brussels sprouts, kohlrabi); these seem to have a protective effect against cancer.

Carotenoids Pigment substances (more than 600) in plants, about 50 of which are precursors to vitamin A; the most potent carotenoid is beta-carotene.

Phytonutrients Compounds found in fruits and vegetables that block formation of cancerous tumors and disrupt the process of cancer.

Nitrosamines Potentially cancer-causing compounds formed when nitrites and nitrates—which are used to prevent the growth of harmful bacteria in processed meats—combine with other chemicals in the stomach.

Carcinogens Substances that contribute to the formation of cancers.

Tips for a Healthy Cancer-Fighting Diet

Increase intake of phytonutrients, fiber, cruciferous vegetables, and more antioxidants by

- Eating a predominantly vegetarian diet
- Eating more fruits and vegetables every day (six to eight servings per day maximize anticancer benefits)
- Increasing the consumption of broccoli, cauliflower, kale, turnips, cabbage, kohlrabi, Brussels sprouts, hot chili peppers, red and green peppers, carrots, sweet potatoes, winter squash, spinach, garlic, onions, strawberries, tomatoes, pineapple, and citrus fruits in your regular diet
- Eating vegetables raw or quickly cooked by steaming or stir-frying
- Substituting tea, fruit and vegetable juices for coffee and soda
- Eating whole-grain breads
- Including calcium in the diet (or from a supplement)
- Including soy products in the diet
- Using whole-wheat flour instead of refined white flour in baking
- Using brown (unpolished) rice instead of white (polished) rice

Decrease daily fat intake by 20 percent of total caloric intake by

- Limiting consumption of beef, poultry, or fish to no more than 3 to 6 ounces (about the size of a deck of cards) once or twice a week
- Trimming all visible fat from meat and removing skin from poultry prior to cooking
- Decreasing the amount of fat and oils used in cooking
- Substituting low-fat for high-fat dairy products
- Using salad dressings sparingly
- Using only half to three-quarters of the amount of fat required in baking recipes
- Limiting fat intake to mostly monounsaturated (olive oil, canola oil, nuts, and seeds) and omega-3 fats (fish, flaxseed, and flaxseed oil)
- Eating fish once or twice a week
- Including flaxseed oil in the diet

Try It

Make a copy of these "Cancer-Fighting Diet" tips and each week incorporate into your lifestyle two additional dietary behaviors from the above list.

---

than 440,000 unnecessary deaths in the United States each year. The World Health Organization estimates that smoking causes 3 million deaths worldwide annually. The average life expectancy for a chronic smoker is about 15 years less than for a nonsmoker. The most prevalent carcinogenic exposure in the workplace is cigarette smoke. At least 28 percent of all cancer is tied to smoking, and 87 percent of lung cancer is tied to smoking. Use of smokeless tobacco can lead to nicotine addiction and dependence as well as increased risk for mouth, larynx, throat, and esophageal cancers.

Avoiding Excessive Sun Exposure

"Safe sun" exposure, up to 15 minutes of unprotected exposure per day is beneficial to health; but too much exposure to ultraviolet radiation (both UVB and UVA rays) is a major contributor to skin cancer. The most common sites of skin cancer are those exposed to the sun most often (face, neck, and backs of the hands). The three types of skin cancer are:

1. Basal cell carcinoma
2. Squamous cell carcinoma
3. Malignant melanoma

Nearly 90 percent of the almost 1 million cases of basal cell or squamous cell skin cancers reported yearly in the United States could have been prevented by protecting the skin from the sun's rays. ACS data indicate that **melanoma** is the most deadly, causing approximately 8,119 deaths in 2007. One in every six Americans will develop some type of skin cancer eventually.

One to two blistering sunburns can double the lifetime risk for melanoma, even more so if the sunburn took place prior to age 18, when cells divide at a much faster rate than later in life. Furthermore, nothing is healthy about a "healthy tan." Tanning of the skin is the body's natural reaction to permanent and irreversible damage from too much exposure to the sun. Even brief exposures to sunlight add up to a greater risk for skin cancer and premature aging. The tan fades at the end of the summer season, but the underlying skin damage does not disappear. People with sensitive skin in particular should avoid sun exposure between 10:00 a.m. and 4:00 p.m.

The stinging sunburn comes from ultraviolet B (UVB) rays, which also are thought to be the main cause of premature wrinkling and skin aging, roughened/leathery/sagging skin, and skin cancer. Unfortunately, the damage may not become evident until up to 20 years later. In contrast, skin that has not been overexposed to the sun remains smooth and unblemished, and, over time, shows less evidence of aging.

Sun lamps and tanning parlors provide mainly ultraviolet A (UVA) rays. Once thought to be safe, they are now known to damage skin and have been linked to melanoma, the most serious form of skin cancer. As little as 15 to 30 minutes of exposure to UVA can be as dangerous as a day spent in the sun.

Sunscreen lotion should be applied about 30 minutes before lengthy exposure to the sun, because the skin takes that long to absorb the protective ingredients. A **sun protection factor (SPF)** of at least 15 is recommended. SPF 15 means that the skin takes 15 times longer to burn than with no lotion. If you ordinarily get a mild sunburn after 20 minutes of noonday sun, an SPF 15 allows you to remain in the sun about 300 minutes before burning. Sunscreens with stronger SPF factors are not necessarily better. They should be applied just as often and they block only an additional 3 to 4 percent ultraviolet rays. An SPF 15 is adequate for most people. When swimming or sweating, you should reapply waterproof sunscreens more often, because all sunscreens lose strength when they are diluted.

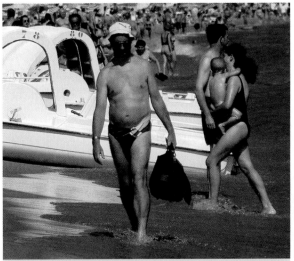

Sunburns and tanning pose a risk for skin cancer from overexposure to the sun's ultraviolet rays.

CRITICAL THINKING

You have learned about many of the risk factors for major cancer sites. • How will this information affect your health choices in the future? • Will it be valuable to you, or will you quickly forget all you have learned and remain in a contemplation stage at the end of this course?

Even better than sunscreen, is wearing protective clothing, including long-sleeved shirts, long pants, and a hat with a two- to three-inch brim all the way around. This sun-protection strategy is even more critical for fair-skinned individuals who burn readily or turn red after only a few minutes of unprotected sun exposure, have a large number of moles, or have a personal or family history of skin cancer risk.

Monitoring Estrogen, Radiation Exposure, and Potential Occupational Hazards

Estrogen use has been linked to endometrial cancer in some studies, although other evidence contradicts those findings. And even though exposure to radiation increases the risk for cancer, the benefits of X-rays may outweigh the risk involved, and most medical facilities use the lowest dose possible to keep the risk to a minimum. Occupational hazards, such as asbestos fibers, nickel and uranium dusts, chromium compounds, vinyl chloride, and bischlormethyl ether, increase the risk for cancer. Cigarette smoking magnifies the risk from occupational hazards.

Physical Activity

An active lifestyle seems to have a protective effect against cancer. Although the mechanism is not clear, physical fitness and cancer mortality in men and women may have a graded and consistent inverse relationship.

A daily 30-minute moderate-intensity exercise program lowers the risk for colon cancer and may lower the risk for cancers of the breast and reproductive system. Research has shown that regular exercise lowers the risk for breast cancer in women by up to 30 percent. In addition, growing evidence suggests that the body's autoimmune system may play a role in preventing cancer. Moderate exercise improves the autoimmune system. And women who are active throughout life cut their risk for endometrial cancer by about 40 percent. Those who started exercise in adulthood cut their risk by about 25 percent.[23]

KEY TERMS

Melanoma The most virulent, rapidly spreading form of skin cancer.

Sun protection factor (SPF) Degree of protection offered by ingredients in sunscreen lotion; at least SPF 15 is recommended.

© Fitness & Wellness, Inc.

Among women diagnosed with breast cancer, women who walk two to three miles per hour one to three times per week are 20 percent less likely to die of the disease. Those who walk three to five times per week cut their risk in half.[24] Researchers believe that the decreased levels of circulating ovarian hormones through physical activity decrease breast cancer risk.

Other data suggest that in men 65 or older, exercising vigorously at least three times per week decreases the risk for advanced or fatal prostate cancer by 70 percent.[25] In addition, growing evidence suggests that the body's autoimmune system may play a role in preventing cancer, and that moderate exercise improves the autoimmune system.

Other Risk Factors for Cancer

Contributions to cancer of many of the other much publicized factors are not as significant as those just pointed out. Intentional food additives, saccharin, processing agents, pesticides, and packaging materials currently used in the United States and other developed countries seem to have minimal consequences. High levels of stress and poor coping may affect the autoimmune system negatively and thereby render the body less effective in dealing with the various cancers.

Genetics plays a role in susceptibility in about 10 percent of all cancers. Most of the effect is seen in the early childhood years. Some cancers are a combination of genetic and environmental liability; genetics may add to the environmental risk for certain types of cancers. "Environment" means more than pollution and smoke. It incorporates diet, lifestyle-related events, viruses, and physical agents such as X-rays and exposure to the sun.

Early Detection

Fortunately, many cancers can be controlled or cured through early detection. The real problem comes when cancerous cells spread, because they are difficult to wipe out then. Therefore, effective prevention, and early detection, is crucial. Herein lies the importance of periodic screening. At home, once a month, women should practice breast self-examination (BSE), and men, testicular self-examination (TSE). Men should pick a regular day each month (for example, the first day of the month) to practice TSE, and women should perform BSE two or three days after the menstrual period is over. Once a month you should also conduct a skin self-examination to detect possible skin cancers. Pay particular attention to areas that are constantly exposed to the sun. Note any changes in the size, texture, or color of moles, warts, or other skin marks. If you notice any change, contact your physician.

Scientific evidence and testing procedures for prevention and early detection of cancer do change. Studies continue to provide new information. The intent of cancer prevention programs is to educate and guide individuals toward a lifestyle that will help prevent cancer and enable early detection of malignancy. Regular physical examinations by your doctor should include the ACS recommendations for the early detection of cancer in asymptomatic people.

BEHAVIOR MODIFICATION PLANNING

Lifestyle Factors That Decrease Cancer Risk

Factor	Function
Physical activity	Controls body weight, may influence hormone levels, strengthens the immune system.
Fiber	Contains anti-cancer substances, increases stool movement, blunts insulin secretion.
Fruits and vegetables	Contain phytonutrients and vitamins that thwart cancer.
Recommended weight	Helps control hormones that promote cancer.
Healthy grilling	Prevents formation of heterocyclic amines (HCAs) and polycyclic aromatic hydrocarbons (PAHs), both carcinogenic substances.
Tea	Contains polyphenols that neutralize free radicals, including epigallocatechin gallate (EGCG), which protects cells and the DNA from damage believed to cause cancer.
Spices	Provide phytonutrients and strengthen the immune system.
Vitamin D	Disrupts abnormal cell growth.
Monounsaturated fat	May contribute to cancer cell destruction.

Try It

In your Online Journal or class notebook, note ways you can incorporate all of these factors into your everyday lifestyle.

Warning Signals for Cancer

Everyone should become familiar with the following warning signs of cancer and bring them to a physician's attention if any are present:

1. Change in bowel or bladder habits.
2. Sore that does not heal.
3. Unusual bleeding or discharge.
4. Thickening or lump in breast or elsewhere.
5. Indigestion or difficulty in swallowing.
6. Obvious change in wart or mole.
7. Nagging cough or hoarseness.

Treatment of cancer always should be left to specialized physicians and cancer clinics. Current treatment modalities include surgery, radiation, radioactive substances, chemotherapy, hormones, and immunotherapy.

Chronic Lower Respiratory Disease

Chronic lower respiratory disease (CLRD) encompasses diseases that limit air flow, such as chronic obstructive pulmonary disease, emphysema, and chronic bronchitis (all diseases of the respiratory system). The incidence of CLRD increases proportionately with cigarette smoking (and other forms of smoked tobacco) and exposure to certain types of industrial pollution. In the case of emphysema, genetic factors also may play a role.

Accidents

Even though most people do not consider accidents to be a health problem, accidents rank as the fourth leading cause of death in the United States, affecting the total well-being of millions of Americans each year. Accident prevention and personal safety also are part of a health enhancement program aimed at achieving a higher quality of life. Proper nutrition, exercise, abstinence from cigarette smoking, and stress management are of little help if the person is involved in a disabling or fatal accident caused by distraction, a single reckless decision, or not wearing safety belts properly.

Accidents do not always just happen. We sometimes cause accidents. Other times we are victims of accidents. Although some factors in life—earthquakes, tornadoes, and airplane crashes, for example—are completely beyond our control, more often than not personal safety and accident prevention are a matter of common sense. Many accidents result from poor judgment and a confused mental state. Frequently accidents happen when we are upset, not paying attention to the task with which we are involved, or abusing alcohol and other drugs.

Alcohol abuse is the number-one cause of all accidents. Alcohol intoxication is the leading cause of fatal automobile accidents. Other drugs commonly abused in society alter feelings and perceptions, cause mental confusion, and impair judgment and coordination, greatly increasing the risk for accidental morbidity and mortality.

Substance Abuse

Chemical dependencies presently encompass some of the most self-destructive behaviors in society. Abused substances include alcohol, hard drugs, and cigarettes (the latter has been discussed already in this chapter). Problems associated with substance abuse include drunken or impaired driving, mixing drug prescriptions, family difficulties, and drugs to improve athletic performance (anabolic steroids). Although all forms of substance abuse are recognized to be unhealthy, the following information focuses on alcohol and on the illegal drugs marijuana, cocaine, methamphetamine, heroin, and MDMA (Ecstasy).

Alcohol

Alcohol use represents one of the most significant health-related drug problems in the United States today. Estimates indicate that 7 in 10 adults, or more than 100 million Americans 18 years and older, are drinkers. Approximately 20 million of them abuse alcohol or are alcohol dependent and will struggle

---

KEY TERMS

Chronic lower respiratory disease (CLRD) A group of diseases that limit air flow, such as chronic obstructive pulmonary disease, emphysema, and chronic bronchitis (all diseases of the respiratory system).

with **alcoholism** throughout life. Among younger people, about 10.8 million between the ages of 12 and 20 are binge drinkers.

Alcohol intake impedes peripheral vision, impairs the ability to see and hear, decreases reaction time, hinders concentration and motor performance (including increased swaying), and causes impaired judgment of distance and speed of moving objects. Further, it lessens fear, increases risk-taking behaviors, stimulates urination, and induces sleep. A single large dose of alcohol also may decrease sexual function. One of the most unpleasant, dangerous, and life-threatening effects of drinking is the **synergistic action** of alcohol when combined with other drugs, particularly central nervous system depressants.

Long-term manifestations of alcohol abuse can be serious and life threatening. These conditions include **cirrhosis** of the liver (often fatal); greater risk for oral, esophageal, and liver cancer; **cardiomyopathy;** high blood pressure; greater risk for strokes; inflammation of the esophagus, stomach, small intestine, and pancreas; stomach ulcers; sexual impotence; malnutrition; brain cell damage and consequent loss of memory; depression, psychosis, and hallucinations. Additional information on the physiologic effects of alcohol is given in Chapter 9.

Illegal Drugs

Approximately 60 percent of the world's production of illegal drugs is consumed in the United States. An estimated 35 million people in the United States used an illegal drug within the past year and 112 million people have used them at least once in their lives. Each year we spend more than $65 billion on illegal drugs.

According to the U.S. Department of Education, today's drugs are stronger and more addictive, posing a greater risk than ever before. Drugs lead to physical and psychological dependence. If used regularly, they integrate into the body's chemistry, raising drug tolerance and forcing the person to increase the dosage constantly for similar results. In addition to the serious health problems caused by drug abuse, more than half of all adolescent suicides are drug related.

Furthermore, almost 50 million Americans, reported nonmedical use of psychotherapeutic drugs at some point in their lifetime. Psychotherapeutic drugs include any prescription pain reliever, tranquilizer, stimulant, or sedative; not including over-the-counter drugs. The risks associated with psycho-

therapy drug misuse or abuse vary depending on the drug. Some of the risks include respiratory depression or cessation, decreased or irregular heart rate, high body temperature, seizures, and cardiovascular failure. Abuse of prescription drugs, or using them in a manner other than exactly as prescribed, can lead to addictive behavior.

Marijuana

Marijuana (pot or grass) is the most widely used illegal drug in the United States. Approximately 25 million people in the country use marijuana regularly. Earlier studies in the 1960s indicated that the potential effects of marijuana were exaggerated and that the drug was relatively harmless. The drug as it is used today, however, is as much as 10 times stronger than it was when the initial studies were conducted. Long-term harmful effects of marijuana use include atrophy of the brain leading to irreversible brain damage, as well as decreased resistance to infectious diseases, chronic bronchitis, lung cancer, and possible sterility and impotence.

Cocaine

Similar to marijuana, for many years cocaine was thought to be a relatively harmless drug. This misconception came to an abrupt halt in the 1980s when two well-known athletes, Len Bias (basketball) and Don Rogers (football), died suddenly following cocaine overdose. Currently, there are an estimated 2.4 million chronic cocaine users and 5.5 million occasional cocaine users in the United States. In 2005, almost 1 million people tried the drug for the first time.

Sustained cocaine snorting can lead to a constant runny nose, nasal congestion and inflammation, and perforation of the nasal septum. Long-term consequences of cocaine use in general include loss of appetite, digestive disorders, weight loss, malnutrition, insomnia, confusion, anxiety, and cocaine psychosis (characterized by paranoia and hallucinations). Large overdoses of cocaine can end in sudden death from respiratory paralysis, cardiac arrhythmias, and severe convulsions. For individuals who lack an enzyme used in metabolizing cocaine, as few as two to three lines of cocaine may be fatal.

Methamphetamine

Methamphetamine or "meth" is a more potent form of amphetamine and has become the fastest-growing drug threat in the United States. More than 10.4 million Americans have tried this powerfully addictive drug. Typically it comes as a white, odorless, bitter-tasting powder that dissolves readily in water or alcohol. The drug is a potent central nervous system stimulant that produces a general feeling of well-being, decreases appetite, increases motor activity, and decreases fatigue and the need for sleep.

Methamphetamine is easily manufactured with over-the-counter ingredients in clandestine "meth labs." The risk for injury in a meth lab is high because potentially explosive environmental contaminants are discarded during production of the drug. Users of methamphetamine experience increases in body temperature, blood pressure, heart rate, and breathing rate; a decrease in appetite; hyperactivity; tremors; and violent behavior. High doses produce irritability, paranoia, irreversible damage to blood vessels in the brain (causing strokes), and risk for sudden death from hyperthermia and convulsions if not treated at once.

Chronic abusers experience insomnia, confusion, hallucinations, inflammation of the heart lining, schizophrenia-like mental disorder, and brain-cell damage similar to that caused by strokes. Physical changes to the brain may last months or perhaps permanently. Over time, methamphetamine use may reduce brain levels of dopamine, which can lead to symptoms of Parkinson's disease. In addition, users frequently are involved in violent crime, homicide, and suicide. Using methamphetamines during pregnancy may cause prenatal complications, premature delivery, and abnormal physical and emotional development of the child.

Heroin

For the first time in decades, heroin use is on the increase. Approximately 3.5 million Americans ages 12 and older reported trying heroin at least once. Common nicknames for heroin include Diesel, Dope, Dynamite, White Death, Nasty Boy, China White, H. Harry, Gumball, Junk, Brown Sugar, Smack, Tootsie Roll, Black Tar, and Chasing the Dragon. The most serious health threat to heroin users today is that they have no way of determining the strength of the drug purchased on the street, thus placing them at a constant risk for overdose and death. An estimated 15 percent of all drug-related hospital emergency room cases involve heroin use.

Heroin use induces a state of euphoria that comes within seconds of intravenous injection or within 5 to 15 minutes when other methods of administration are used. The drug is a sedative, so during the initial rush the person has a sense of relaxation and does not feel any pain. In users who inhale the drug, the rush may be accompanied by nausea, vomiting, intense itching, and at times severe asthma attacks. As the rush wears off, users become drowsy and confused and have reduced cardiac function and breathing rate.

A heroin overdose can cause convulsions, coma, and death. During an overdose, heart rate, breathing, blood pressure, and body temperature drop dramatically. These physiological responses can induce vomiting, tighten the muscles, and cause breathing to stop. Death is often the result of lack of oxygen or choking to death on vomit.

Within four to five hours after the drug is taken, withdrawal sets in. Heroin withdrawal is painful and may last up to two weeks but could go on several months. Symptoms of withdrawal for long-term users include red/raw nostrils, bone and muscle pains, muscle spasms and cramps, sweating, hot and cold flashes, runny nose and eyes, drowsiness, sluggishness, slurred speech, loss of appetite, nausea, diarrhea, restlessness, and violent yawning. Heroin use also can kill a developing fetus or cause a spontaneous abortion.

Symptoms of long-term use of heroin include hallucinations, nightmares, constipation, sexual difficulties, impaired vision, reduced fertility, boils, collapsed veins, and significantly elevated risk for lung, liver, and cardiovascular diseases, including bacterial infections in blood vessels and heart valves. Additives in street heroin can clog vital blood vessels because they do not dissolve in the body and therefore can lead to infections and death of cells in vital organs. Sudden infant death syndrome (SIDS) is seen more frequently in children born to addicted mothers.

MDMA (Ecstasy)

MDMA, also known as "Ecstasy," became popular among teenagers and young adults in the United States in the mid-1980s. Prior to 1985, few Americans abused this drug. MDMA is named for its chemical

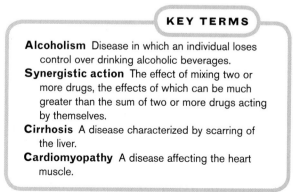

KEY TERMS

Alcoholism Disease in which an individual loses control over drinking alcoholic beverages.

Synergistic action The effect of mixing two or more drugs, the effects of which can be much greater than the sum of two or more drugs acting by themselves.

Cirrhosis A disease characterized by scarring of the liver.

Cardiomyopathy A disease affecting the heart muscle.

structure: 3,4-methylenedioxymethamphetamine. Besides ecstasy, other street names for the drug are X-TC, E, Adam, and love drug. More than 11.5 million persons aged 12 and older have reported using ecstasy at least once.

Although MDMA usually is swallowed in the form of one or two pills in doses of 50–240 mg, it also can be smoked, snorted, or occasionally injected. Because the drug is often prepared with other substances, users have no way of knowing the exact potency of the drug or additional substances found in each pill.

MDMA has a reputation among young people for being fun and harmless as long as it is used sensibly. MDMA, however, is not a harmless drug. Users may experience rapid eye movement, faintness, blurred vision, chills, sweating, nausea, muscle tension, and teeth-grinding. Individuals with heart, liver, or kidney disease or high blood pressure are especially at risk because MDMA increases blood pressure, heart rate, and body temperature; thus, it may lead to kidney failure, a heart attack, a stroke, and seizures.

Other evidence suggests that a pregnant woman using MDMA may find long-term learning and memory difficulties in her child. Other long-term side effects, lasting for weeks after use, include confusion, depression, sleep disorders, anxiety, aggression, paranoia, and impulsive behavior. Verbal and visual memory may be significantly impaired for years after prolonged use.

Treatment for Chemical Dependency

Recognizing the hazards of chemical use, families, teams, and communities can assist each other in preventing problems, as well as help those who already have problems with chemical use. Treating chemical dependency (including alcohol) seldom is accomplished without professional guidance and support. To secure the best available assistance, people in need should contact a physician, your institution's counseling center, or obtain a referral from a local mental health clinic (see Yellow Pages in the phone book).

Sexually Transmitted Infections

As the name implies, **sexually transmitted infections (STIs)** are infections spread through sexual contact. STIs have reached epidemic propor-

tions in the United States. Of the more than 25 known STIs, some are still incurable. The American Social Health Association projected that 25 percent of all Americans will acquire at least one STI during their lifetime. Each year, more than 19 million people in the United States are newly infected with STIs, and almost half of them are seen in young people between the ages of 15 and 24.[26]

HIV/AIDS

AIDS (acquired immunodeficiency syndrome) is the most frightening of all STIs because it has no cure and in most cases is fatal. It is the end result of **human immunodeficiency virus (HIV),** which spreads among individuals who engage in risky behavior such as having unprotected sex or sharing hypodermic needles. When a person becomes infected with HIV, the virus multiplies and attacks and destroys white blood cells. These cells are part of the immune system, whose function is to fight off infections and diseases in the body. As the number of white blood cells killed increases, the body's immune system breaks down gradually or may be destroyed totally. Without a functioning immune system, a person becomes susceptible to **opportunistic infections** or cancers ordinarily not seen in healthy people.

HIV is a progressive infection. At first, people who become infected with HIV might not know they are infected. An incubation period of weeks, months, or years may pass during which no symptoms appear. The virus may live in the body 10 years or longer before symptoms emerge. HIV infection can produce neurological abnormalities, leading to depression, memory loss, slower mental and physical response time, and sluggishness in limb movements that may progress to a severe disorder known as HIV dementia.

As the infection progresses to the point at which certain diseases develop, the person is said to have AIDS. HIV itself doesn't kill. Nor do people die from AIDS. AIDS is the term used to define the final stage of HIV infection. Death is caused by a weakened immune system that is unable to fight off opportunistic diseases.

No one has to become infected with HIV. At present, once infected, a person cannot become uninfected. There is no second chance. Everyone must protect themselves against this chronic infection. If people do not—and are so ignorant as to believe it cannot happen to them—they are putting themselves and their partners at risk.

HIV is transmitted by the exchange of cellular body fluids—blood, semen, vaginal secretions, and maternal milk. These fluids may be exchanged during sexual intercourse, by using hypodermic needles that infected individuals have used previously, between a pregnant woman and her developing fetus, in babies from infected mothers during childbirth, less frequently during breast feeding, and, rarely, from a blood transfusion or an organ transplant.

People do not get HIV because of who they are but, rather, because of what they do. HIV and AIDS threaten anyone, anywhere: men, women, children, teenagers, young people, older adults, whites, blacks, Hispanics, homosexuals, heterosexuals, bisexuals, druggies, Americans, Africans, Asians, Europeans. Nobody is immune to HIV.

You cannot tell if people are infected with HIV or have AIDS simply by looking at them or taking their word. Not you, not a nurse, not even a doctor can tell, without an HIV antibody test. Therefore, every time you engage in risky behavior, you run the risk for contracting HIV. The two most basic risky behaviors are (a) having unprotected vaginal, anal, or oral sex with an HIV-infected person, and (b) sharing hypodermic needles or other drug paraphernalia with someone who is infected.

Estimates by the Centers for Disease Control and Prevention indicate that through the end of 2005, a cumulative total of 952,629 AIDS cases had been diagnosed in the United States, and 550,394 people had died from the diseases caused by HIV. About 70 percent of the people who died are in the 25–44 age group. Of the reported AIDS cases, 761,723 were in males.

Although initially more than half of all AIDS cases in the United States occurred in homosexual or bisexual men, HIV infection is now spreading at a faster rate in heterosexuals. Many heterosexuals practice unprotected sex because they don't believe it can happen to their segment of the population. HIV is an epidemic that does not discriminate by sexual orientation.

As with any other serious illness, AIDS patients deserve respect, understanding, and support. Rejection and discrimination are traits of immature, hateful, and ignorant people. Education, knowledge, and responsible behaviors are the best ways to minimize fear and discrimination.

Guidelines for Preventing STIs

With all the grim news about STIs, the good news is that you can do things to prevent their spread and take precautions to keep yourself from becoming a victim. The facts are in: The best preventive technique is a mutually monogamous sexual relationship—sex with only one person who has sexual relations only with you. That one behavior will remove you almost completely from any risk for developing an STI.

Unfortunately, in today's society, trust is an elusive concept. You may be led to believe you are in a monogamous relationship when your partner actually (a) may be cheating on you and gets infected, (b) ends up having a one-night stand with someone who is infected, (c) got the virus several years ago before the present relationship and still isn't aware of the infection, (d) may not be honest with you and chooses not to tell you about the infection, or (e) is shooting up drugs and becomes infected. In any of these cases, HIV can be passed on to you.

Because your future and your life are at stake and because you may never know if your partner is infected, you should give serious and careful consideration to postponing sex until you believe you have found a lifetime monogamous relationship. In doing so, you will not have to live with the fear of catching HIV or other STIs or deal with an unplanned pregnancy.

As strange as this may seem to some, many people postpone sexual activity until they are married. This is the best guarantee against HIV. Young people should understand that married life will provide plenty of time for fulfilling and rewarding sex. If you choose to delay sex, do not let peers pressure you into having sex. Some people would have you believe you are not a real man or woman if you don't have sex. Manhood and womanhood are not proven during sexual intercourse but, instead, through ma-

> **KEY TERMS**
>
> **Sexually transmitted infections (STIs)** Communicable infections spread through sexual contact.
>
> **Acquired immunodeficiency syndrome (AIDS)** End stage of HIV infection, manifested by any of a number of diseases that arise when the body's immune system is compromised by HIV.
>
> **Human immunodeficiency virus (HIV)** Virus that leads to acquired immunodeficiency syndrome (AIDS).
>
> **Opportunistic infections** Diseases that arise in the absence of a healthy immune system that would fight them off in healthy people.

ture, responsible, and healthy choices. Other people lead you to believe that love doesn't exist without sex. Sex in the early stages of a relationship is not the product of love but is simply the fulfillment of a physical, and often selfish, drive. A loving relationship develops over a long time with mutual respect for each other.

Teenagers are especially susceptible to peer pressure leading to premature sexual intercourse. As a result, more than a million teens become pregnant each year, with a 43 percent pregnancy rate for all girls at least once as a teenager. Too many young people wish they had postponed sex and silently admire those who do. Sex lasts only a few minutes. The consequences of irresponsible sex may last a lifetime. In some cases they are fatal. Then there are those who enjoy bragging about their sexual conquests and mock people who choose to wait. In essence, many of these conquests are only fantasies expounded in an attempt to gain popularity with peers.

Sexual promiscuity never leads to a trusting, loving, and lasting relationship. Mature people respect others' choices. If someone does not respect your choice to wait, he or she certainly does not deserve your friendship or, for that matter, anything else. There is no greater sex than that between two loving and responsible individuals who mutually trust and admire each other. Contrary to many beliefs, these relationships are possible. They are built upon unselfish attitudes and behaviors.

As you look around, you will find people who have these values. Seek them out and build your friendships and future around people who respect you for who you are and what you believe. You don't have to compromise your choices or values. In the end, you will reap the greater rewards of a fulfilling and lasting relationship, free of AIDS and other STIs.

Also, be prepared so that you will know your course of action before you get into an intimate situation. Look for common interests and work to-gether toward them. Express your feelings openly: "I'm not ready for sex; I just want to have fun and kissing is fine with me." If your friend does not accept your answer and is not willing to stop the advances, be prepared with a strong response. Statements such as "Please stop" or "Don't!" are for the most part ineffective. Use a firm statement such as, "No, I'm not willing to do it" or "I've already thought about this, and I'm not going to have sex." If this still doesn't work, label the behavior rape: "This is rape, and I'm going to call the police."

What about those who do not have—or do not desire—a monogamous relationship? Risky behaviors that significantly increase the chances of contracting an STI, including HIV infection, are:

- Multiple or anonymous sexual partners such as a pick-up or prostitute
- Anal sex with or without a condom
- Vaginal or oral sex with someone who shoots drugs or engages in anal sex
- Sex with someone you know who has several sex partners
- Unprotected sex (without a condom) with an infected person
- Sexual contact of any kind with anyone who has symptoms of AIDS or who is a member of a group at high risk for AIDS
- Sharing toothbrushes, razors, or other implements that could become contaminated with blood with anyone who is, or might be, infected with the HIV virus

Avoiding risky behaviors that destroy quality of life and life itself is a critical component of a healthy lifestyle. Learning the facts so you can make responsible choices can protect you and those around you from startling and unexpected conditions. Using alcohol moderately (or not at all), refraining from substance abuse, and preventing sexually transmitted infections are keys to averting both physical and psychological damage.

---

www WEB INTERACTIVE

Create a Diet to Lower Your Cholesterol. This interactive website will provide personalized guidelines on how to eat healthy and decrease your risk for heart disease, based on your height, weight, age, gender, and activity level. **http://www.nhlbisupport.com/chd1/create.htm**

Cancer Prevention. Follow these seven steps to reduce your risk of cancer. **http://mayoclinic.com/health/cancer-prevention/CA00024**

Log on to academic.cengage.com/login and take a wellness inventory to assess the behaviors that might benefit most from healthy change.

1. Is your diet fundamentally low in saturated fats, trans fats, processed meats, and do you meet the daily suggested amounts of fruits, vegetables, and fiber?

2. Are you familiar with basic lifestyle guidelines to prevent cancer?

3. Is your life free of addictive behavior? If not, will you commit right now to seek professional help at your institutions' counseling center? Addictive behavior destroys health and lives, don't let it end yours.

4. Do you believe in a mutually monogamous sexual relationship as the best way to prevent STIs? If not, do you always take precautions to practice safer sex?

Log on to academic.cengage.com/login to assess your understanding of this chapter's topics by taking the chapter pre-test and exploring the modules recommended in your Personalized Study Plan.

1. Coronary heart disease
   a. is the single leading cause of death in the United States.
   b. is the leading cause of sudden cardiac deaths.
   c. is a condition in which the arteries that supply the heart muscle with oxygen and nutrients are narrowed by fatty deposits.
   d. accounts for approximately 20 percent of all deaths.
   e. All of the above are correct choices.

2. The risk for heart disease increases with
   a. high LDL cholesterol.
   b. high HDL cholesterol.
   c. lack of homocysteine.
   d. low levels of hs-CRP.
   e. all of the above factors.

3. Type 2 diabetes is related closely to
   a. low BMI.
   b. obesity and lack of physical activity.
   c. genetically low homocysteine.
   d. increased insulin sensitivity.
   e. all of the above factors.

4. Metabolic syndrome is related to
   a. low HDL cholesterol.
   b. high triglycerides.
   c. increased blood-clotting mechanism.
   d. an abnormal insulin response to carbohydrates.
   e. all of the above.

5. Cancer can be defined as
   a. a process whereby some cells invade and destroy the immune system.
   b. an uncontrolled growth and spread of abnormal cells.
   c. the spread of benign tumors throughout the body.
   d. the interference of normal body functions through blood flow disruption caused by angiogenesis.
   e. All are correct choices.

6. Cancer
   a. is primarily a preventable disease.
   b. is often related to tobacco use.
   c. has been linked to dietary habits.
   d. has a risk that increases with obesity.
   e. All are correct choices.

7. A cancer prevention diet should include
   a. ample amounts of fruits and vegetables.
   b. cruciferous vegetables.
   c. phytonutrients.
   d. soy products.
   e. all of the above.

8. The biggest carcinogenic exposure in the workplace is to
   a. asbestos fibers.
   b. cigarette smoke.
   c. biological agents.
   d. nitrosamines.
   e. pesticides.

9. Treatment of chemical dependency is
   a. primarily accomplished by the individual alone.
   b. most successful when there is peer pressure to stop.
   c. best achieved with the help of family members.
   d. seldom accomplished without professional guidance.
   e. usually done with the help of friends.

CONTINUED

10. The best way to protect yourself against sexually transmitted infections is

   a. through the use of condoms with a spermicide.
   b. by knowing about the people who have previously had sex with your partner.
   c. through a mutually monogamous sexual relationship.
   d. by having sex only with an individual who has no symptoms of STIs.
   e. All of the above choices provide equal protection against STIs.

Correct answers can be found at the back of the book.

Managing Cardiovascular Disease and Cancer Risks

Name _____ Date _____

Course _____ Section _____

I. Cardiovascular Disease

	Yes	No
1. I accumulate between 30 and 60 minutes of physical activity at least five days per week.	☐	☐

Total number of daily steps: [_____] Total minutes of daily physical activity: [_____]

	Yes	No
2. I exercise aerobically a minimum of three times a week in the appropriate target zone for at least 20 minutes per session.	☐	☐
3. I am at or slightly below the health fitness recommended percent body fat (see Chapter 2, Table 2.12, page 51), or my BMI is below 25.	☐	☐
4. My blood lipids are within normal range.	☐	☐
5. I get 25 (women) to 38 (men) grams of fiber in my daily diet.	☐	☐

Fiber is present in whole grains, fruits and vegetables (including peaches, strawberries, potatoes, spinach, and tomatoes), wheat and bran cereals, rice, popcorn, and whole-wheat bread.

	Yes	No
6. I eat more than five servings of fruits and vegetables every day.	☐	☐
7. I limit saturated fat, trans fats, and cholesterol in my daily diet.	☐	☐
8. I am not a diabetic.	☐	☐
9. My blood pressure is normal.	☐	☐
10. I do not smoke cigarettes or use tobacco in any other form.	☐	☐
11. I manage stress adequately in daily life.	☐	☐
12. I do not have a personal or family history of heart disease.	☐	☐

Evaluation

A "no" answer to any of the above items increases your risk for cardiovascular disease. The greater the number of "no" responses, the higher the risk for developing cardiovascular disease.

Please indicate lifestyle changes you will implement or maintain to decrease your personal risk for cardiovascular disease.

_____

_____

_____

_____

_____

II. Cancer Prevention Questionnaire: Cancer Risk: Are You Taking Control?

Today, scientists think most cancers may be related to lifestyle and environment—what you eat and drink, whether you smoke, and where you work and play. The good news, then, is that you can help reduce your own cancer risk by taking control of things in your daily life.

15 Steps to a Healthier Life and Reduced Cancer Risk

	Yes	No
1. Are you eating more cruciferous vegetables?		
They include broccoli, cauliflower, Brussels sprouts, all cabbages, and kohlrabi.	☐	☐
2. Are high-fiber foods included in your diet?	☐	☐
3. Do you choose foods with vitamin A?		
Fresh foods with beta-carotene—including carrots, peaches, apricots, squash, and broccoli—are the best source, not vitamin pills.	☐	☐
4. Is vitamin C included in your diet?		
You'll find it naturally in lots of fresh fruits and vegetables including grapefruit, cantaloupe, oranges, strawberries, red and green peppers, broccoli, and tomatoes.	☐	☐
5. Do you eat sufficient selenium-bearing foods (fish, Brazil nuts, whole grains) so you obtain at least 100 mcg of selenium per day (but no more than 400 mcg per day)?	☐	☐
6. Are you physically active, exercise, and monitor calorie intake to avoid weight gain?	☐	☐
7. Are you cutting overall fat intake?		
This is done by eating lean meat, fish, skinned poultry, and low-fat dairy products.	☐	☐
8. Do you limit salt-cured, smoked, and nitrite-cured foods?		
Choose bacon, ham, hot dogs, or salt-cured fish only occasionally if you like them a lot.	☐	☐
9. Are you a nonsmoker?	☐	☐
10. If you smoke, have you tried quitting?	☐	☐
11. Do you abstain from all other forms of tobacco?	☐	☐
12. If you drink alcohol, are you moderate in your intake?	☐	☐
13. Do you get up to 15 minutes of daily "safe sun" exposure (face, arms, and hands) during peak daylight hours (10:00 a.m. to 4:00 p.m.), but yet you respect the sun's rays (your skin does not turn red, and you do not sunburn)?		
Protect yourself with sunscreen (at least SPF 15) and wear long sleeves and a hat, especially during midday hours if you are going to be exposed to the sun for a prolonged period of time.	☐	☐
14. Do you have a family history of any type of cancer? (If so, you should bring this to the attention of your personal physician.)	☐	☐
15. Are you familiar with the seven warning signals for cancer?	☐	☐

Evaluation

If you answered yes to most of these questions, congratulations. You are taking control of simple lifestyle factors that will help you feel better and reduce your risk for cancer.

Please indicate lifestyle changes you will implement or maintain to decrease your personal risk for cancer:

_____

_____

_____

Relevant Fitness and Wellness Issues

© David P. Hall/Corbis

OBJECTIVES

- Dispel common misconceptions related to physical fitness and wellness
- Give practical advice and tips regarding safety
- Address some concerns specific to women
- Clarify additional concepts regarding nutrition and weight control
- Answer some questions regarding wellness and aging
- Provide guidelines related to fitness/wellness consumer issues

CENGAGENOW Log on to **CengageNOW at academic .cengage.com/login** to find innovative study tools—including pre- and post-tests, personalized study plans, activities, labs, and the personal change planner.

This chapter addresses some of the most frequently asked questions about various facets of physical fitness and wellness. The answers will further clarify concepts discussed throughout the book, as well as put to rest several myths that misinform fitness and wellness participants. "Q" denotes the question, and "A" designates the answer.

Wellness Behavior Modification Issues

Q: If a person were going to do only one thing to improve health, what would it be?

A: This is a common question. It is a mistake to think, though, that you can modify just one factor and enjoy wellness. Wellness requires a constant and deliberate effort to change unhealthy behaviors and reinforce healthy behaviors. While it is difficult to work on many lifestyle changes all at once, being involved in a regular physical activity program and proper nutrition are two behaviors I would work on first. If you use tobacco in any form, or you have any other form of chemical dependency, stop today and seek professional counseling to overcome the addictive behavior. Others behavioral changes should follow, depending on your lifestyle.

Q: Why is it so hard to change?

A: Change is incredibly difficult for most people. Our behaviors are based on our core values. Whether we are trying to increase physical activity, quit smoking, change unhealthy eating habits, or reverse heart disease; it is human nature to resist change even when we know that change will provide substantial benefits.

Furthermore, Dr. Richard Earle, managing director of the Canadian Institute of Stress and the Hans Selye Foundation, explains that people have a tendency toward pessimism. In every spoken language, there is a ratio of three pessimistic adjectives to one positive adjective. Thus, linguistically, psychologically, and emotionally, we focus on what can go wrong and we lose motivation before we even start.

Q: What triggers the desire to change?

A: Motivation comes from within. In most instances, neither pressure, reasoning, or fear will inspire people to take action. Change in behavior is most likely to occur by speaking to people's feelings. Most people start contemplating change when there is a change in core values that will make them feel uncomfortable with the present behavior(s) or lack thereof.

Core values change when feelings are addressed. The challenge is to find ways that will help people understand the problems and solutions in a manner that will influence emotions and not just the thought process. Once the problem behavior is understood and "felt," the person may become uncomfortable with the situation and will be more inclined to address the problem behavior or adoption of a healthy behavior. Discomfort is a great motivator. People tolerate any situation until it becomes too uncomfortable for them. At that point, they seek for ways to make changes in their lives. It is then that the information presented in this book provides the tools to implement a successful plan for change.

Keep in mind that as lifestyle changes are addressed, relationships and friendships may also need to be addressed. You need to distance yourself from those individuals who share your bad habits (smoking, drinking, unhealthy eating, sedentary lifestyle) and associate with people who practice healthy habits. Are you prepared to do so?

Q: Why is it so difficult to change dietary habits?

A: In most developed countries there is an overabundance of food and practically an unlimited number of food choices. With unlimited supply and choices, most people do not have the willpower, stemming from their core values to avoid overconsumption.

Our bodies were not created to go hungry or to overeat. We are uncomfortable overeating and we feel even worse when we have to go hungry. Our health values, however, are not strong enough to prevent overconsumption. The end result: weight gain. Next, we restrict calories (go on a diet), we feel hungry, and we have a difficult time adhering to the diet. Stated quite simply, going hungry is an uncomfortable and unpleasant experience. And people do not like to feel this way.

To avoid this vicious cycle, our dietary habits (and most likely physical activity habits) must change. A question you need to ask yourself is: Do you value health and quality of life more than food overindulgence? If you do not, then the achievement and maintenance of recommended body weight and good health is a mute point. If you desire to avoid disease and increase quality of life, you have to value health more than food overconsumption. If you have spent the last 20 years tasting and "devouring" every food item in sight, it is now time to make healthy choices and consume only moderate amounts (portion control) of food at a time. You do not have to taste and eat everything that is placed before your eyes. If you can make such a change in your eating habits, you may not have to worry about another diet throughout life.

Safety of Exercise Participation and Injury Prevention

Q: Can aerobic exercise make a person immune to heart and blood vessel disease?

A: Scientific evidence clearly indicates that aerobically fit individuals have a much lower incidence of cardiovascular disease. A regular aerobic exercise program by itself, however, is not an absolute guarantee against diseases of the heart and blood vessels. Several factors increase a person's risk for cardiovascular disease.

Though physical inactivity is one of the most significant risk factors, studies have documented that these risk factors have multiple interrelations. Physical inactivity, for instance, often contributes to an increase in (a) body fat, (b) LDL cholesterol, (c) triglycerides, (d) inflammation, (e) stress, (f) blood pressure, and (g) risk for diabetes (see Figure 9.1). As discussed in Chapter 8, most risk factors for cardiovascular disease are preventable and reversible. Overall management of the risk factors is the best way to minimize the risk for cardiovascular disease. Research also indicates that the odds of surviving a heart attack are much higher for people who engage in a regular aerobic exercise program.

Q: What amount of aerobic exercise is optimal to significantly decrease the risk for cardiovascular disease?

A: The amount of exercise required to maintain cardiorespiratory fitness calls for a training session approximately every 48 hours for 20 to 30 minutes in the appropriate target training zone (see Chapter 3). People who accumulate 30 minutes of moderate-intensity physical activity on most days of the week, however, can expect to reap many of the health benefits provided by a regular exercise program, although higher intensity also means higher benefits. The amount of exercise required to offset the risk cannot be pinpointed specifically because of the many individual differences (genetic and lifestyle) between people. Research, however, has shed some light on this subject.

One of the earlier studies indicated that about 300 calories should be expended daily through physical activity to obtain a certain degree of protection against cardiovascular disease.[1] A study among Harvard alumni (see Chapter 1, Figure 1.7) found that expending 2,000 calories per week as a result of physical activity yielded the lowest risk for cardiovascular disease in this group of almost 17,000 people. The 2,000 calories per week represents about 300 calories per daily exercise session.

The work alluded to in Chapter 8 (see Figure 8.5, page 197), conducted at the Aerobics Research Institute in Dallas, indicated that even moderate fitness levels can reduce the incidence of cardiovascular problems substantially.[2] The minimum dose for moderate fitness requires an expenditure of about 150 to 200 calories five to seven times per week (see Table 9.1). Greater protection, however, is achieved at higher energy expenditures and better fitness levels.

Clinical data on individuals with or at risk for coronary heart disease suggest that more than 1,400 calories per week may have to be expended to improve cardiorespiratory fitness, more than 1,500 weekly calories to stop the progression of atherosclerotic lesions, and more than 2,200 calories per week, or the equivalent of five to six hours

---

FIGURE 9.1

Interrelationships among leading cardiovascular risk factors.

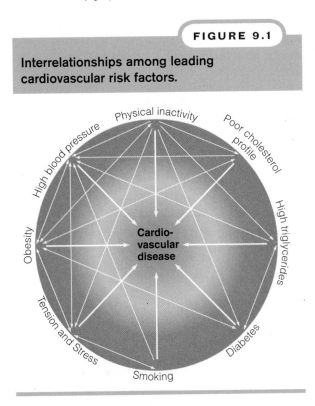

TABLE 9.1

Minimum Amount of Walking (Aerobic Activity) Required for Moderate Fitness Adults

Program 1	Days/Week	Distance (miles)	Time (min)
Women	≥3	2	≤30
Men	≥3	2	≤27
Program 2			
Women	5–6	2	30–40
Men	6–7	2	30–40

From S. N. Blair, *Fitness and Mortality* (Dallas: Aerobics Research Center, 1991).

of weekly exercise, for regression of lesions.[3] As noted in the previous question, neither physical activity nor exercise by itself provides an absolutely risk-free guarantee against cardiovascular disease.

Q: At what age should I start concerning myself with cardiovascular disease?

A: The disease process for cardiovascular disease, as well as cancer, starts early in life as a result of poor lifestyle habits. Studies have shown beginning stages of atherosclerosis and elevated blood lipids in children as young as 10 years old.

Many positive habits can be established early in life within the walls of one's own home. If people are taught at a young age that they should avoid excessive calories, sweets, salt, and alcohol; not use tobacco; and participate in physical activity, their chances of leading a healthier life are much greater than is true with the present generation. When it comes to teaching, some of the best advice that can be given is, "Come and follow me." If you cultivate positive health habits in your own life, your children will be more likely to follow.

Q: Does regular physical activity decrease cancer risk?

A: Regular physical activity has been shown to decrease the risk of developing certain types of cancer, in particular cancers of the colon, breast, endometrium, and prostate gland. Physical activity also prevents type 2 diabetes and obesity. The latter have been linked to colon, pancreatic, gallbladder,

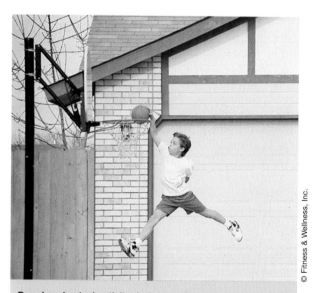

Regular physical activity during youth enhances the likelihood of lifetime participation in an exercise program.

© Fitness & Wellness, Inc.

ovarian, thyroid, cervical, and possibly other types of cancers. The American Cancer Society recommends that you aim for at least 30 minutes of moderate to vigorous physical activity five or more days per week, although 45 to 60 minutes of intentional activity are preferable. For most non–tobacco users, a healthy dietary pattern and regular physical activity are the two most significant lifestyle behaviors that reduce cancer risk.

Q: Does alcohol protect against cardiovascular disease?

A: The health benefits of moderate alcohol consumption have been extensively reported by the media, but also widely exaggerated. The media love to discuss this topic because it appears to be "a vice that's good for you." The research supports the consumption of no more than two alcoholic beverages a day for men and one a day for women as providing modest benefits in decreasing the risk for cardiovascular disease. Not reported in the media, however, is that these modest health benefits do not always apply to African Americans.

The benefits of modest alcohol use can be equated to benefits obtained through a small daily dose of aspirin (about 81 mg per day, or the equivalent of a baby aspirin), or eating a small amount of nuts each day. And aspirin or a few nuts do not lead to impaired judgment or actions that you may later regret or have to live with the rest of your life.

Alcohol is not for everyone. Alcoholism seems to have both a genetic and an environmental component. The reasons why some people can drink for years without becoming addicted, whereas others follow the downward spiral of alcoholism are not understood. The addiction develops slowly. Most people think they are in control of their drinking habits and do not realize they have a problem until they become alcoholics, when they find themselves physically and emotionally dependent on alcohol.

Short- and long-term detrimental consequences of alcohol abuse are discussed in Chapter 8 (pages 215–216). If you don't drink alcohol, don't start. Better ways to take care of your heart are to engage in regular physical activity and adhere to a healthy diet.

Q: What is more important for good health: Aerobic fitness or muscular fitness (good muscular strength)?

A: They are both important. During the initial fitness boom in the 1970s and 1980s, the emphasis was placed almost exclusively on aerobic fitness.

We now know that they both contribute to health, fitness, work capacity, and overall quality of life. Aerobic fitness is important in the prevention of cardiovascular diseases and some types of cancer; whereas muscular fitness will build strong muscles and bones, preventing osteoporosis, and will decrease the risk for low back pain and other musculoskeletal injuries.

Q: What is the best fitness activity?

A: No single physical activity, sport, or exercise contributes to the development of overall fitness (see Chapter 4, Table 4.1). Most people who exercise pick and adhere to a single mode, such as walking, swimming, or jogging. Many activities will contribute to cardiorespiratory development. The extent of contribution to other fitness components, though, varies among the activities. For total fitness, aerobic activities should be supplemented with strength and flexibility programs. Cross-training, that is, selecting different activities for fitness development and maintenance (jogging, water aerobics, spinning), adds enjoyment to the program, decrease the risk of incurring injuries from overuse, and keep exercise from becoming monotonous.

Q: Can too much exercise be detrimental to health?

A: Moderate exercise training provides many health benefits and strengthens immune function. Prolonged and intense exercise, however, can negatively affect immune function and result in increased susceptibility to upper respiratory tract infections (common cold and influenza) and viral infections. The primary concern in this area is with elite endurance athletes who train for lengthy periods of time each day. These athletes are more susceptible to infections during intense training and competition.

Q: Will exercise help me feel better?

A: Yes. Many studies have found that exercise helps people feel better, improves self-esteem and self-confidence, relieves stress, and even alleviates depression. As with the physiological benefits of exercise, regular participation in exercise yields psychological benefits. Hence, a lifetime of physical activity is just as important for mental wellness.

CRITICAL THINKING

What role do physical activity and exercise play in your life? • What impact do these have on your emotional well-being?

Q: How can I tell if I'm exceeding the safe limits for exercising?

A: The best way to determine whether you are exercising too strenuously is to check your heart rate and make sure it doesn't exceed the limits of your target zone. Exercising above this target zone may not be safe for unconditioned or high-risk individuals. You do not need to exercise beyond your target zone to gain the desired benefits for the cardiorespiratory system. Also, if your heart rate has not returned to under 120 beats per minute five minutes after you stopped exercise, you have overexerted yourself. If elevated recovery heart rates persist after you decrease exercise intensity and duration, you may have a medical condition that should be investigated.

In addition, several physical signs will tell you when you are exceeding functional limitations: rapid or irregular heart rate, difficult breathing, nausea, vomiting, lightheadedness, headaches, dizziness, pale skin, flushness, extreme weakness, lack of energy, shakiness, sore muscles, cramps, and tightness in the chest. These are all signs of exercise intolerance—the physical aversion to exercise conducted at intensity levels beyond a person's functional capacity. Learn to listen to your body. If you notice any of these symptoms, seek medical attention before continuing your exercise program.

Q: Should I exercise when I have a cold or the flu?

A: The most important consideration is to use common sense and pay attention to your symptoms. Usually you may continue exercise if your symptoms are a runny nose, sneezing, or a scratchy throat. But if you have a fever or achy muscles, or if you are vomiting, have diarrhea, or have a hacking cough, you should avoid exercise. Following an illness, be sure to ease back gradually into your program. Do not attempt to return at the same intensity and duration that you were used to prior to your illness.

Q: How fast does a person lose the benefits of exercise after stopping an exercise program?

A: How quickly the benefits of exercise are lost differs among the various components of physical fitness and also depends on the condition the person achieves before discontinuing the exercise. Specifically with regard to cardiorespiratory endurance, it has been estimated that four weeks of aerobic training are completely reversed in two consecutive weeks of physical inactivity.

If you have been exercising regularly for months or years, two weeks of inactivity will not hurt you as much as it will someone who has exercised only a few weeks. Generally speaking, within two to three days of aerobic inactivity, the cardiorespiratory system starts to lose some of its capacity. Flexibility can be maintained with two or three stretching sessions per week, and strength is maintained with just one maximal training session per week. If you have to interrupt the program for reasons beyond your control, do not attempt to resume your training at the same level you left off but, instead, build up gradually again.

You should maintain a regular fitness program even during traveling and vacation periods. When traveling, plan ahead and examine your options before you leave home. Many hotels provide in-house fitness facilities. Although the equipment often is limited, it's generally sufficient for an adequate cardiorespiratory and strength workout. Frequent travelers would benefit from joining a nationally franchised health club, a YMCA, or a YWCA. In this manner, you can continue the same exercise program while visiting different cities.

Activities that require a minimum of equipment and no facilities, such as walking, jogging, and rope jumping, are excellent alternatives for the road. If you are going to venture out in a new city, always ask for safe places to walk or jog. Nearby parks or a high school track are usually safe and help you stay away from traffic and stop lights. The strength-training (without equipment) and flexibility exercises provided in Appendixes A and B, pages 258–268, can be used to maintain your strength and flexibility. If you are visiting a resort area, fitness rental equipment, such as bikes and roller blades, is often available.

Q: What type of clothing should I wear when I exercise?

A: The type of clothing you wear during exercise is important. In general, clothing should fit comfortably and allow free movement of the various body parts. Select clothing according to expected air temperature, humidity, and exercise intensity. Avoid nylon and rubberized materials and tight clothes that interfere with the body's cooling mechanism or obstruct normal blood flow. Fabrics made from polypropylene, Capilene, Thermax, and synthetics are best. These types of fabrics wick (draw) moisture away from the skin, enhancing evaporation and cooling the body. Exercise intensity also is important because the harder you exercise, the more heat your body produces.

When exercising in the heat, avoid the hottest time of the day, between 11:00 a.m. and 5:00 p.m. Avoid surfaces such as asphalt, concrete, and artificial turfs because they absorb heat, which then radiates to the body. (Also see the discussion on exercise in hot and humid conditions on pages 233–234).

Only minimal clothing is necessary during exercise in the heat, to allow for maximal evaporation. Clothing should be lightweight, light-colored, loose-fitting, airy, and absorbent. Examples of commercially available products that can be used during exercise in the heat are Asci's Perma Plus, Cool-max, and Nike's Dri-F.I.T. Double-layer acrylic socks are more absorbent than cotton and help to prevent blistering and chafing of the feet. A straw-type hat can be worn to protect the eyes and head from the sun. Clothing for exercise in the cold is discussed on pages 234–235.

A good pair of shoes is vital to prevent lower-limb injuries. You should wear shoes manufactured specifically for your choice of activity. Other considerations for proper footwear include body type, tendency toward pronation or supination, and exercise surfaces. Shoes should have good stability, motion control, and comfortable fit. It's best to purchase shoes in the middle of the day when the feet have expanded and might be one-half size larger. For increased breatheability, choose shoes with nylon or mesh uppers. Generally, salespeople at reputable athletic shoe stores are knowledgeable and can help you select a good shoe that fits your needs. Examine your shoes

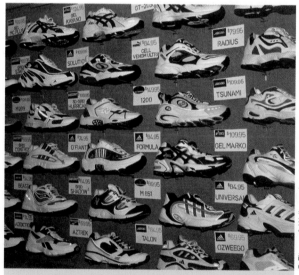

Activity-specific shoes are recommended to prevent injury to the lower extremities.

© Fitness & Wellness, Inc.

after 500 miles or six months and obtain a new pair if they are worn out. Old shoes frequently are responsible for lower-limb injuries.

Q: What time of the day is best for exercise?

A: A person can exercise at almost any time of the day except about two hours following a large meal, or the noon and early afternoon hours on hot and humid days. Many people enjoy exercising early in the morning because it gives them a good boost to start the day. If you have a difficult time sticking to an exercise program, early morning exercise is best because the chances of some other activity or conflict interfering with your exercise time are minimal. Some people prefer the lunch hour for weight-control reasons. By exercising at noon, they do not eat as big a lunch, which helps keep down daily caloric intake. Highly stressed people seem to like the evening hours because of the relaxing effects of exercise.

Q: How long should a person wait after a meal before engaging in strenuous physical exercise?

A: The length of time to wait before exercising after a meal depends on the amount of food eaten. On the average, after a regular meal a person should wait about two hours before participating in strenuous physical activity. Light physical activity, such as a walk, is fine. If anything, it helps burn extra calories and may help the body metabolize fats more efficiently.

Q: How should acute sports injuries be treated?

A: The best treatment always has been prevention. If an activity causes unusual discomfort or chronic irritation, you need to treat the cause by decreasing the intensity, switching activities, substituting equipment, or upgrading clothing, such as buying properly fitted shoes.

In cases of acute injury, the standard treatment is rest, cold application, compression or splinting (or both), and elevation of the affected body part. The applicable acronym is RICE:

R = rest
I = ice application
C = compression
E = elevation

Cold should be applied three to five times a day for 15 to 20 minutes at a time during the first 36 to 48 hours, by submerging the injured area in cold water, using an ice bag, or applying ice massage to the affected part. An elastic bandage or wrap can be used for compression. Elevating the body part

decreases blood flow to it. The purpose of these treatment modalities is to minimize swelling in the area, which hastens recovery time.

After the first 36 to 48 hours, heat can be used if the injury shows no further swelling or inflammation. If you have doubts regarding the nature or seriousness of the injury (such as suspected fracture), you should seek a medical evaluation.

Obvious deformities (such as in fractures, dislocations, or partial dislocations) call for splinting, cold application with an ice bag, and medical attention. Never try to reset any of these conditions by yourself, as muscles, ligaments, and nerves could be damaged further. These injuries should be treated by specialized medical personnel. A quick reference guide for the signs or symptoms and treatment of exercise-related problems is provided in Table 9.2.

Q: What causes muscle soreness and stiffness?

A: Muscle soreness and stiffness are common in individuals who (a) begin an exercise program or participate after a long layoff from exercise, (b) exercise beyond their customary intensity and duration, and (c) perform eccentric training. The acute soreness that sets in during the first few hours after exercise is related to general fatigue caused by chemical waste products that build up in the exercised muscles.

The delayed-onset muscle soreness (DOMS) that appears several hours after exercise (usually 12 hours or so later) and lasts two to four days may be related to microscopic tears in muscle tissue, muscle spasms that increase fluid retention and thereby stimulate the pain nerve endings, and overstretching or tearing of connective tissue in and around muscles and joints.

Two types of contraction accompany muscular activity with movement (also see the Chapter 3 discussion on mode of training—concentric muscle contraction and eccentric muscle contraction—pages 71–73). **Concentric muscle contraction** is a dynamic contraction in which the muscle shortens as it develops tension. **Eccentric muscle contraction** is a dynamic contraction in

---

KEY TERMS

Concentric muscle contraction A dynamic contraction in which the muscle shortens as it develops tension.

Eccentric muscle contraction A dynamic contraction in which the muscle lengthens as it develops tension.

TABLE 9.2

Reference Guide for Exercise-Related Problems

Injury	Signs/Symptoms	Treatment*
Bruise (contusion)	Pain, swelling, discoloration	Cold application, compression, rest
Dislocations/Fractures	Pain, swelling, deformity	Splinting, cold application, seek medical attention
Heat cramps	Cramps, spasms and muscle twitching in the legs, arms, and abdomen	Stop activity, get out of the heat, stretch, massage the painful area, drink plenty of fluids
Heat exhaustion	Fainting, profuse sweating, cold/clammy skin, weak/rapid pulse, weakness, headache	Stop activity, rest in a cool place, loosen clothing, rub body with cool/wet towel, drink plenty of fluids, stay out of heat for 2–3 days
Heat stroke	Hot/dry skin, no sweating, serious disorientation, rapid/full pulse, vomiting, diarrhea, unconsciousness, high body temperature	Seek immediate medical attention, request help and get out of the sun, bathe in cold water/spray with cold water/rub body with cold towels, drink plenty of cold fluids
Joint sprains	Pain, tenderness, swelling, loss of use, discoloration	Cold application, compression, elevation, rest, heat after 36 to 48 hours (if no further swelling)
Muscle cramps	Pain, spasm	Stretch muscle(s), use mild exercises for involved area
Muscle soreness and stiffness	Tenderness, pain	Mild stretching, low-intensity exercise, warm bath
Muscle strains	Pain, tenderness, swelling, loss of use	Cold application, compression, elevation, rest, heat after 36 to 48 hours (if no further swelling)
Shin splints	Pain, tenderness	Cold application prior to and following any physical activity, rest, heat (if no activity is carried out)
Side stitch	Pain on the side of the abdomen below the rib cage	Decrease level of physical activity or stop altogether, gradually increase level of fitness
Tendinitis	Pain, tenderness, loss of use	Rest, cold application, heat after 48 hours

*Cold should be applied 3 to 4 times a day for 15 minutes. Heat can be applied 3 times a day for 15 to 20 minutes.

which the muscle fibers lengthen while developing tension.

For example, during the arm-curl exercise, the elbow flexor muscles (biceps, brachioradialis, and brachialis) shorten as the weight is brought toward the shoulder (concentric contraction). On the way down, the muscles contract eccentrically as they lengthen while the person lowers the weight slowly to the starting position.

As you place your foot on the ground when running, the muscles contract eccentrically to absorb the weight of the body as you strike the ground. This eccentric contraction is followed by a concentric contraction of the leg as you push off the ground to propel the body forward.

Unlike running, cycling requires only concentric contractions of the leg muscles as you pedal the bicycle. Pushing down on the pedal produces a concentric contraction of the quadriceps muscles.

If you use toe clips, pulling the pedal back up to the top of the circle produces a concentric contraction of the hamstring muscles.

Eccentric training has been shown to produce more muscle soreness than concentric training does. A hard running workout, therefore, produces greater muscle soreness than a hard cycling workout of similar intensity and duration.

To prevent soreness and stiffness, the recommended approach is to warm up gradually before physical activity and to stretch adequately after exercise. Do not attempt to do too much too quickly. If you become sore and stiff, you have overdone your workout. In these cases, mild stretching, low-intensity exercise to stimulate blood flow, and a warm bath can bring relief.

Stretching may be of greatest significance following exercise. Tired muscles tend to contract to a length that is shorter than normal. Byproducts of exercise metabolism also may cause muscle spasms. Post-exercise stretching thus can help return a muscle to its normal length.

Q: What causes muscle cramps, and what should be done when they occur?

A: Muscle cramps are caused by the body's depletion of essential electrolytes or a breakdown in coordination between opposing muscle groups. If you have a muscle cramp, first attempt to stretch the muscle(s) involved. In the case of the calf muscle, for example, pull your toes up toward the knees. After stretching the affected muscles, rub them down gently, and finally do some mild exercises requiring the use of those specific muscles.

In pregnant and lactating women and people who get very little calcium in the diet, muscle cramps often are caused by a lack of this nutrient. Calcium supplements are recommended in these cases and usually relieve the problem. Tight clothing also can cause cramps because it restricts blood flow to active muscle tissue.

Q: Why is exercising in hot and humid conditions unsafe?

A: When a person exercises, only 30 to 40 percent of the energy the body produces is used for mechanical work or movement. The rest of the energy (60 to 70 percent) is converted into heat. If this heat cannot be dissipated properly because the weather is too hot or the relative humidity is too high, body temperature increases and, in extreme cases, can result in death.

The specific heat of body tissue (the heat required to raise the temperature of the body by $1°C$) is .38 calories per pound of body weight per $1°C$ (.38 cal/lb/$°C$). This indicates that if no body heat is dissipated, a 150-pound person has to burn only 57 calories ($150 \times .38$) to increase total body temperature by $1°C$. If this person were to engage in an exercise session requiring 300 calories (about 3 miles running) without dissipating any heat, the inner body temperature would increase by $5.3°C$, the equivalent of going from 98.6 to $108.1°F$.

This example clearly illustrates the need for caution when exercising in hot or humid weather. If the weather is too hot or the relative humidity is too high, body heat cannot be lost through evaporation because the atmosphere already is saturated with water vapor. In one instance, a football casualty occurred when the outdoor temperature was only $64°F$, but the relative humidity was 100 percent. As a general rule, a person must take care when air temperature is above $90°F$ and relative humidity is above 60 percent.

The American College of Sports Medicine has recommended that individuals should not engage in strenuous physical activity when the readings of a wet bulb globe thermometer exceed $82.4°F$. With this type of thermometer, the wet bulb is cooled by evaporation, and on dry days it shows a lower temperature than the regular (dry) thermometer. On humid days, the cooling effect is less because of less evaporation; hence, the difference between the wet and dry readings is not as great.

Following are symptoms of and first-aid measures for the three major signs of trouble when exercising in the heat:

1. *Heat cramps.* Symptoms include cramps and spasms and muscle twitching in the legs, arms, and abdomen. To relieve heat cramps, stop exercising, get out of the heat, stretch slowly, massage the painful area, and drink plenty of fluids (water, fruit drinks, or electrolyte beverages).

2. *Heat exhaustion.* Symptoms include fainting, dizziness, profuse sweating, cold, clammy skin, weakness, headache, and a rapid, weak pulse. If you develop any of these symptoms, stop and find a cool place to rest. Drink cool water only if conscious. Loosen or remove clothing, and rub your body with a cool/wet towel or ice packs. Place yourself in a supine position with legs elevated 8 to 12 inches. If you are not fully recovered in 30 minutes, seek immediate medical attention.

3. *Heat stroke.* Symptoms include serious disorientation; warm, dry skin; no sweating; rapid, full pulse; vomiting; diarrhea; unconsciousness; and high body temperature. As the body temperature climbs, unexplained anxiety sets in. When the body temperature reaches $104°F$ to $105°F$, the individual may feel a cold sensation in the trunk of the body, goose bumps, nausea, throbbing in the temples, and numbness in the extremities. Most people become incoherent after this stage. When body temperature reaches $105°F$ to $106°F$, disorientation, loss of fine motor control, and muscular weakness set in. If the temperature exceeds $106°F$, serious neurologic injury and death may be imminent.

Heat stroke requires immediate emergency medical attention. Request help and get out of the sun and into a cool, humidity-controlled environment. While you're waiting to be taken to the hospital's emergency room, you should be placed in a semi-seated position, and your body should be sprayed with cool water and rubbed with cool towels. If possible, cold packs should be placed in areas with abundant blood supply, such as the head, neck, armpits, and groin. Fluids should not be given if you are unconscious.

In any case of heat-related illness, if the person refuses water, vomits, or starts to lose consciousness, call for an ambulance immediately. Proper initial treatment of heat stroke is critical.

Q: What are the recommended guidelines for fluid replacement during prolonged aerobic exercise?

A: The main objective of fluid replacement during prolonged aerobic exercise is to maintain the blood volume so circulation and sweating can continue at normal levels. Adequate water replacement is the most important factor in preventing heat disorders. Drinking about 6 to 8 ounces of cool water every 15 to 20 minutes during exercise seems to be ideal to prevent dehydration. Cold fluids are absorbed more rapidly from the stomach.

Commercial fluid-replacement solutions (e.g., Powerade®, All-Sport®, Gatorade®) contain about

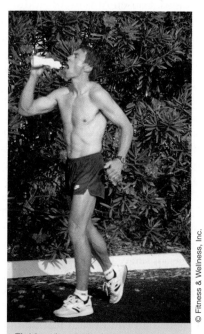

Fluid and carbohydrate replacement is essential during prolonged exercise.

© Fitness & Wellness, Inc.

6 to 8 percent glucose, which seems to be optimal for fluid absorption and performance in most cases. Commercially prepared sports drinks are recommended especially when exercise will be strenuous and carried out for more than an hour. For exercise lasting less than an hour, water is sufficient to replace fluid loss. The sports drinks you select should be based on your personal preference. Try different drinks at 6 to 8 percent glucose concentration to see which drink you tolerate best and suits your taste as well. The sugar in these products does not become available to the muscles until about 30 minutes after drinking a glucose solution.

Drinks high in fructose or with a glucose concentration above 8 percent will actually slow water absorption when you exercise in the heat. Most soft drinks (cola, noncola) contain between 10 and 12 percent glucose, an amount that is too high for proper rehydration in these circumstances.

For long-distance events, researchers recommend that 30 to 60 grams of carbohydrate (120 to 240 calories) be consumed every hour. This is best accomplished by drinking 8 ounces of a 6 to 8 percent carbohydrate sports drink every 15 minutes. The percentage of the carbohydrate drink is determined by dividing the amount of carbohydrate (in grams) by the amount of fluid (in mL) and multiplying by 100. For example, 18 grams of carbohydrate in 240 mL (8 oz) of fluid yields a drink at 7.5 percent ($18 \div 240 \times 100$).

Q: What precautions must a person take when exercising in the cold?

A: The two factors to consider when you exercise in the cold are frostbite and hypothermia. In contrast to hot and humid conditions, exercising in the cold usually is not health threatening because clothing for heat conservation can be selected and exercise itself increases the production of body heat.

Most people actually overdress for exercise in the cold. Because exercise increases body temperature, a moderate workout on a cold day makes you feel that it is 20°F to 30°F warmer than the actual temperature. Overdressing for exercise can make the clothes damp from excessive perspiration. The risk for **hypothermia** increases when a person is wet or not moving around sufficiently to increase body heat. Initial warning signs of hypothermia include shivering, loss of coordination, and difficulty in speaking. With a continued drop in body temperature, shivering stops, the muscles weaken and stiffen, and the person feels elated or intoxicated and eventually loses consciousness. To prevent hypothermia, use common sense, dress properly, and be aware of environmental conditions.

The popular belief that exercising in cold temperatures (32°F and lower) freezes the lungs is false because the air is warmed properly in the air passages before it reaches the lungs. The threat is not the cold; it's the wind velocity—which affects the chill factor greatly.

For example, exercising at a temperature of 25°F with adequate clothing is not too cold, but if the wind is blowing at 25 miles per hour, the chill factor lowers the actual temperature to 15°F. This effect is even worse if a person is wet and exhausted. On windy days, exercise (jog, cycle) against the wind on the way out and with the wind when you return.

Even though the lungs are not at risk when you exercise in the cold, your face, head, hands, and feet should be protected, because they are subject to frostbite. Watch for numbness and discoloration—signs of frostbite. In cold temperatures, as much as 50 percent of the body's heat can be lost through an unprotected head and neck. A wool or synthetic cap, hood, or hat will help to hold in body heat. Mittens are better than gloves because they keep the fingers together so the surface area from which to lose heat is less. Inner linings of synthetic material are recommended because they wick moisture away from the skin. Avoid cotton next to the skin because, once it gets wet—whether from perspiration, rain, or snow—cotton loses its insulating properties.

Wearing several layers of lightweight clothing is preferable to wearing one single, thick layer because warm air is trapped between layers of clothes, enabling greater heat conservation. As body temperature increases, you can remove layers as necessary. For prolonged or long-distance workouts (cross-country skiing or long runs), take a small backpack to carry any clothing you remove. You also can carry extra warm and dry clothes in case you stop exercising away from shelter. If you remain outdoors following exercise, added clothing and continuous body movement are essential.

The first layer of clothes should wick moisture away from the skin. Polypropylene, Capilene, and Thermax are recommended. Next, a layer of wool, dacron, or polyester fleece insulates well even when wet. Lycra tights or sweat pants help to protect the legs. The outer layer should be waterproof, wind-resistant, and breatheable. A synthetic material such as Gore-Tex is best so moisture still can escape from the body. A ski mask or face mask helps to protect the face. In extremely cold conditions, petroleum jelly can be used to protect exposed skin such as the nose, cheeks, or around the eyes.

Special Considerations for Women

Q: What are the physiological differences between men and women as related to exercise?

A: Men and women have several basic differences that affect their physical performance. On the average, men are about 3 to 4 inches taller and 25 to 30 pounds heavier than women. The average body fat in college males is about 12 percent to 16 percent, whereas in college females it is 22 percent to 26 percent.

Maximal oxygen uptake (aerobic capacity) is about 15 percent to 30 percent greater in men, caused primarily by their lower body fat content (essential fat), higher **hemoglobin** concentration, and larger heart size. The higher hemoglobin concentration allows men to carry more oxygen during exercise, which is advantageous during aerobic events. A larger heart pumps more blood with each stroke, thereby increasing the amount of oxygenated blood available to the working muscles.

The quality of muscle in men and women is the same. Men, however, are stronger because they have more muscle mass and a greater capacity for muscle hypertrophy, the muscle's ability to increase in size. The larger capacity for muscle hypertrophy is related to sex-specific hormones. Strength differences are significantly less, though, when taking into consideration body size and composition.

Men also have wider shoulders, longer extremities, and a 10 percent greater bone width, except for pelvic width. Notwithstanding all these gender differences in physiological characteristics, the two sexes respond to training in a similar way.

KEY TERMS

Hypothermia A breakdown in the body's ability to generate heat, resulting in body temperature below 95°F.

Hemoglobin Protein-iron compound in red blood cells that transports oxygen in the blood.

Q: If the potential for muscle hypertrophy in women is not as great, why do so many women body builders develop such heavy musculature?

A: The idea that strength training allows women to develop muscle hypertrophy to the same extent as men do is as false as the notion that playing basketball will turn women into giants. Masculinity and femininity are established by genetic inheritance, not by the amount of physical activity. Variations in the extent of masculinity and femininity are determined by individual differences in hormonal secretions of androgen, testosterone, estrogen, and progesterone.

Women with a bigger than average build often are inclined to participate in sports because of their natural physical advantage. As a result, many women have associated participation in sports and strength training with large muscle size.

As the number of women who participate in sports has increased, the misconception that strength training in women leads to large increases in muscle size has abated somewhat. For example, per pound of body weight, women gymnasts are considered to be among the strongest athletes in the world. These athletes engage regularly in intense strength-training programs. Yet, of all women, female gymnasts have some of the most well-toned and graceful figures.

In recent years, improved body appearance has become the rule rather than the exception for women who participate in strength-training programs. Some of the most attractive female movie stars and participants in beauty pageants train with weights to improve their personal image.

At the same time, you may ask, "If weight training doesn't masculinize women, why do so many women body builders develop such heavy musculature?" In the sport of body building, the athletes follow intense training routines consisting of two or more hours of constant weight lifting with short rest intervals between sets.

Many times, body-building training routines call for back-to-back exercises using the same muscle groups. The objective of this type of training is to pump extra blood into the muscles, which makes the muscles appear much bigger than they really are in a resting condition. Based on the intensity and the length of the training session, the muscles can remain filled with blood and appear measurably larger for several hours after completing the training session. Therefore, in real life, these women are not as muscular as they seem when they are "pumped up" for a contest.

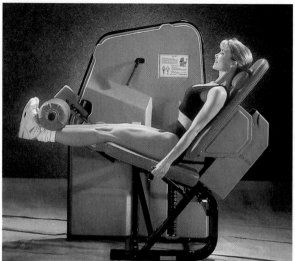

Contrary to some beliefs, high levels of strength do not lead to large muscle size in women.

© Nautilus Sports/Medical Industries, Inc.

In the sport of body building, a big point of controversy is the use of **anabolic steroids** and human growth hormones, by women as well as men. These hormones produce detrimental and undesirable side effects, which some women deem tolerable (for example, hypertension, fluid retention, smaller breasts, deepening of the voice, facial whiskers, and growth of body hair). Use of anabolic steroids in general, except for medical reasons and when monitored carefully by a physician, can have serious health consequences.

Use of anabolic steroids by women body builders is widespread. According to several sports medicine physicians and women body builders, a very high percentage of women body builders have used steroids. Furthermore, according to several women's track-and-field coaches, many women athletes in this sport around the world have used anabolic steroids and other performance-enhancing drugs to be competitive at the international level.

Undoubtedly, women who take steroids will build heavy musculature and, if they take the steroids long enough, will show masculinizing effects. As a result, the International Federation of Body Building has a mandatory drug-testing program for women participating in the Miss Olympia contest. When drugs are not used to promote development, improved body image is the rule rather than the exception in women who participate in body building, strength training, and sports in general.

Q: Does participation in exercise hinder menstruation?

A: In some instances highly trained athletes develop **oligomenorrhea** or **amenorrhea** during training and competition. These conditions are often seen in extremely lean women with disordered eating behaviors who engage in strenuous physical training over a sustained time. Amenorrhea is often associated with lower estrogen levels. Lack of estrogen leads to bone loss and a subsequent increase in risk for osteoporosis (also see the question on osteoporosis on pages 238–241).

Primary amenorrhea exists when a girl has reached the age of 16 without menstruating or she has gone two years following the development of secondary sex characteristics without the onset of menses. Secondary amenorrhea is defined as cessation of menses following normal menstrual cycles.

At present we do not know whether the disorders are caused by physical stress or emotional stress related to high-intensity training, excessively low body fat, or other factors. Intense training and decreased caloric intake (often seen in athletes in an attempt to improve performance) appears to hinder the release of hormones needed for normal menses.

The combination of disordered eating, secondary amenorrhea, and bone mineral disorders is known as the **female athlete triad** (see Figure 9.2). The triad is seen most often in highly trained young women who participate in sports. It is also referred to as the female triad because it is seen in some non-athlete women who are very lean and extremely active. A woman can have one, two, or all three parts of the triad.

The American College of Sports Medicine has issued a position statement on the female athlete triad indicating that these disorders can lead to decreased physical capacity, illness, and premature death.[4] These conditions are by no means irreversible. Women who stop menstruating because of heavy exercise training should seek the advice of a physician. A gradual increase in daily caloric intake, slight weight gain, decreased exercise training, maintenance of adequate calcium intake, and possible estrogen replacement therapy are all recommended to treat the female athlete triad.

Q: Does exercise help relieve dysmenorrhea?

A: Although exercise has not been shown to either cure or aggravate **dysmenorrhea,** it has been shown to help relieve menstrual cramps because it improves circulation to the uterus. Particularly, stretching exercises of the muscles in the pelvic region seem to reduce and prevent painful menstruation that is not the result of a disease.

Q: Is exercising safe during pregnancy?

A: Exercise is beneficial during pregnancy. According to the American College of Obstetricians and Gynecologists (ACOG), in the absence of contraindications, healthy pregnant women are encouraged to participate in regular moderate-intensity physical activities to continue to derive health benefits during pregnancy.[5] Pregnant women, however, should consult with their respective physicians to ensure that there are no contraindications to exercise during pregnancy (see box).

As a general rule, healthy pregnant women can also accumulate 30 minutes of moderate-intensity physical activity on most, if not all, days of the week. Physical activity strengthens the body and helps prepare for the challenges of labor and childbirth. The

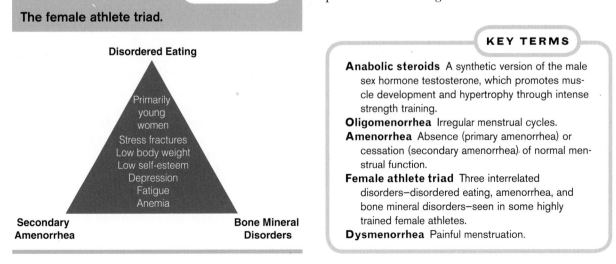

FIGURE 9.2

The female athlete triad.

Disordered Eating

Primarily young women

Stress fractures
Low body weight
Low self-esteem
Depression
Fatigue
Anemia

Secondary Amenorrhea

Bone Mineral Disorders

KEY TERMS

Anabolic steroids A synthetic version of the male sex hormone testosterone, which promotes muscle development and hypertrophy through intense strength training.

Oligomenorrhea Irregular menstrual cycles.

Amenorrhea Absence (primary amenorrhea) or cessation (secondary amenorrhea) of normal menstrual function.

Female athlete triad Three interrelated disorders—disordered eating, amenorrhea, and bone mineral disorders—seen in some highly trained female athletes.

Dysmenorrhea Painful menstruation.

average labor and delivery lasts 10–12 hours. In most cases, labor and delivery are highly intense, with repeated muscular contractions interspersed with short rest periods. Proper conditioning will better prepare the body for childbirth. Moderate exercise during pregnancy also helps to prevent back pain and excessive weight gain, and it speeds up recovery following childbirth.

The most common recommendations for exercise during pregnancy for healthy pregnant women with no additional risk factors are as follows:

1. Do not start a new or more rigorous exercise program without proper medical clearance.

2. Accumulate 30 minutes of moderate-intensity physical activities on most days of the week.

3. Instead of using heart rate to monitor intensity, exercise at an intensity level that is perceived between "moderate" and "somewhat hard." An exertion above "somewhat hard" is not recommended during pregnancy.

4. Gradually switch from weight-bearing and high-impact activities such as jogging and aerobics, to non–weight-bearing/lower-impact activities such as walking, stationary cycling, swimming, and water aerobics. The latter activities minimize the risk of injury and may allow exercise to continue throughout pregnancy.

5. Avoid exercising at an altitude above 6,000 feet (1,800 meters) or scuba diving, because these may compromise availability of oxygen to the fetus.

6. Women who are accustomed to vigorous exercise may continue in the early stages of pregnancy but should gradually decrease the amount, intensity, and exercise mode as pregnancy advances (most healthy pregnant women, however, slow down during the first few weeks of pregnancy because of morning sickness and fatigue).

7. Pay attention to the body's signals of discomfort and distress and never exercise to exhaustion. When fatigued, slow down or take a day off. Do not stop exercising altogether unless you experience any of the contraindications for exercise listed in the box on the next page.

8. To prevent fetal injury, avoid activities that involve potential contact, loss of balance, or cause even mild trauma to the abdomen. Examples of these activities are basketball, soccer, volleyball, Nordic or water skiing, ice skating, road cycling, horseback riding, and motorcycle riding.

9. Do not exercise for weight-loss purposes during pregnancy.

10. Get proper nourishment (pregnancy requires between 150 and 300 extra calories per day) and eat a small snack or drink some juice 20 to 30 minutes prior to exercise.

11. Prevent dehydration by drinking a cup of fluids 20 to 30 minutes before exercise and drink 1 cup of liquid every 15 to 20 minutes during exercise.

12. During the first three months in particular, do not exercise in the heat. Wear clothing that allows for proper dissipation of heat. A body temperature above 102.6°F (39.2°C) can harm the fetus.

13. After the first trimester, avoid exercises that require lying on the back. This position can block blood flow to the uterus and the baby.

14. Perform stretching exercises gently because hormonal changes during pregnancy increase the laxity of muscles and connective tissue. Although these changes facilitate delivery, they also make women more susceptible to injuries during exercise.

Q: What is **osteoporosis,** and how can it be prevented?

A: Osteoporosis, literally meaning "porous bones," is a condition in which bones lack the minerals required to keep them strong. In osteoporosis, bones—primarily of the hip, wrist, and spine—become so weak and brittle that they fracture readily. The process begins slowly in the third and fourth decades of life. Women are especially susceptible after menopause because of the accompanying loss of **estrogen,** which increases the rate at which bone mass is broken down.

Based on estimates, approximately 8 million women and 2 million men in the United States have osteoporosis. Postmenopausal women are at the greatest risk. About 30 percent of these women have osteoporosis, but only about 2 percent are actually diagnosed and treated for the condition.[6] The chances of a post-menopausal woman developing osteoporosis are much greater than her chances of developing breast cancer or incurring a heart attack or a stroke. Another 34 million people aged 50 and older have **osteopenia** (low bone mass). The latter figure represent 55 percent of this segment of the population.

Osteoporosis is the leading cause of serious morbidity and functional loss in the elderly population. One of every two women and one in eight men over age 50 will have an osteoporotic-related fracture at some point in their lives. Up to 20 per-

Contraindications to Exercise During Pregnancy

Stop exercise and seek medical advice if you experience any of the following symptoms:

- Unusual pain or discomfort, especially in the chest or abdominal area
- Cramping, primarily in the pelvic or lower back areas
- Muscle weakness, excessive fatigue, or shortness of breath
- Abnormally high heart rate or a pounding (palpitations) heart rate
- Decreased fetal movement
- Insufficient weight gain
- Amniotic fluid leakage
- Nausea, dizziness, or headaches
- Persistent uterine contractions
- Vaginal bleeding or rupture of the membranes
- Swelling of ankles, calves, hands, or face

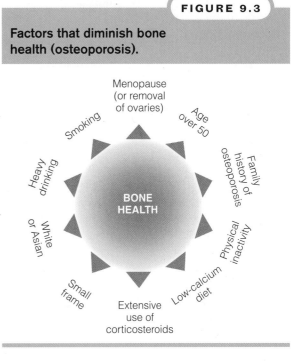

FIGURE 9.3

Factors that diminish bone health (osteoporosis).

cent of people who have a hip fracture die within a year because of complications related to the fracture. As alarming as these figures are, they do not convey the pain and loss of quality of life in people who suffer the crippling effects of osteoporotic fractures.

Although osteoporosis is viewed primarily as a women's disease, more than 30 percent of all men will be affected by age 75. About 100,000 of the yearly 300,000 hip fractures in the United States occur in men.

The genetic component is strong, but osteoporosis is preventable. Maximizing bone density at a young age and subsequently decreasing the rate of bone loss later in life are critical to preventing osteoporosis.

Normal hormone levels prior to menopause and adequate calcium intake and physical activity throughout life cannot be overemphasized. These factors are all crucial to prevent osteoporosis. The absence of any one of these three factors leads to bone loss for which the other two factors never completely compensate. Smoking, excessive use of alcohol, and corticosteroid drugs also accelerate the rate of bone loss in women and men alike. Osteoporosis is also more common in whites, Asians, and small-frame people. Figure 9.3 depicts these variables.

Bone health begins at a young age. Some experts have called osteoporosis a "pediatric disease." Bone density can be promoted early in life by making sure the diet has sufficient calcium and participating in weight-bearing activities. Adequate

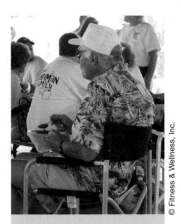

© Fitness & Wellness, Inc.

Osteoporosis is the leading cause of serious morbidity and functional loss in older adults.

KEY TERMS

Osteoporosis Softening, deterioration, or loss of bone.

Estrogen Female sex hormone; essential for bone formation and conservation of bone density.

Osteopenia Low bone mass.

TABLE 9.3

Recommended Daily Calcium Intake

Age	Amount (gr)
1–5	800
6–10	800–1,200
11–24	1,200–1,500
25–50 Women	1,000
25–64 Men	1,000
PMW* on HRT**	1,000
PMW not on HRT	1,500
>65	1,200–1,500

*PMW = Postmenopausal women

**HRT = Hormone replacement therapy

calcium intake in both women and men is also associated with a reduced risk for colon cancer.[7] The Recommended Daily Allowance (RDA) for calcium is between 1,000 and 1,300 mg per day, but leading researchers in this area recommend higher intakes (see Table 9.3). Although the recommended daily intakes can be met easily through diet alone, some experts recommend calcium supplements even for children before puberty.

To obtain your daily calcium requirement, get as much calcium as possible from calcium-rich foods, including calcium-fortified foods. If, like most people, you don't get enough, take calcium supplements.

Supplemental calcium can be obtained in the form of calcium citrate and calcium carbonate. Calcium citrate seems to be equally well absorbed with or without food, whereas calcium carbonate is not well absorbed without food. Thus if your supplement contains calcium carbonate, always take the supplement with meals. Do not take more than 500 mg at a time, because larger amounts are not well absorbed. And don't forget vitamin D, which is vital for calcium absorption.

Avoid taking calcium supplements with an iron-rich meal or in conjunction with an iron-containing multivitamin. Unfortunately, calcium interferes with iron absorption; thus, it is best to separate the intake of these two minerals. The benefit of taking a calcium supplement (calcium citrate) without food is that in a young menstruating woman who needs iron, calcium won't interfere with its absorption.

Table 9.4 provides a list of selected foods and their calcium content. Along with adequate calcium intake, taking 400 to 800 IU of vitamin D

TABLE 9.4

Calcium-Rich Foods

Food	Amount	Calcium (mg)	Calories
Beans, red kidney, cooked	1 cup	70	218
Beet, greens, cooked	½ cup	82	19
Bok choy (Chinese cabbage)	1 cup	158	20
Broccoli, cooked, drained	1 cup	72	44
Burrito, bean (no cheese)	1	57	225
Cottage cheese, 2% low-fat	½ cup	78	103
Ice milk (vanilla)	½ cup	102	100
Instant breakfast, nonfat milk	1 cup	407	216
Kale, cooked, drained	1 cup	94	36
Milk, nonfat, powdered	1 tbs	52	15
Milk, skim	1 cup	296	88
Oatmeal, instant, fortified, plain	½ cup	109	70
Okra, cooked, drained	½ cup	74	23
Orange juice, fortified	1 cup	300	110
Soy milk, fortified, fat free	1 cup	400	110
Spinach, raw	1 cup	56	12
Turnip greens, cooked	1 cup	197	29
Tofu (some types)	½ cup	138	76
Yogurt, fruit	1 cup	372	250
Yogurt, low-fat, plain	1 cup	448	155

daily is the recommendation for optimal calcium absorption. People over age 50 may require 800 to 1,000 IU. About 40 percent of these adults are deficient in vitamin D.

Excessive protein intake could also affect the body's absorption of calcium. The more protein that we eat, the higher is the calcium content in the urine (that is, the more calcium excreted). This might be the reason that countries with a high protein intake, including the United States, also have the highest rates of osteoporosis. Nonetheless, you should aim to achieve the RDA for protein, because people who consume too little protein (under 35 grams per day), lose more bone mass than those who eat too much (more than

100 grams per day). The RDA for protein is about 50 grams per day for women and 63 for men.

Vitamin B$_{12}$ may also be a key nutrient in the prevention of osteoporosis. Several reports have shown an association between low vitamin B$_{12}$ and lower bone mineral density in both men and women. Vitamin B$_{12}$ is found primarily in dairy products, meats, poultry, fish, and some fortified cereals.

Soft drinks, coffee, and alcoholic beverages can also contribute to a loss in bone density if consumed in large quantities. The damage may not be caused directly by these food items but, rather, because they take the place of dairy products in the diet.

Exercise plays a key role in preventing osteoporosis by decreasing the rate of bone loss following menopause. Active people are able to maintain bone density much more effectively than their inactive counterparts. A combination of weight-bearing exercises, such as walking or jogging and strength training, is especially helpful.

The benefits of exercise go beyond maintaining bone density. Exercise strengthens muscles, ligaments, and tendons—all of which provide support to the bones (skeleton). Exercise also improves balance and coordination, which can help prevent falls and injuries.

Current studies indicate that on the average, people who are active have denser bone mineral than inactive people do. Similar to other benefits of participating in exercise, there is no such thing as "bone in the bank." To have good bone health, people need to participate in a regular lifetime exercise program.

Prevailing research also tells us that estrogen is the most important factor in preventing bone loss. Lumbar bone density in women who have always had regular menstrual cycles exceeds that of women with a history of oligomenorrhea and amenorrhea interspersed with regular cycles. Furthermore, the lumbar density of these two groups of women is higher than that of women who have never had regular menstrual cycles.

For instance, athletes with amenorrhea (who have lower estrogen levels) have lower bone mineral density than even nonathletes with normal estrogen levels. Studies have shown that amenorrheic athletes at age 25 have the bones of women older than age 50. Over the last few years, it has become clear that sedentary women with normal estrogen levels have better bone mineral density than active amenorrheic athletes. Many experts believe the best predictor of bone mineral content is the history of menstrual regularity.

As a baseline, women age 65 and older should have a bone density test to establish the risk for osteoporosis. Younger women who are at risk for osteoporosis should discuss a bone density test with their physician at menopause. The test can also be used to monitor changes in bone mass over time and to predict the risk of future fractures. Bone density tests are painless scans requiring only small amounts of radiation to determine bone mass of the spine, hip, wrist, heel, or fingers. The amount of radiation is so low that technicians administering the test can sit right next to the person receiving it. The procedure often takes less than 10 minutes.

Following menopause, every woman should consider some type of therapy to prevent bone loss. The various therapy modalities available should be discussed with a physician.

Hormone Replacement Therapy

For decades, hormone-replacement therapy (HRT) was the most common treatment modality to prevent bone loss following menopause. A large study (16,000 healthy women, ages 50 to 79) was terminated three years early because the results showed that taking estrogen and progestin, a common form of HRT, actually increased the risk for disease.[8] The study was the first major long-term (eight-year) clinical trial investigating the association between HRT and age-related diseases that included cardiovascular disease, cancer, and osteoporosis. Although the risk for hip fractures and colorectal cancer decreased, the risk of developing breast cancer, blood clots, strokes, and heart attacks increased.

HRT may still be the most effective treatment for the relief of acute (short-term) symptoms of menopause, such as hot flashes, mood swings, sleep difficulties, and vaginal dryness. Researchers and physicians, however, must now determine how long women can remain on HRT, how to best taper off treatment to provide maximal physical and emotional relief, and how to protect women from osteoporosis and other age-related diseases. Women who believed that HRT would help them strengthen their bones and ward off age-related diseases must now seek other treatments.

New alternative treatments to prevent bone loss are being developed. Miacalcin, a synthetic form of the hormone calcitonin, is approved by the U.S.

Food and Drug Administration (FDA) for women who have osteoporosis and are at least five years postmenopausal. Calcitonin is a thyroid hormone that helps maintain the body's delicate balance of calcium by taking calcium from the blood and depositing it in the bones. Though it is effective in preventing bone loss, it does not help much in rebuilding bone. The drug seems to have no side effects. It is available in injectable and nasal spray forms.

Two promising nonhormonal drugs, alendronate (Fosamax) and risedronate (Actonel), prevent bone loss and even actually help to increase bone mass. Alendronate is recommended for women who already have osteoporosis. Alendronate is used primarily for bone health and does not provide benefits to the cardiovascular system. Although the research is limited, this drug seems to be safe and effective.

Selective estrogen receptor modulators (SERMs) are also used to prevent bone loss. These compounds have a positive effect on blood lipids and pose no risk to breast and uterine tissue. SERMs, however, do not help increase bone density. One SERM currently used to prevent osteoporosis is raloxifene (Evista).

Q: Do women have special needs for iron?

A: Iron is a key element of hemoglobin in blood. The RDA of iron for adult women is between 15 and 18 mg per day (8 to 11 mg for men). Inadequate iron intake is often seen in children, teenagers, women of childbearing age, and endurance athletes. If iron absorption does not compensate for losses or dietary intake is low, iron deficiency develops.

As many as 50 percent of American women have a deficiency of iron. Over time, excessive depletion of iron stores in the body leads to iron-deficiency anemia, a condition in which the concentration of hemoglobin in the red blood cells is lower than it should be; this leads to fatigue and headaches, among other symptoms.

Physically active individuals, women in particular, have a greater than average need for iron. Heavy training creates a demand for iron that is higher than the recommended intake because small amounts of iron are lost through sweat, urine, and stools. Mechanical trauma, caused by the pounding of the feet on the pavement during extensive jogging, may also lead to destruction of iron-containing red blood cells.

A large percentage of female endurance athletes are reported to have iron deficiency. The blood **ferritin** levels of women who participate in intense physical training should be checked frequently.

The rates of iron absorption and iron loss vary from person to person. In most cases, though, people can get enough iron by eating more iron-rich foods such as beans, peas, green leafy vegetables, enriched grain products, egg yolk, fish, and lean meats. Although organ meats, such as liver, are especially good sources, they also are high in cholesterol. A list of foods high in iron is given in Table 9.5.

TABLE 9.5

Iron-Rich Foods

Food	Amount	Iron (mg)	Calories	Cholesterol	Calories from Fat
Beans, red kidney, cooked	1 cup	4.4	218	0	4%
Beef, ground lean	3 oz	3.0	186	81	48%
Beef, sirloin	3 oz	2.5	329	77	74%
Beef, liver, fried	3 oz	7.5	195	345	42%
Beet greens, cooked	½ cup	1.4	13	0	–
Broccoli, cooked, drained	1 sm stalk	1.1	36	0	–
Burrito, bean	1	2.4	307	14	28%
Egg, hard-cooked	1	1.0	72	250	63%
Farina (Cream of Wheat), cooked	½ cup	6.0	51	0	–
Instant breakfast, whole milk	1 cup	8.0	280	33	26%
Peas, frozen, cooked, drained	½ cup	1.5	55	0	–
Shrimp, boiled	3 oz	2.7	99	128	9%
Spinach, raw	1 cup	1.7	14	0	–
Vegetables, mixed, cooked	1 cup	2.4	116	0	–

Nutrition and Weight Control

Q: What is the difference between a calorie and a kilocalorie (kcal)?

A: A calorie is the unit of measure indicating the energy value of food to the person who consumes it. It is also used to express the amount of energy a person expends in physical activity. Technically, a kilocalorie (kcal), or large calorie, is the amount of heat necessary to raise the temperature of 1 kilogram of water 1 degree centigrade. For simplicity, people call it a calorie rather than a kcal. For example, if the caloric value of a food is 100 calories (that is, 100 kcal), the energy in this food would raise the temperature of 100 kilograms of water 1 degree centigrade. Similarly, walking 1 mile would burn about 100 calories (again, 100 kcal).

Q: What constitutes ideal body weight?

A: There is no such thing as "ideal" body weight. Health/fitness professionals prefer to use the terms "recommended" or "healthy" body weight. Let's examine the question in more detail. For instance, 25 percent body fat is the recommended health fitness standard for a 40-year-old man. For the average "apparently healthy" individual, this body fat percentage does not constitute a threat to good health. Due to genetic and lifestyle conditions, however, if a person this same age at 25 percent body fat is prediabetic and prehypertensive with abnormal blood lipids (cholesterol and triglycerides—see Chapter 8), weight (fat) loss and a lower percent body fat may be recommended. Thus, what will work as recommended weight for most individuals, may not be the best standard for individuals with disease risk factors. The current recommended or healthy weight standards (based on percent body fat or body mass index [BMI]) are established at the point where there appears to be a lower incidence for overweight-related conditions for most people. Individual differences have to be taken into consideration when making a final recommendation, especially in people with risk factors or a personal and family history of chronic conditions.

Q: What is more important for weight loss: A negative caloric balance (diet) or increasing physical activity?

A: Most of the research shows that weight loss is more effective when cutting back on calories (dieting) as opposed to only increasing physical activity

or exercise. Weight loss is accelerated, nonetheless, when physical activity is added to dieting. Body composition changes, however, are much more effective when dieting and exercise are combined while attempting to lose body weight. Most of the weight loss when dieting with exercise comes in the form of body fat and not lean body tissue, a desirable outcome. Weight-loss maintenance, however, in most cases is only possible with 60 to 90 minutes of sustained *daily* physical activity or exercise.

Q: Is low-intensity aerobic exercise more effective in burning fat for weight loss purposes?

A: Without a question, vigorous-intensity aerobic exercise is more effective. True, during low-intensity exercise a greater percentage of the energy is derived from fat. It is also true that an even greater percentage of the energy comes from fat when doing absolutely nothing (resting/sleeping). And when one does nothing, as in a sedentary lifestyle, one doesn't burn many calories.

Let's examine this issue. During resting conditions, the human body is a very efficient "fat-burning machine." That is, most of the energy, approximately 70 percent, is derived from fat and only 30 percent from carbohydrates. But we burn few calories at rest, about 1.5 calories per minute as compared with 3 to 4 calories during low-intensity exercise and 8 to 10 calories per minute during vigorous-intensity exercise. As we begin to exercise, and subsequently increase the intensity of exercise, we progressively rely more on carbohydrates and less on fat for energy, until we reach maximal intensity when 100 percent of the energy is derived from carbohydrates. Even though a lower percentage of the energy is derived from fat during vigorous-intensity exercise, the total caloric expenditure is so much greater (twice as high or more), that overall the total fat burned is still higher than during moderate intensity.

A word of caution, nonetheless: Do not start vigorous-intensity exercise without several weeks of proper and gradual conditioning. Even worse if such exercise is a high impact activity. If you participate in high impact activities from the onset, you increase the risk of injury and may have to stop exercising altogether.

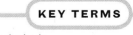

KEY TERMS

Ferritin Iron stored in the body.

Q: Can a healthy diet reduce cancer risk?

A: Much research is currently under way to examine the effects of foods in preventing and fighting off cancer. There is strong scientific evidence that a healthy diet and maintenance of recommended body weight reduce cancer risk. The current state of knowledge, however, cannot indicate that a certain dietary pattern will absolutely reduce your cancer risk. Years of research will be required to unravel most of this knowledge. Moreover, science may never be able to provide conclusive evidence that a certain diet will prevent cancer in most cases. Many of the foods that are currently recommended in a cancer-prevention diet, nonetheless, are similar to those encouraged to decrease disease risk and enhance health and overall well-being. If you are truly adhering to healthy dietary guidelines (see the Behavior Modification Planning box on page 136), you are most likely eating the right foods to decrease your cancer risk.

Q: Are fruits and vegetables less nutritious today?

A: The notion that the soil is depleted of nutrients is one of those myths that has been hard to rectify. The following are comments from Dr. Gary Banuelos, a soil scientist with the USDA Research Service in Fresno, California:[9]

Fruits, vegetables, and grains will not grow, cannot be sold, and will not be bought if they contain insufficient nutrition. If there's an inadequate amount of nutrients in the soil, plants may die because of insect infestation or disease, or cannot be sold because of poor appearance.

Many other scientists have echoed these words. Promoters of this myth are either misinformed or are not telling you the truth. Most of the time they are trying to promote supplements for personal financial gain.

Q: Are organic foods better than conventional foods?

A: Concerns over pesticides in foods has led many people to turn to organic foods. Currently, less than 2 percent of imported food products is inspected by the FDA and domestic food is seldom inspected at all. Health risks from pesticide exposure from foods are relatively small for healthy adults. The health benefits of produce far outweigh the risks. Children, older adults, pregnant and lactating women, and people with a weak immune system, however, may be vulnerable to some types of pesticides.

Organic crops have to be grown without the use of conventional pesticides, artificial fertilizers, human waste, or sewage sludge, and have been processed without ionizing radiation or food additives. Organic livestock is raised under certain grazing conditions, using organic feed, and without the use of antibiotics and growth hormones.

While pesticide residues in organic foods are substantially lower than conventionally grown foods, organic foods can also be contaminated with bacteria, pathogens, and heavy metals that pose major health risks. The soil itself may become contaminated or if the produce comes in contact with feces of grazing cattle, wild animals or birds, farm workers, or any other source, potentially harmful microorganisms can contaminate the produce. The best safeguard to protect yourself is to follow the food safety recommendations, items 9 to 14, under the 2005 Dietary Guidelines for Americans provided in Chapter 5, pages 139–140.

Q: Fish is known to be heart healthy. Should we worry about mercury toxicity concerns?

A: Fish and shellfish contain high-quality protein, omega-3 fatty acids, and other essential nutrients. Fish is lower in saturated fat and cholesterol than meat or poultry. Data indicate that eating as little as 6 ounces of fatty fish per week reduces the risk of premature death from heart disease as well as overall death rates. Fish also appears to have anti-inflammatory properties that can help treat chronic inflammatory kidney disease, osteoarthritis, rheumatoid arthritis, Crohn's disease, and autoimmune disorders like asthma and lupus. Thus, fish is one of the healthiest foods we can consume.

Potential contaminants in fish, in particular mercury, have created concerns among some people. Mercury, a natural occurring trace mineral, can be released into the air from industrial pollution. As mercury falls into streams and oceans, it accumulates in the aquatic food chain. Larger fish accumulate larger amounts of mercury because they eat medium and small-size fish. Of particular concern are shark, swordfish, king mackerel, pike, bass, and tilefish that have higher levels. Farm-raised salmon also has slightly higher levels of polychlorinated biphenyls (PCBs), which the Environmental Protection Agency (EPA) lists as a "probable human carcinogen."

The American Heart Association recommends consuming fish twice a week. The risk for adverse effects from eating fish is extremely low and primarily theoretical in nature. For most people, eating two servings (up to 6 ounces) of fish per week poses no health threat. Pregnant and nursing women, and young children, however, should avoid mercury in fish.

The best recommendation is to balance the risks against the benefits. If you are concerned, consume no more than 12 ounces per week of a variety of fish and shellfish that are lower in mercury, including canned light tuna, wild salmon, shrimp, pollock, catfish, and scallops. Seafood is among the best foods one can consume for good health.

Q: In many instances, why don't the different fats listed on food labels add up to the total amount of fat listed on the labels?

A: Trans fatty acids have been listed on the label separately as "trans fat." They constitute only a small part of the total fat in most foods. As of 2006, however, food labels have to include the trans fat content. Glycerol is also included in the total amount of fat because it is used as a building block for fatty acids (triglycerides).

Hydrogen is often added to monounsaturated and polyunsaturated fats to increase shelf life and to solidify them so they are more spreadable. During this process, called "partial hydrogenation," the position of hydrogen atoms may be changed along the carbon chain, transforming the fat into a **trans fatty acid.**

Margarine and spreads, crackers, cookies, dairy products, meats, and fast foods often contain trans fatty acids. Trans fatty acids are not essential and provide no known health benefit. Health-conscious people minimize intake of these types of fats, because diets high in trans fatty acids create an inflammatory response that contributes to heart disease and cancer. Paying attention to food labels is important, because the words "partially hydrogenated" and "trans fat" indicate that the product carries a health risk just as high as that of saturated fat.

Q: Are "natural" supplements to boost metabolism safe?

A: Supplements to boost metabolism contain stimulants that are harmful to individuals sensitive to such substances. These stimulants can also cause damage to people with metabolic disorders, heart disease, and high blood pressure. A physician or registered dietitian should be consulted prior to taking such supplements.

Q: Do athletes or individuals who train for long periods need a special diet?

A: In general, athletes do not require special supplementation or any other special type of diet. Unless the diet is deficient in basic nutrients, no special, secret, or magic diet will help people perform better or develop faster as a result of what they eat. As long as the diet is balanced, based on a large variety of nutrients from the basic food groups, athletes do not require additional supplements. Even in strength training and body building, protein in excess of 20 percent of total daily caloric intake is not necessary.

The main difference between a sedentary person and a highly active individual is in the total number of calories required daily and the amount of carbohydrate intake during bouts of prolonged physical activity. During training, people consume more calories because of the greater energy expenditure required as a result of intense physical training.

A regular diet should be altered to include about 70 percent carbohydrates (carbohydrate loading) during several days of heavy aerobic training or when a person is going to participate in a long-distance event of more than 90 minutes (marathons, triathlons, road cycling races). For events shorter than 90 minutes, carbohydrate loading does not seem to enhance performance.

Q: Are there specific nutrient requirements for optimal development and recovery following exercise?

A: Carbohydrates with some protein appear to be best. Protein is recommended prior to and immediately following high-intensity aerobic or strength-training exercise. Intense exercise causes microtears in muscle tissue and the presence of amino acids (the building blocks of proteins) in the blood contributes to the healing process and subsequent development and strengthening of the muscle fibers. Protein consumption along with carbohydrates also accelerates glycogen replenishment in the body after intense or prolonged exercise. Thus, carbohydrates provide energy for exercise and replenishment of glycogen stores after exercise, while protein optimizes muscle repair,

> **KEY TERMS**
>
> **Trans fatty acid** Solidified fat formed by adding hydrogen to monounsaturated and polyunsaturated fats to increase shelf life.

growth, glycogen replenishment, and recovery following exercise. Aim for a ratio of 4 to 1 grams of carbohydrates to protein. For example, you may consume a snack that contains 40 grams of carbohydrates (160 calories) and 10 grams of protein (40 calories). Examples of good recovery foods include milk and cereal, a tuna fish sandwich, a peanut butter and jelly sandwich, or pasta with turkey meat sauce.

Exercise and Aging

Q: What is the relationship between aging and physical work capacity?

A: The elderly population constitutes the fastest growing segment of the U.S. population. The number of Americans 65 and older increased from 3.1 million in 1900 (4.1 percent of the population) to more than 34 million (12.8 percent) in 1996. By the year 2030, more than 70 million people, or 22 percent of the population in the United States, are expected to be older than age 65.

The main objective of fitness programs for older adults is to help them improve their **functional fitness** and contribute to healthy aging. This implies the ability to maintain **functional independence** and to avoid disability. Older adults are encouraged to participate in programs that will help develop cardiorespiratory endurance, muscu-

lar strength and endurance, muscular flexibility, agility and balance, and motor coordination.

Data on individuals who have taken part in systematic physical activity throughout life indicate that these groups of people maintain a higher level of functional capacity and do not experience the typical declines in later years. From a functional point of view, typical sedentary Americans are about 25 years older than their chronological age indicates. Thus, an active 60-year-old person can have a work capacity similar to that of a sedentary 35-year-old.

Unhealthy behaviors precipitate premature aging. For sedentary people, productive life ends at about age 60. Most of these people hope to live to be 65 or 70 and often must cope with serious physical ailments. These people stop living at age 60 but choose to be buried at age 70! (See the theoretical model in Figure 9.4.)

A healthy lifestyle allows people to live a vibrant life—physically, intellectually, emotionally, socially active, and functionally independent existence—to age 95. When death comes to active people, it usually is rather quick and not as a result of prolonged illness (see Figure 9.4). Such are the rewards of a wellness way of life.

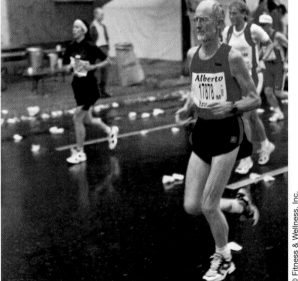

Exercise enhances quality of life and longevity.

© Fitness & Wellness, Inc.

FIGURE 9.4

Relationships among physical work capacity, aging, and lifestyle habits.

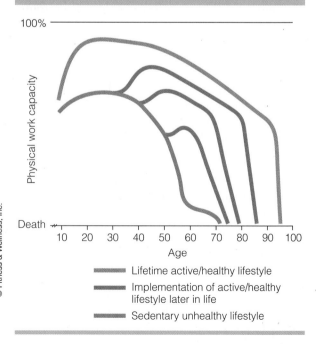

Lifetime active/healthy lifestyle

Implementation of active/healthy lifestyle later in life

Sedentary unhealthy lifestyle

Regular participation in physical activity provides both physiologic and physical benefits to older adults.[10] Cardiorespiratory endurance training helps to increase functional capacity, decrease the risk for disease, improve health status, and increase life expectancy. Strength training decreases the rate of strength and muscle mass loss commonly associated with aging. Among the psychological benefits are preserved cognitive function, reduced symptoms and behaviors related to depression, and improved self-confidence and self-esteem.

CRITICAL THINKING

Have you ever considered how you would like to feel and what type of activities you would like to carry on after age 65? • What will it take for you to accomplish your goals?

Q: Do older adults respond to physical training?

A: The trainability of older men and women alike and the effectiveness of physical activity in enhancing health have been demonstrated in prior research. Older adults who increase their physical activity experience significant changes in cardiorespiratory endurance, strength, and flexibility. The extent of the changes depends on their initial fitness level and the types of activities they select for their training (walking, cycling, strength training, and so on).

Improvements in maximal oxygen uptake in older adults are similar to those of younger people, although older people seem to require a longer training period to achieve these changes. Declines in maximal oxygen uptake average about 1 percent per year between ages 25 and 75. A slower rate of decline is seen in people who maintain a lifetime aerobic exercise program.

Results of research on the effects of aging on the cardiorespiratory system of male exercisers versus nonexercisers showed that the maximal oxygen uptake of regular exercisers was almost twice that of the nonexercisers.[11] The study revealed a decline in maximal oxygen uptake, between ages 50 and 68, of only 13 percent in the active group compared with 41 percent in the inactive group. These changes indicate that about one-third of the loss in maximal oxygen uptake results from aging and two-thirds of the loss comes from inactivity.

Blood pressure, heart rate, and body weight also were remarkably better in the exercising group.

Furthermore, aerobic training seems to decrease high blood pressure in the older participants at the same rate as in young, hypertensive people.

Muscle strength declines by 10 to 20 percent between the ages of 20 and 50, but between ages 50 and 70 it drops by another 25 to 30 percent. Through strength training, frail adults in their 80s or 90s can double or triple their strength in just a few months. The amount of muscle hypertrophy achieved, however, decreases with age. Strength gains close to 200 percent have been found in previously inactive adults older than 90. In fact, research has shown that regular strength training improves balance, gait, speed, functional independence, morale, depression symptoms, and energy intake.[12]

Although muscle flexibility drops by about 5 percent per decade of life, 10 minutes of stretching every other day can prevent most of this loss as a person ages. Improved flexibility enhances mobility skills. The latter promotes independence because it helps older adults successfully perform **activities of daily living.**

In terms of body composition, inactive adults continue to gain body fat after age 60 despite the tendency toward lower body weight. The increase in body fatness is most likely caused by a decrease in basal metabolic rate and physical activity along with increased caloric intake above that required to maintain daily energy requirements.

Older adults who wish to initiate or continue an exercise program are strongly encouraged to have a complete medical exam, including a stress electrocardiogram test (see Chapter 8). Recommended activities for older adults include calisthenics, walking, jogging, swimming, cycling, and water aerobics.

Older people should avoid isometric and very high intensity strength-training exercises. Activities that require all-out effort or require participants to hold their breath (Valsalva maneuver) tend to

KEY TERMS

Functional fitness The physical capacity of the individual to meet ordinary and unexpected demands of daily life safely and effectively.

Functional independence Ability to carry out activities of daily living without assistance from other individuals.

Activities of daily living Everyday behaviors that people normally do to function in life (cross the street, carry groceries, lift objects, do laundry, sweep floors).

lessen blood flow to the heart and cause a significant increase in blood pressure and the load placed on the heart. Older adults should participate in activities that require continuous and rhythmic muscular activity (about 40 to 60 percent of functional capacity). These activities do not cause large increases in blood pressure or place an intense overload on the heart.

Fitness/Wellness Consumer Issues

Q: How do I protect myself from quackery and fraud in the fitness/wellness industry?

A: The rapid growth in fitness and wellness programs during the last three decades has spurred **quackery** and **fraud.** The promotion of fraudulent products has deceived consumers into adopting "miraculous," quick, and easy ways toward total well-being.

Today's market is saturated with "special" foods, diets, supplements, pills, cures, equipment, books, and videos that promise quick, dramatic results. Advertisements for these products often are based on testimonials, unproven claims, secret research, half-truths, and quick-fix statements that the uneducated consumer wants to hear. In the meantime, the organization or enterprise making the claims stands to reap a large profit from consumers' willingness to pay for astonishing and spectacular solutions to problems related to their unhealthy lifestyle.

Television, magazine, and newspaper advertisements are not necessarily reliable. For instance, one piece of equipment sold through television and newspaper advertisements promised to "bust the gut" through five minutes of daily exercise that appeared to target the abdominal muscle group. This piece of equipment consisted of a metal spring attached to the feet on one end and held in the hands on the other end. According to handling and shipping distributors, the equipment was "selling like hotcakes," and companies could barely keep up with consumers' demands.

Three problems became apparent to the educated consumer. First, there is no such thing as spot-reducing; therefore, the claims could not be true. Second, five minutes of daily exercise burn hardly any calories and, therefore, have no effect on weight loss. Third, the intended abdominal (gut) muscles were not really involved during the exercise. The exercise engaged mostly the gluteal

and lower-back muscles. This piece of equipment now can be found at garage sales for about a tenth of its original cost!

Although people in the United States tend to be firm believers in the benefits of physical activity and positive lifestyle habits as a means to promote better health, most do not reap these benefits because they simply do not know how to put into practice a sound fitness and wellness program that will give them the results they want. Unfortunately, many uneducated wellness consumers are targets of deception by organizations making fraudulent claims for their products.

Deception is not limited to advertisements. Deceit is found all around us. One can find it in newspaper and magazine articles, trade books, radio, and television shows. To make a profit, popular magazines occasionally exaggerate health claims or leave out pertinent information to avoid offending advertisers. Some publishers print books on diets or self-treatment approaches that have no scientific foundation. Consumers should even be cautious about news reports of the latest medical breakthroughs. Reporters have been known to overlook important information or give certain findings greater credence than they deserve.

Precautions must also be taken when seeking health advice on the Internet. The Internet is full of both credible and dubious information. The following tips can help as you conduct a search on the Internet:

- Look for credentials of the person or organization sponsoring the website.
- Check when the site was last updated. Credible sites are updated often.
- Check the appearance of the information on the site. It should be presented in a professional manner. If every sentence ends with an exclamation point, you have good cause for suspicion.
- Be cautious if the website's sponsor is trying to sell a product. If so, be leery of opinions posted on the site. They could be biased, given that the company's main objective is to sell a product. Credible companies trying to sell a product on the Internet usually reference their sources of health information and provide additional links that support their product.
- Compare the content of a website with other credible sources. The content should compare favorably with that of other reputable sites or publications.

- Note the address and contact information for the company. A reliable company will list more than a PO box, an 800 number, and the company's e-mail address. When only the latter information is provided, consumers may never be able to locate the company for questions, concerns, or refunds.
- Be on the alert for companies that claim to be innovators while criticizing competitors or the government for being closed-minded or trying to keep them from doing business.
- Watch for advertisers that use valid medical terminology in an irrelevant context or use vague pseudomedical jargon to sell their product.

Not all people who promote fraudulent products know they are doing so. Some may be convinced that the product is effective. If you have questions or concerns about a health product, you may write to the National Council Against Health Fraud (NCAHF), PO Box 141, Fort Lee, NJ 07021. The purpose of this organization is to provide consumers with responsible, reliable, evidence-driven health information. The organization also monitors deceitful advertising, investigates complaints, and offers public information regarding fraudulent health claims. You may also report any type of quackery to the NCAHF on its website at http://www.ncahf.org/. The site contains an updated list of reliable and unreliable health websites for the consumer.

Other consumer protection organizations offer to follow up on complaints about quackery and fraud. The existence of these organizations, however, should not give the consumer a false sense of security. The overwhelming number of complaints made each year to these organizations makes it impossible for them to follow up on each case individually.

The FDA's Center for Drug Evaluation Research, for example, has developed a priority system to determine which health fraud product it should regulate first. Products are rated on how great a risk they pose to the consumer. With this in mind, you can use the following list of organizations to make an educated decision before you spend your money. You can also report consumer fraud to these organizations:

- *Better Business Bureau (BBB).* The BBB can tell you whether other customers have lodged complaints about a product, a company, or a salesperson. You can find a listing for the local office in the business section of the phone book, or you can check its website at http://www.betterbusinessbureau.com/.
- *Consumer Product Safety Commission (CPS).* This independent federal regulatory agency targets products that threaten the safety of American families. Unsafe products can be researched and reported on its website at http://www.cpsc.gov/.
- *U.S. Food and Drug Administration (FDA).* The FDA regulates safety and labeling of health products and cosmetics. You can search for the office closest to you in the federal government listings (blue pages) of the phone book.

Another way to get informed before you make your purchase is to seek the advice of a reputable professional. Ask someone who understands the product but does not stand to profit from the transaction. As examples, a physical educator or an exercise physiologist can advise you regarding exercise equipment; a registered dietitian can provide information on nutrition and weight control programs; a physician can offer advice on nutritive supplements. Also, be alert to those who bill themselves as "experts." Look for qualifications, degrees, professional experience, certifications, and reputation.

Keep in mind that if it sounds too good to be true, it probably is. Fraudulent promotions often rely on testimonials or scare tactics and promise that their products will cure a long list of unrelated ailments. They use words such as quick-fix, time-tested, newfound, miraculous, special, secret, all natural, mail-order only, and money-back guarantee. Deceptive companies move often enough that customers have no way of contacting the company to ask for a reimbursement.

When claims are made, ask where the claims are published. Refereed scientific journals are the most reliable sources of information. When a researcher submits information for publication in a refereed journal, at least two qualified and reputable professionals in the field conduct blind reviews of the manuscript. A blind review means that the author does not know who will review the manuscript and the reviewers do not know who submitted the manuscript. Acceptance for publication is based on this input and relevant changes.

KEY TERMS

Quackery/fraud The conscious promotion of unproven claims for profit.

Q: What guidelines should I follow when looking for a reputable health/fitness facility?

A: As you follow a lifetime wellness program, you may want to consider joining a health/fitness facility. Or, if you have mastered the contents of this book and your choice of fitness activity is one you can pursue on your own (walking, jogging, cycling), you may not need to join a health club. Barring injuries, you may continue your exercise program outside the walls of a health club for the rest of your life. You also can conduct strength-training and stretching programs in your own home (see Chapters 3 and 4 and Appendices A, B, and C).

To stay up-to-date on fitness and wellness developments, you probably should buy a reputable and updated fitness/wellness book every four or five years. You also might subscribe to a credible health, fitness, nutrition, or wellness newsletter to stay current. You can also surf the Web—but be sure that the websites you are searching are from credible and reliable organizations.

Joining a health fitness facility provides the opportunity to exercise in a safe environment under qualified supervision. Most likely you will have state-of-the-art equipment available for exercise and other beneficial health and wellness activities. The social component of exercising at a health/fitness center can enhance exercise compliance. If you are contemplating membership in a fitness facility:

- Make sure that the facility complies with the standards established by the American College of Sports Medicine (ACSM) for health and fitness facilities. These standards are given in Figure 9.5.
- Examine all exercise options in your community—health clubs/spas, YMCAs, gyms, colleges, schools, community centers, senior centers, and the like.
- Check to see if the facility's atmosphere is pleasurable and nonthreatening to you. Will you feel comfortable with the instructors and other people who go there? Is it clean and well kept up? If the answer is no, this may not be the right place for you.
- Analyze costs versus facilities, equipment, and programs. Take a look at your personal budget. Will you really use the facility? Will you exercise there regularly? Many people obtain memberships and permit dues to be withdrawn automatically from a local bank account, yet seldom attend the fitness center.

FIGURE 9.5

American College of Sports Medicine standards for health and fitness facilities.

1. A facility must have an appropriate emergency plan.
2. A facility must offer each adult member a pre-activity screening that is relevant to the activities that will be performed by the member.
3. Each person who has supervisory responsibility must be professionally competent.
4. A facility must post appropriate signs in those areas of a facility that present potential increased risk.
5. A facility that offers services or programs to youth must provide appropriate supervision.
6. A facility must conform to all relevant laws, regulations, and published standards.

SOURCE: Adapted from *ACSM's Health/Fitness Facility Standards and Guidelines* (Champaign, IL: Human Kinetics, 1997).

- Find out what types of facilities are available: walking/running track, basketball/tennis/racquetball courts, aerobic exercise room, strength-training room, pool, locker rooms, saunas, hot tubs, handicapped access, and so on.
- Check the aerobic and strength-training equipment available. Does the facility have treadmills, bicycle ergometers, stair climbers, cross-country skiing simulators, free weights, strength-training machines? Make sure the facilities and equipment meet your activity interests.
- Consider the location. Is the facility close, or do you have to travel several miles to get there? Distance often discourages participation.
- Check on times the facility is accessible. Is it open during your preferred exercise time (for example, early morning or late evening)?
- Work out at the facility several times before becoming a member. Are people standing in line to use the equipment, or is it readily available during your exercise time?
- Inquire about the instructors' qualifications. Do the fitness instructors have college degrees or professional certifications from organizations such as the ACSM or the International Dance Exercise Association (IDEA)? These organizations have rigorous standards to ensure professional preparation and quality of instruction.
- Consider the approach to fitness (including all health-related components of fitness). Is it well rounded? Do the instructors spend time with members, or do members have to seek them out constantly for help and instruction?

care expenses and time under medical supervision, and a longer more productive life. Without question, these benefits altogether translate into one great benefit: a higher quality of life. That is, the freedom to live life to its fullest without functional and health limitations. People go through life wishing that they could live without functional limitations. The power, nevertheless, is within each one of us to do so. And such is only accomplished by taking action today and living a wellness way of life for the rest of our lives.

What's Next?

The objective of this book is to provide you with the basic information necessary to implement your personal healthy lifestyle program. Your activities over the last few weeks or months may have helped you develop positive habits that you should try to carry on throughout life.

Now that you are about to finish this course, the real challenge will be a lifetime commitment to fitness and wellness. Adhering to the program in a structured setting is a lot easier. Fitness and wellness is a continual process. As you proceed with the program, keep in mind that the greatest benefit is a higher quality of life.

Most people who adopt a wellness way of life recognize this new quality after only a few weeks into the program. For some people—especially individuals who have led a poor lifestyle for a long time—establishing positive habits and gaining feelings of well-being might take a few months. In the end, however, everyone who applies the principles of fitness and wellness will reap the desired benefits.

CRITICAL THINKING

What impact has this course had on your personal fitness and healthy lifestyle program? • Have you implemented changes that are improving your quality of life?

Being diligent and taking control of yourself will provide you a better, happier, healthier, and more productive life. Be sure to maintain a program based on your needs and what you enjoy doing most. This will make the journey easier, and you'll have more fun along the way. Once you reach the top, you will know there is no looking back. Improving your longevity and quality of life now is in your hands. It will require persistence and commitment, but only you can take control of your lifestyle and thereby reap the benefits of wellness.

www WEB INTERACTIVE

Lifescan Health Risk Appraisal. This website was created by Bill Hettler, M.D., of the National Wellness Institute and features a series of questions to help you identify what specific lifestyle factors can impair your health and longevity.
http://wellness.uwsp.edu/other/lifescan/

Select Your Health Quiz. Test your general health and medical knowledge; select Health and choose from the over twenty health conditions.
http://www.ivillage.com/quiz

ASSESS YOUR BEHAVIOR

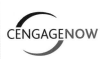

Log on to **academic.cengage.com/login** *and take a wellness inventory to assess the behaviors that might benefit most from healthy change.*

1. Has your level of physical activity increased, compared with the beginning of the term?

2. Do you participate in a regular exercise program that includes cardiorespiratory endurance, muscular strength, and muscular flexibility training?

3. Is your diet healthier now, compared with a few weeks ago?

4. Are you able to take pride in the lifestyle changes that you have implemented over the last several weeks? Have you rewarded yourself for your accomplishments?

CENGAGENOW

*Log on to **academic.cengage.com/login** to assess your understanding of this chapter's topics by taking the chapter pre-test and exploring the modules recommended in your Personalized Study Plan.*

1. A regular aerobic exercise program
   a. makes a person immune to heart disease.
   b. significantly decreases the risk for cardiovascular disease.
   c. decreases HDL cholesterol.
   d. increases triglycerides.
   e. All are correct choices.

2. Which of the following is *not* a sign that you have exceeded your functional limitations during exercise?
   a. Dizziness
   b. Difficult breathing
   c. Tightness in the chest
   d. Irregular heart rate
   e. All of the above are signs of overexertion.

3. The standard treatment for an acute injury is
   a. rest.
   b. cold application.
   c. compression.
   d. elevation.
   e. All choices apply.

4. Which of the following recommendations is false regarding exercise during pregnancy?
   a. Women who are accustomed to strenuous exercise may continue to do so in the early stages of pregnancy.
   b. After the first trimester, women should avoid exercises that require lying on the back.
   c. Exercise above 6,000 feet of altitude is not recommended.
   d. Women are encouraged to exercise above a "somewhat hard" exertion level.
   e. Women may accumulate 30 minutes of moderate-intensity physical activities on most days of the week.

5. From a functional point of view, typical sedentary people in the United States are about _____ years older than their chronological age indicates.
   a. 2
   b. 8
   c. 15
   d. 25
   e. 50

6. A person suffering from heat stroke
   a. requires immediate medical attention.
   b. should be placed in a cool, humidity-controlled environment.
   c. should be sprayed with cool water and rubbed with cool towels.
   d. should not be given fluids if unconscious.
   e. All of the above are correct choices.

7. Drinking about a cup of cool water every _____ minutes seems to be ideal to prevent dehydration during exercise in the heat.
   a. 5
   b. 15 to 20
   c. 30
   d. 30 to 45
   e. 60

8. Improvements in maximal oxygen uptake in older adults (compared with younger adults) as a result of cardiorespiratory endurance training are
   a. similar.
   b. higher.
   c. lower.
   d. difficult to determine.
   e. nonexistent.

9. Osteoporosis is
   a. a crippling disease.
   b. more prevalent in women.
   c. higher in people who were calcium deficient at a young age.
   d. linked to heavy drinking and smoking.
   e. All are correct choices.

10. To protect yourself from consumer fraud when buying a new product,
    a. get as much information as you can from the salesperson.
    b. obtain details about the product from another salesperson.
    c. ask someone who understands the product but does not stand to profit from the transaction.
    d. obtain all the research information from the manufacturer.
    e. All choices are correct.

Correct answers can be found at the back of the book.

Fitness and Wellness Lifestyle Self-Evaluation

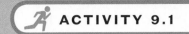

Name _____   Date _____

Course _____   Section _____

I. Explain the exercise program that you implemented in this course. Express your feelings about the outcomes of this program and how well you accomplished your fitness goals.

_____

_____

_____

_____

_____

_____

_____

_____

_____

_____

II. List nutritional or dietary changes that you were able to implement this term and the effects of these changes on your body composition and personal wellness.

_____

_____

_____

_____

_____

_____

_____

_____

_____

_____

_____

III. List other lifestyle changes that you were able to make this term that may decrease your risk for disease. In a few sentences, explain how you feel about these changes and their impact on your overall well-being.

_____

_____

_____

_____

_____

_____

_____

_____

_____

_____

V. Indicate your total number of daily steps at the beginning of this course: ⬚

Indicate your current total number of daily steps: ⬚

VI. Briefly evaluate this course and its impact on your quality of life. Indicate what you feel will be needed for you to continue to adhere to an active and healthy lifestyle.

_____

_____

_____

_____

_____

_____

_____

_____

_____

_____

_____

_____

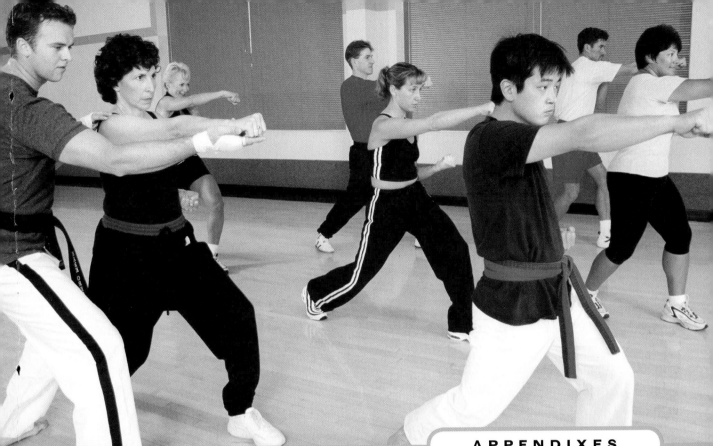

© Rob & Sas/Corbis

Strength-Training Exercises
Strength-Training Exercises Without Weights

EXERCISE 1
STEP-UP

Action: Step up and down using a box or chair approximately 12 to 15 inches high. Conduct one set using the same leg each time you go up and then conduct a second set using the other leg. You could also alternate legs on each step-up cycle. You may increase the resistance by holding a child or some other object in your arms (hold the child or object close to the body to avoid increased strain in the lower back.)

Muscles Developed: Gluteal muscles, quadriceps, gastrocnemius, and soleus.

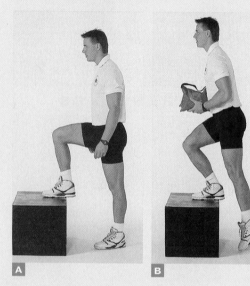

Photos © Fitness & Wellness, Inc.

EXERCISE 2
ROWING TORSO

Action: Raise your arms laterally (abduction) to a horizontal position and bend your elbows to 90°. Have a partner apply enough pressure on your elbows to gradually force your arms forward (horizontal flexion) while you try to resist the pressure. Next, reverse the action, horizontally forcing the arms backward as your partner applies sufficient forward pressure to create resistance.

Muscles Developed: Posterior deltoid, rhombus, and trapezius.

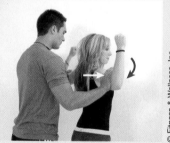

© Fitness & Wellness, Inc.

EXERCISE 3
Push-Up

Action: Maintaining your body as straight as possible, flex the elbows, lowering the body until you almost touch the floor, then raise yourself back up to the starting position. If you are unable to perform the push-up as indicated, you can decrease the resistance by supporting the lower body with the knees rather than the feet (see illustration c).

Muscles Developed: Triceps, deltoid, pectoralis major, erector spinae, and abdominals

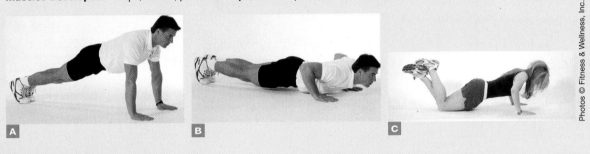

Photos © Fitness & Wellness, Inc.

EXERCISE 4
ABDOMINAL CRUNCH AND BENT-LEG CURL-UP

Action: Start with your head and shoulders off the floor, arms crossed on your chest, and knees slightly bent (the greater the flexion of the knee, the more difficult the curl-up). Now curl up to about 30° (abdominal crunch—see illustration b) or curl all the way up (bent-leg curl-up), then return to the starting position without letting the head or shoulders touch the floor, or allowing the hips to come off the floor. If you allow the hips to raise off the floor and the head and shoulders to touch the floor, you will most likely "swing up" on the next sit-up, which minimizes the work of the abdominal muscles. If you cannot curl up with the arms on the chest, place the hands by the side of the hips or even help yourself up by holding on to your thighs (illustrations d and e). Do not perform the curl-up exercise with your legs completely extended, as this will cause strain on the lower back.

Muscles Developed: Abdominal muscles (crunch) and hip flexors (complete curl-up)

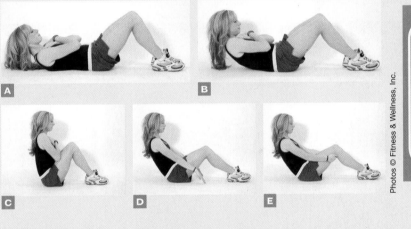

Photos © Fitness & Wellness, Inc.

NOTE: The bent-leg curl-up exercise should be used only by individuals of at least average fitness without a history of lower back problems. New participants and those with a history of lower back problems should use the abdominal crunch exercise in its place.

EXERCISE 5
LEG CURL

Action: Lie on the floor face down. Cross the right ankle over the left heel. Apply resistance with your right foot, while you bring the left foot up to 90° at the knee joint. (Apply enough resistance so that the left foot can only be brought up slowly.) Repeat the exercise, crossing the left ankle over the right heel.

Muscles Developed:
Hamstrings (and quadriceps)

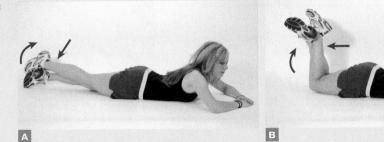

Photos © Fitness & Wellness, Inc.

EXERCISE 6
MODIFIED DIP

Action: Place your hands on a box or gymnasium bleacher. The feet are supported and held in place by an exercise partner. Dip down at least a 90° angle at the elbow joint and then return to the starting position.

Muscles Developed: Triceps, deltoid, and pectoralis major

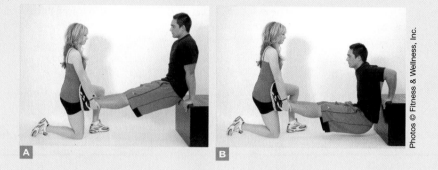

Photos © Fitness & Wellness, Inc.

EXERCISE 7
PULL-UP

Action: Suspend yourself from a bar with a pronated grip (thumbs in). Pull your body up until your chin is above the bar, then lower the body slowly to the starting position. If you are unable to perform the pull-up as described, either have a partner hold your feet to push off and facilitate the movement upward—see illustrations c and d.

Muscles Developed: Biceps, brachioradialis, brachialis, trapezius, and latissimus dorsi

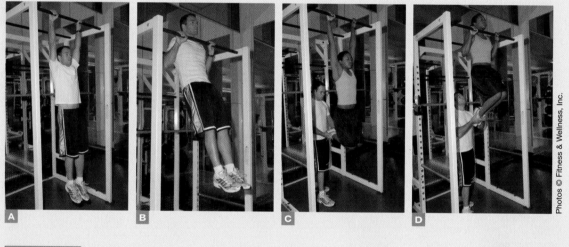

Photos © Fitness & Wellness, Inc.

EXERCISE 8
ARM CURL

Action: Using a palms-up grip, start with the arm completely extended (a), and with the aid of a sandbag or bucket filled (as needed) with sand or rocks, curl up as far as possible (b), then return to the initial position. Repeat the exercise with the other arm.

Muscles Developed: Biceps, brachioradialis, and brachialis

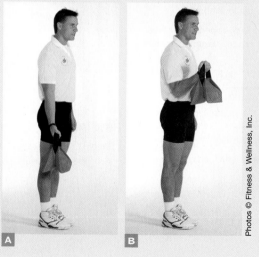

Photos © Fitness & Wellness, Inc.

EXERCISE 9
HEEL RAISE

Action: From a standing position with feet flat on the floor or at the edge of a step (a), raise and lower your body weight by moving at the ankle joint only (b). For added resistance, have someone else hold your shoulders down as you perform the exercise.

Muscles Developed: Gastrocnemius and soleus

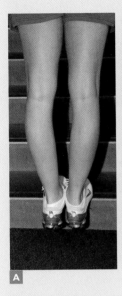
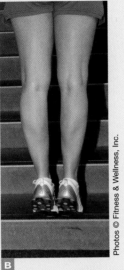

Photos © Fitness & Wellness, Inc.

EXERCISE 10
LEG ABDUCTION AND ADDUCTION

Action: Both participants sit on the floor. The person on the left places the feet on the inside of the other participant's feet. Simultaneously, the person on the left presses the legs laterally (to the outside—abduction), while the one on the right presses the legs medially (adduction). Hold the contraction for 5 to 10 seconds. Repeat the exercise at all three angles, and then reverse the pressing sequence. The person on the left places the feet on the outside and presses inward, while the one on the right presses outward.

Muscles Developed: Hip abductors (rectus femoris, sartorius, gluteus medius and minimus), and adductors (pectineus, gracilis, adductor magnus, adductor longus, and adductor brevis)

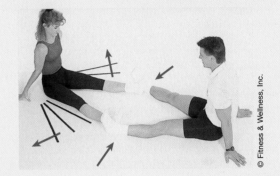

© Fitness & Wellness, Inc.

EXERCISE 11
REVERSE CRUNCH

Action: Lie on your back with arms to the sides and knees and hips flexed at 90° (a). Now attempt to raise the pelvis off the floor by lifting vertically from the knees and lower legs (b). This is a challenging exercise that may be difficult for beginners to perform.

Muscles Developed: Abdominals

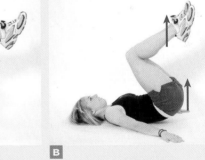

Photos © Fitness & Wellness, Inc.

EXERCISE 12
PELVIC TILT

Action: Lie flat on the floor with the knees bent at about a 90° angle (a). Tilt the pelvis by tightening the abdominal muscles, flattening your back against the floor, and raising the lower gluteal area ever so slightly off the floor (b). Hold the final position for several seconds.

Areas Stretched: Low back muscles and ligaments.

Areas Strengthened: Abdominal and gluteal muscles

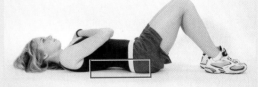
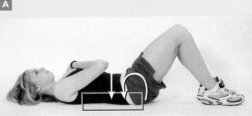

Photos © Fitness & Wellness, Inc.

APPENDIX A

EXERCISE 13
LATERAL BRIDGE

Action: Lie on your side with legs bent (a: easier version) or straight (b: harder version) and support the upper body with your arm. Straighten your body by raising the hip off the floor, and hold the position for several seconds. Repeat the exercise with the other side of the body.

Muscles Developed: Abdominals (obliques and transversus abdominus) and quadratus lumborum (lower back)

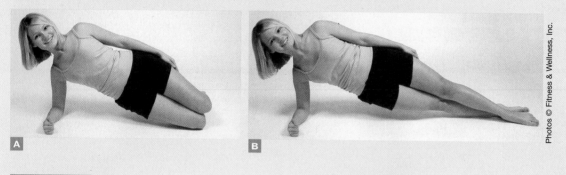

Photos © Fitness & Wellness, Inc.

EXERCISE 14
PRONE BRIDGE

Action: Starting in a prone position on a floor mat, balance yourself on the tips of your toes and elbows while attempting to maintain a straight body from heels to toes (do not arch your back—see illustration a). You can increase the difficulty of this exercise by placing your hands in front of you and straightening the arms (see illustration b).

Muscles Developed: Anterior and posterior muscle groups of the trunk and pelvis

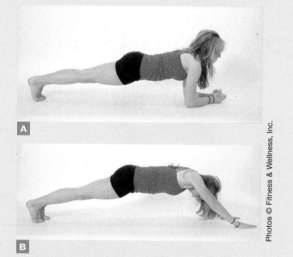

Photos © Fitness & Wellness, Inc.

EXERCISE 15
SUPINE BRIDGE

Action: Lie face up on the floor with the knees bent at about 120°. Do a pelvic tilt (Exercise 12, page 261) and maintain the pelvic tilt while you raise the hips off the floor until the upper body and upper legs are in a straight line. Hold this position for up to 5 seconds.

Areas Strengthened: Gluteal and abdominal flexor muscles

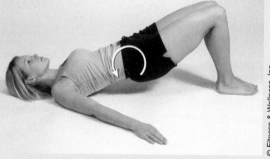

© Fitness & Wellness, Inc.

Strength-Training Exercises With Weights

EXERCISE 16
ARM CURL

Action: Use a supinated or palms-up grip, and start with the arms almost completely extended (a). Now curl up as far as possible (b), then return to the starting position.

Muscles Developed: Biceps, brachioradialis, and brachialis

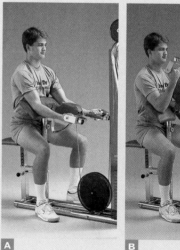
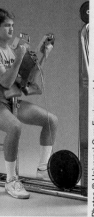

Photos © Universal Gym Equipment, Inc.

EXERCISE 17
BENCH PRESS

Action: Lie down on the bench with the head by the weight stack, the bench press bar above the chest, and place the feet on the bench (a). Grasp the bar handles and press upward until the arms are completely extended (b), then return to the original position. Do not arch the back during this exercise.

Muscles Developed: Pectoralis major, triceps, and deltoid

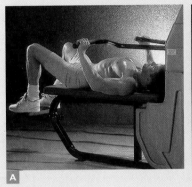
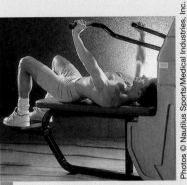

A   B

Photos © Nautilus Sports/Medical Industries, Inc.

EXERCISE 18
ABDOMINAL CRUNCH

Action: Sit in an upright position and grasp the handles over your shoulders and crunch forward. Slowly return to the original position.

Muscles Developed: Abdominals

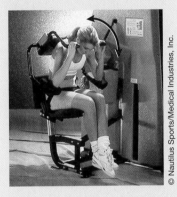

© Nautilus Sports/Medical Industries, Inc.

EXERCISE 19
LEG PRESS

Action: From a sitting position with the knees flexed at about 90° and both feet on the footrest (a), extend the legs fully (b), then return slowly to the starting position.

Muscles Developed: Quadriceps and gluteal muscles

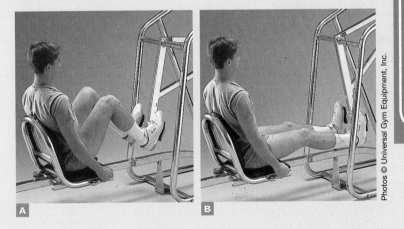

A   B

Photos © Universal Gym Equipment, Inc.

EXERCISE 20
LEG CURL

Action: Lie with the face down on the bench, legs straight, and place the back of the feet under the padded bar (a). Curl up to at least 90° (b), and return to the original position.

Muscles Developed: Hamstrings

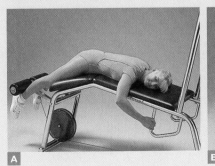
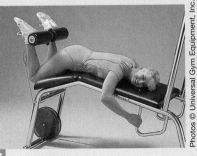

A   B

Photos © Universal Gym Equipment, Inc.

APPENDIX A

Action: Starting from a sitting position, hold the exercise bar with a wide grip (a). Pull the bar down in front of you until it reaches the base of the neck (b), then return to the starting position.

Muscles Developed: Latissimus dorsi, pectoralis major, and biceps

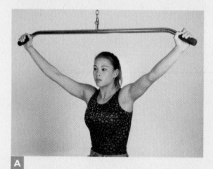

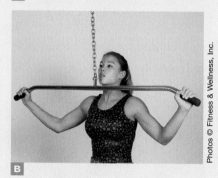

Photos © Fitness & Wellness, Inc.

Action: Start with your feet either flat on the floor or the front of the feet on an elevated block (a), then raise and lower yourself by moving at the ankle joint only (b). If additional resistance is needed, you can use a squat strength-training machine.

Muscles Developed: Gastrocnemius and soleus

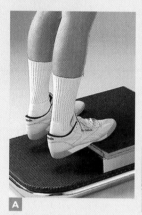
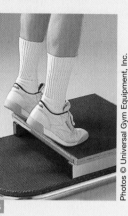

Photos © Universal Gym Equipment, Inc.

Action: Using a palms-down grip, grasp the bar slightly closer than shoulder width, and start with the elbows almost completely bent (a). Extend the arms fully (b), then return to starting position.

Muscles Developed: Triceps

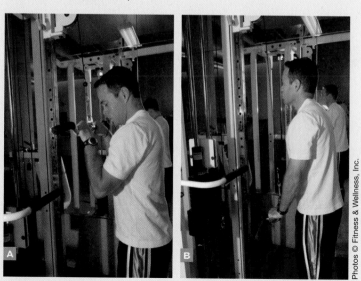

Photos © Fitness & Wellness, Inc.

Action: Sit upright into the machine and place the elbows behind the padded bars. Rotate the torso as far as possible to one side and then return slowly to the starting position. Repeat the exercise to the opposite side.

Muscles Developed: Internal and external obliques (abdominal muscles)

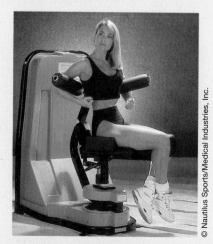

© Nautilus Sports/Medical Industries, Inc.

EXERCISE 25
SEATED BACK

Action: Sit in the machine with your trunk flexed and the upper back against the shoulder pad. Place the feet under the padded bar and hold on with your hands to the bars on the sides (a). Start the exercise by pressing backward, simultaneously extending the trunk and hip joints (b). Slowly return to the original position.

Muscles Developed: Erector spinae and gluteus maximus

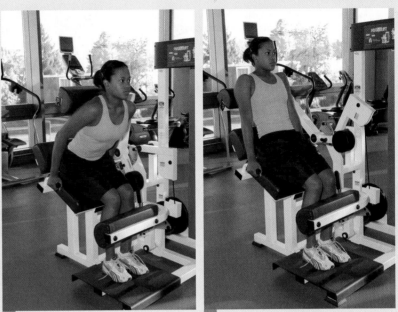

Photos © Fitness & Wellness, Inc.

EXERCISE 26
ROWING TORSO

Action: Sit in the machine with your arms in front of you, elbows bent and resting against the padded bars (a). Press back as far as possible, drawing the shoulder blades together (b). Return to the original position.

Muscles Developed: Posterior deltoid, rhomboids, and trapezius

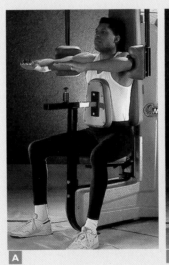
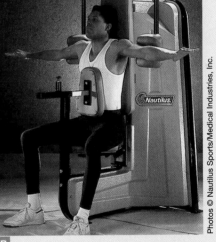

Photos © Nautilus Sports/Medical Industries, Inc.

APPENDIX A

EXERCISE 27
BACK EXTENSION

Action: Place your feet under the ankle rollers and the hips over the padded seat. Start with the trunk in a flexed position and the arms crossed over the chest (a). Slowly extend the trunk to a horizontal position (b), hold the extension for 2 to 5 seconds, then slowly flex (lower) the trunk to the original position.

Muscles Developed: Erector spinae, gluteus maximus, and quadratus lumborum (lower back)

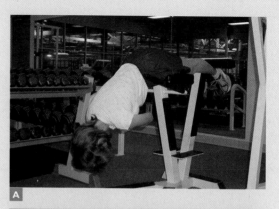

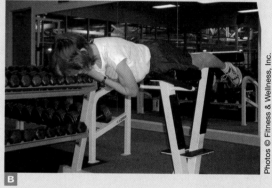

Photos © Fitness & Wellness, Inc.

Flexibility Exercises

EXERCISE 28
LATERAL HEAD TILT

Action: Slowly and gently tilt the head laterally. Repeat several times to each side.

Areas Stretched: Neck flexors and extensors and ligaments of the cervical spine

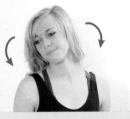

EXERCISE 29
ARM CIRCLES

Action: Gently circle your arms all the way around. Conduct the exercise in both directions.

Areas Stretched: Shoulder muscles and ligaments

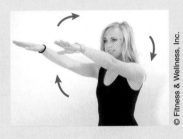
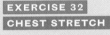

EXERCISE 30
SIDE STRETCH

Action: Stand straight up, feet separated to shoulder width, and place your hands on your waist. Now move the upper body to one side and hold the final stretch for a few seconds. Repeat on the other side.

Areas Stretched: Muscles and ligaments in the pelvic region

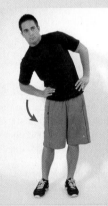

EXERCISE 31
BODY ROTATION

Action: Place your arms slightly away from your body and rotate the trunk as far as possible, holding the final position for several seconds. Conduct the exercise for both the right and left sides of the body. You can also perform this exercise by standing about 2 feet away from the wall (back toward the wall), and then rotate the trunk, placing the hands against the wall.

Areas Stretched: Hip, abdominal, chest, back, neck, and shoulder muscles; hip and spinal ligaments

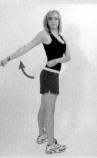

EXERCISE 32
CHEST STRETCH

Action: Place your hand on the shoulders of your partner, who will in turn push you down by your shoulders. Hold the final position for a few seconds.

Areas Stretched: Chest (pectoral) muscles and shoulder ligaments

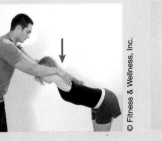

EXERCISE 33
SHOULDER HYPEREXTENSION STRETCH

Action: Have a partner grasp your arms from behind by the wrists and slowly push them upward. Hold the final position for a few seconds.

Areas Stretched: Deltoid and pectoral muscles, and ligaments of the shoulder joint

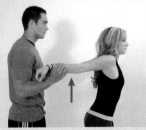

© Fitness & Wellness, Inc.

APPENDIX B

EXERCISE 34
SHOULDER ROTATION STRETCH

Action: With the aid of surgical tubing or an aluminum or wood stick, place the tubing or stick behind your back and grasp the two ends using a reverse (thumbs-out) grip. Slowly bring the tubing or stick over your head, keeping the elbows straight. Repeat several times (bring the hands closer together for additional stretch).

Areas Stretched: Deltoid, latissimus dorsi, and pectoral muscles; shoulder ligaments

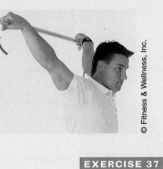

© Fitness & Wellness, Inc.

EXERCISE 35
QUAD STRETCH

Action: Lie on your side and move one foot back by flexing the knee. Grasp the front of the ankle and pull the ankle toward the gluteal region. Hold for several seconds. Repeat with the other leg.

Areas Stretched: Quadriceps muscle, and knee and ankle ligaments

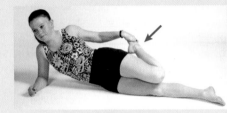

© Fitness & Wellness, Inc.

EXERCISE 36
HEEL CORD STRETCH

Action: Assume a push-up position, then bend one knee and stretch the opposite heel cord. Hold the stretched position for a few seconds. Alternate legs. You may also perform this exercise leaning against a wall or standing at the edge of a step, then stretch the heel downward.

Areas Stretched: Heel cord (Achilles tendon), gastrocnemius, and soleus muscles

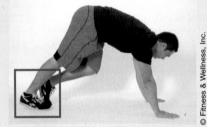

© Fitness & Wellness, Inc.

EXERCISE 37
ADDUCTOR STRETCH

Action: Stand with your feet about twice shoulder width and place your hands slightly above the knee. Flex one knee and slowly go down as far as possible, holding the final position for a few seconds. Repeat with the other leg.

Areas Stretched: Hip adductor muscles

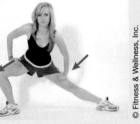

© Fitness & Wellness, Inc.

EXERCISE 38
SITTING ADDUCTOR STRETCH

Action: Sit on the floor and bring your feet in close to you, allowing the soles of the feet to touch each other. Now place your forearms (or elbows) on the inner part of the thigh and push the legs downward, holding the final stretch for several seconds.

Areas Stretched: Hip adductor muscles

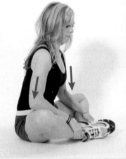

© Fitness & Wellness, Inc.

EXERCISE 39
SIT-AND-REACH STRETCH

Action: Sit on the floor with legs together and gradually reach forward as far as possible. Hold the final position for a few seconds. This exercise may also be performed with the legs separated, reaching to each side as well as to the middle.

Areas Stretched: Hamstrings and lower back muscles, and lumbar spine ligaments

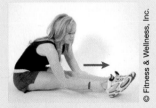

© Fitness & Wellness, Inc.

EXERCISE 40
TRICEPS STRETCH

Action: Place the right hand behind your neck. Grasp the right arm above the elbow with the left hand. Gently pull the elbow backward. Repeat the exercise with the opposite arm.

Areas Stretched: Back of upper arm (triceps muscle) and shoulder joint

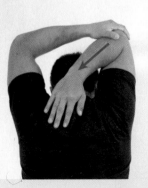

© Fitness & Wellness, Inc.

Exercises for the Prevention and Rehabilitation of Low Back Pain

EXERCISE 41
SINGLE-KNEE TO CHEST STRETCH

Action: Lie down flat on the floor. Bend one leg at approximately 100° and gradually pull the opposite leg toward your chest. Hold the final stretch for a few seconds. Switch legs and repeat the exercise.

Areas Stretched: Lower back and hamstring muscles, and lumbar spine ligaments

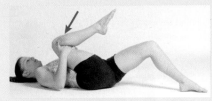

© Fitness & Wellness, Inc.

EXERCISE 42
DOUBLE-KNEE TO CHEST STRETCH

Action: Lie flat on the floor and then slowly curl up into a fetal position. Hold for a few seconds.

Areas Stretched: Upper and lower back and hamstring muscles; spinal ligaments

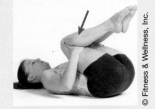

© Fitness & Wellness, Inc.

EXERCISE 43
UPPER AND LOWER BACK STRETCH

Action: Sit on the floor and bring your feet in close to you, allowing the soles of the feet to touch each other. Hold on to your feet and gently bring your head and upper chest toward your feet.

Areas Stretched: Upper and lower back muscles and ligaments

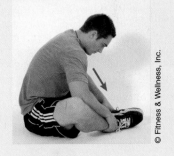

© Fitness & Wellness, Inc.

EXERCISE 44
SIT-AND-REACH-STRETCH

See Exercise 39 in Appendix B.

EXERCISE 45
GLUTEAL STRETCH

Action: Sit on the floor, bend the right leg and place your right ankle slightly above the left knee. Grasp the left thigh with both hands and gently pull the leg toward your chest. Repeat the exercise with the opposite leg.

Areas Stretched: Buttock area (gluteal muscles)

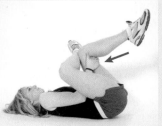

© Fitness & Wellness, Inc.

EXERCISE 46
BACK EXTENSION

Action: Lie face down on the floor with the elbows by the chest, forearms on the floor, and the hands beneath the chin. Gently raise the trunk by extending the elbows until you reach an approximate 90° angle at the elbow joint. Be sure that the forearms remain in contact with the floor at all times. Hold the stretched position for a few seconds. DO NOT extend the back beyond this point. Hyperextension of the lower back may lead to or aggravate an already existing back problem.

Area Stretched: Abdominal region

Additional Benefit: Restore lower back curvature

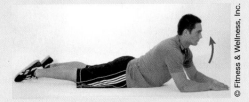

© Fitness & Wellness, Inc.

EXERCISE 47
TRUNK ROTATION AND LOWER BACK STRETCH

Action: Sit on the floor and bend the left leg, placing the left foot on the outside of the right knee. Place the right elbow on the left knee and push against it. At the same time, try to rotate the trunk to the left (counterclockwise). Hold the final position for a few seconds. Repeat the exercise with the other side.

Areas Stretched: Lateral side of the hip and thigh; trunk, and lower back

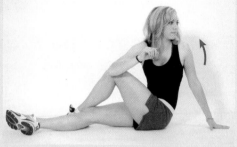

© Fitness & Wellness, Inc.

EXERCISE 48
HIP FLEXORS STRETCH

Action: Kneel down on an exercise mat, a soft surface, or place a towel under your knees. Raise the left knee off the floor and place the left foot about 3 feet in front of you. Place your left hand over your left knee and the right hand over the back of the right hip. Keeping the lower back flat, slowly move forward and downward as you apply gentle pressure over the right hip. Repeat the exercise with the opposite leg forward.

Areas Stretched: Flexor muscles in front of the hip joint

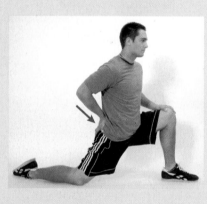

EXERCISE 49
CAT STRETCH

Action: Kneel on the floor and place your hands in front of you (on the floor) about shoulder width apart. Relax your trunk and lower back (a). Now arch the spine and pull in your abdomen as far as you can and hold this position for a few seconds (b). Repeat the exercise 4–5 times.

Areas Stretched: Low back muscles and ligaments

Areas Strengthened: Abdominal and gluteal muscles

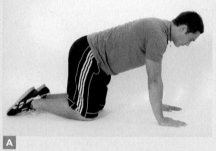

A

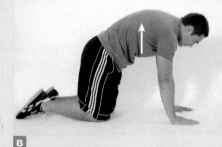

B

Photos © Fitness & Wellness, Inc.

EXERCISE 50
PELVIC CLOCK

Action: Lie face up on the floor with the knees bent at about 120°. Fully extend the hips as in the supine bridge (Exercise 15, page 262). Now progressively rotate the hips in a clockwise manner (2 o'clock, 4 o'clock, 6 o'clock, 8 o'clock, 10 o'clock, and 12 o'clock), holding each position in an isometric contraction for about 1 second. Repeat the exercise counterclockwise.

Areas Strengthened: Gluteal, abdominal, and hip flexor muscles

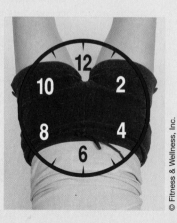

© Fitness & Wellness, Inc.

EXERCISE 51
PELVIC TILT

See Exercise 12 in Appendix A, page 261.

EXERCISE 52
ABDOMINAL CRUNCH OR BENT-LEG CURL-UP

See exercise on page 259.

It is important that you do not stabilize your feet when performing either of these exercises, because doing so decreases the work of the abdominal muscles. Also, remember not to "swing up" but, rather, to curl up as you perform these exercises.

Contraindicated Exercises

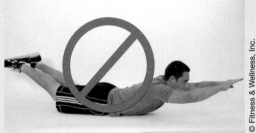

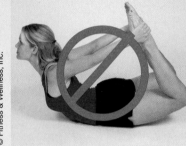

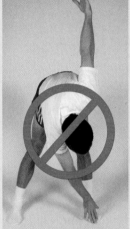

SWAN STRETCH

Excessive strain on the spine; may harm intervertebral disks.

Alternative: Flexibility Exercise 46, page 269

CRADLE

Excessive strain on the spine, knees, and shoulders.

Alternatives: Flexibility Exercises 46, 35, and 33, pages 269, 268, and 267

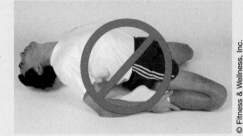

WINDMILL

Excessive strain on the spine and knees.

Alternatives: Flexibility Exercises 39 and 47, pages 268 and 270

HURDLER STRETCH

Excessive strain on the bent knee.

Alternatives: Flexibility Exercises 35 and 39, page 268

THE HERO

Excessive strain on the knees.

Alternatives: Flexibility Exercises 35 and 48, pages 268 and 270

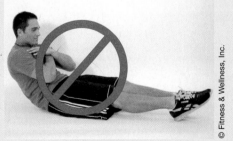

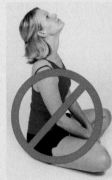

HEAD ROLL

May injure neck disks.

Alternative: Flexibility Exercise 28, page 267

STRAIGHT-LEG SIT-UP

ALTERNATING BENT-LEG SIT-UP

These exercises strain the lower back.

Alternatives: Strength Exercises 4 and 18, pages 259 and 263

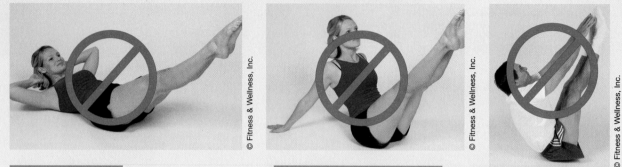

© Fitness & Wellness, Inc.

© Fitness & Wellness, Inc.

© Fitness & Wellness, Inc.

DOUBLE-LEG LIFT

UPRIGHT DOUBLE-LEG LIFT

V-SIT

All three of these exercises cause excessive strain on the spine and may harm disks.

Alternatives: Strength Exercises 4 and 18, pages 259 and 263

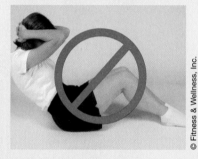

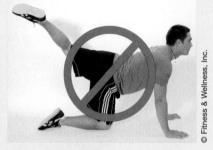

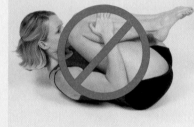

© Fitness & Wellness, Inc.

© Fitness & Wellness, Inc.

© Fitness & Wellness, Inc.

SIT-UP WITH HANDS BEHIND THE HEAD

Excessive strain on the neck.

Alternatives: Strength Exercises 4 and 18, pages 259 and 263

DONKEY KICK

Excessive strain on the back, shoulders, and neck.

Alternatives: Flexibility Exercises 46, 48, and 28, pages 269, 270 and 267

KNEE TO CHEST

Excessive strain on the knee.

Alternatives: Flexibility Exercises 41 and 42, page 269

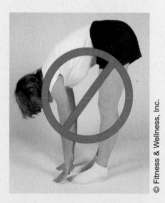

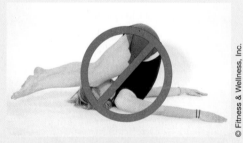

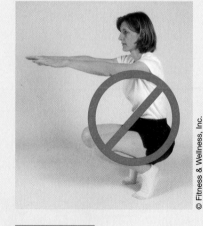

© Fitness & Wellness, Inc.

© Fitness & Wellness, Inc.

© Fitness & Wellness, Inc.

YOGA PLOW

Excessive strain on the spine, neck, and shoulders.

Alternatives: Flexibility Exercises 39, 41, 42, 43, and 45, pages 268 and 269

STANDING TOE TOUCH

Excessive strain on the knee and lower back.

Alternative: Flexibility Exercise 39, page 268

FULL SQUAT

Excessive strain on the knees.

Alternatives: Flexibility Exercise 35, Strength Exercises 1, 19, pages 268, 258, and 263

Selective Nutrient Content of Common Foods

Food Description	Qty	Measure	Energy (cal)	Protein (g)	Carb (g)	Dietary Fiber (g)	Fat (g)	Sat Fat (g)	Trans Fat (g)	Cholesterol (mg)
Almonds, dry roasted, no salt added	¼	cup(s)	206	8	7	4	18	1.40	–	0
Apples, raw medium, w/peel	1	item(s)	72	<1	19	3	<1	0.04	–	0
Applesauce, sweetened, canned	½	cup(s)	97	<1	25	2	<1	0.04	–	0
Apricot, fresh w/o pits	4	item(s)	67	2	16	3	1	0.04	–	0
Apricot, halves w/skin, canned in heavy syrup	½	cup(s)	107	1	28	2	<1	0.01	–	0
Asparagus, boiled, drained	½	cup(s)	20	2	4	2	0.19	0.06	–	0
Avocado, California, whole, w/o skin or pit	1	item(s)	284	3	15	12	26	3.59	–	0
Bacon, cured, broiled, pan fried, or roasted	2	slice(s)	68	5	<1	0	5	1.73	0	14
Bagel chips, plain	3	item(s)	130	3	19	1	5	0.50	–	0
Bagel, plain, enriched, toasted	1	item(s)	195	7	38	2	1	0.16	0	0
Banana, fresh whole, w/o peel	1	item(s)	105	1	27	3	<1	0.13	–	0
Beans, black, boiled	½	cup(s)	114	8	20	7	<1	0.12	–	0
Beans, Fordhook lima, frozen, boiled, drained	½	cup(s)	88	5	16	5	<1	0.07	–	0
Beans, mung, sprouted, boiled, drained	½	cup(s)	13	1	3	<1	<1	0.02	–	0
Beans, red kidney, canned	½	cup(s)	109	7	20	8	<1	0.06	–	0
Beans, refried, canned	½	cup(s)	119	7	20	7	2	0.60	–	10
Beans, yellow snap, string or wax, boiled, drained	½	cup(s)	22	1	5	2	<1	0.04	–	0
Beef, chuck, arm pot roast, lean & fat, ¼″ fat, braised	3	ounce(s)	282	23	0	0	20	7.97	–	84
Beef, corned, canned	3	ounce(s)	213	23	0	0	13	5.25	–	73
Beef, ground, lean, broiled, well	3	ounce(s)	238	24	0	0	15	5.89	–	86
Beef, ground, regular, broiled, medium	3	ounce(s)	246	20	0	0	18	6.91	–	77
Beef, liver, pan fried	3	ounce(s)	149	23	4	0	4	1.27	0.17	324
Beef, rib steak, small end, lean, ¼″ fat, broiled	3	ounce(s)	188	24	0	0	10	3.84	–	68
Beef, rib, whole, lean & fat, ¼″ fat, roasted	3	ounce(s)	320	19	0	0	27	10.71	–	72
Beef, short loin, T-bone steak, lean, ¼″ fat, broiled	3	ounce(s)	174	23	0	0	9	3.05	–	50
Beer	12	fluid ounce(s)	118	1	6	<1	<1	0.00	0	0
Beer, light	12	fluid ounce(s)	99	1	5	0	0	0.00	0	0
Beets, sliced, canned, drained	½	cup(s)	26	1	6	1	<1	0.02	–	0
Biscuits	1	item(s)	121	3	16	1	5	1.40	0	<1
Blueberries, raw	½	cup(s)	41	1	10	2	<1	0.02	–	0

Food Description	Qty	Measure	Energy (cal)	Protein (g)	Carb (g)	Dietary Fiber (g)	Fat (g)	Sat Fat (g)	Trans Fat (g)	Cholesterol (mg)
Bologna, beef	1	slice(s)	90	3	1	0	8	3.50	—	20
Bologna, turkey	1	slice(s)	50	3	1	0	4	1.00	—	20
Brazil nuts, unblanched, dried	¼	cup(s)	230	5	4	3	23	5.30	—	0
Bread, cracked wheat	1	slice(s)	65	2	12	1	1	0.23	—	0
Bread, French	1	slice(s)	69	2	13	1	1	0.16	—	0
Bread, mixed grain	1	slice(s)	65	3	12	2	1	0.21	—	0
Bread, pita	1	item(s)	165	5	33	1	1	0.10	—	0
Bread, pumpernickel	1	slice(s)	80	3	15	2	1	0.14	—	0
Bread, rye	1	slice(s)	83	3	15	2	1	0.20	—	0
Bread, white	1	slice(s)	67	2	13	1	1	0.18	—	0
Bread, whole wheat	1	slice(s)	128	4	24	3	2	0.37	—	0
Broccoli, chopped, boiled, drained	½	cup(s)	27	2	6	3	<1	0.06	—	0
Brownie, prepared from mix	1	item(s)	112	1	12	1	7	1.76	—	18
Brussels sprouts, boiled, drained	½	cup(s)	28	2	6	2	<1	0.08	—	0
Bulgur, cooked	½	cup(s)	76	3	17	4	<1	0.04	—	0
Buns, hamburger, plain	1	item(s)	120	4	21	1	2	0.47	—	0
Butter	1	tablespoon(s)	108	<1	<1	0	12	6.13	—	32
Buttermilk, low fat	1	cup(s)	98	8	12	0	2	1.34	—	10
Cabbage, boiled, drained, no salt added	1	cup(s)	33	2	7	3	1	0.08	—	0
Cabbage, raw, shredded	1	cup(s)	17	1	4	2	<1	0.01	—	0
Cake, angel food, from mix	1	slice(s)	129	3	29	<1	<1	0.02	—	0
Cake, butter pound, ready to eat, commercially prepared	1	slice(s)	291	4	37	<1	15	8.67	—	166
Cake, carrot, cream cheese frosting, from mix	1	slice(s)	484	5	52	1	29	5.43	—	60
Cake, chocolate, chocolate icing, commercially prepared	1	slice(s)	235	3	35	2	10	3.05	—	27
Cake, devil's food cupcake, chocolate frosting	1	item(s)	120	2	20	1	4	1.80	—	19
Cake, white, coconut frosting, from mix	1	slice(s)	399	5	71	1	12	4.36	—	1
Candy, Almond Joy bar	1	item(s)	240	2	29	2	13	9.00	0	3
Candy, Life Savers	1	item(s)	8	0	2	0	<1	0.00	0	0
Candy, M&M's peanut chocolate candy, small bag	1	item(s)	250	5	30	2	13	5.00	—	5
Candy, M&M's plain chocolate candy, small bag	1	item(s)	240	2	34	1	10	6.00	—	5
Candy, milk chocolate bar	1	item(s)	483	8	53	2	28	16.69	—	22
Candy, Milky Way bar	1	item(s)	270	2	41	1	10	5.00	—	5
Candy, Reese's peanut butter cups	2	piece(s)	250	5	25	1	14	5.00	0	3
Candy, Special Dark chocolate bar	1	item(s)	220	2	24	3	13	8.00	0	3
Candy, Starburst fruit chews, original fruits	1	package	240	0	48	0	5	1.00	—	0

Food Description	Qty	Measure	Energy (cal)	Protein (g)	Carb (g)	Dietary Fiber (g)	Fat (g)	Sat Fat (g)	Trans Fat (g)	Cholesterol (mg)
Candy, York peppermint patty	1	item(s)	170	1	34	1	3	2.00	0	0
Cantaloupe	½	cup(s)	27	1	7	1	<1	0.04	—	0
Carrots, raw	½	cup(s)	25	1	6	2	<1	0.02	0	0
Carrots, sliced, boiled, drained	½	cup(s)	27.29	0.59	6.41	2.33	0.14	0.02	—	0
Cashews, dry roasted	¼	cup(s)	197	5	11	1	16	3.14	—	0
Catsup/ketchup	1	tablespoon(s)	14	<1	4	<1	<1	0.01	—	0
Cauliflower, boiled, drained	½	cup(s)	14	1	3	2	<1	0.04	—	0
Celery, stalk	2	item(s)	11	1	2	1	<1	0.03	—	0
Cereal, All-Bran	1	cup(s)	160	8	46	20	2	0.00	0	0
Cereal, All-Bran Buds	1	cup(s)	212	6	73	42	3	—	0	0
Cereal, Bran Flakes, Post	1	cup(s)	133	4	32	7	1	0.00	—	0
Cereal, Cap'n Crunch	1	cup(s)	144	2	30	1	2	0.53	—	0
Cereal, Cheerios	1	cup(s)	110	3	22	3	2	0.00	—	0
Cereal, Complete wheat bran flakes	1	cup(s)	120	4	31	7	1	—	0	0
Cereal, Corn Flakes	1	cup(s)	100	2	24	1	0	0.00	0	0
Cereal, Corn Pops	1	cup(s)	120	1	28	0	0	0.00	0	0
Cereal, Cracklin' Oat Bran	1	cup(s)	266	5	47	7	9	2.70	0	0
Cereal, Cream of Wheat, instant, prepared	½	cup(s)	61	2	13	<1	<1	0.01	0	0
Cereal, Frosted Flakes	1	cup(s)	160	1	37	1	0	0.00	0	0
Cereal, Frosted Mini-Wheats	5	item(s)	180	5	41	5	1	0.00	0	0
Cereal, granola, prepared	½	cup(s)	299	9	32	5	15	2.76	—	0
Cereal, Kashi puffed	1	cup(s)	70	3	13	2	1	0.00	—	0
Cereal, Life	1	cup(s)	160	4	33	3	2	0.35	—	0
Cereal, Multi-Bran Chex	1	cup(s)	200	4	49	7	2	0.00	0	0
Cereal, Nutri-Grain golden wheat	1	cup(s)	133	4	31	5	1	0.00	—	0
Cereal, oatmeal, cooked w/water	½	cup(s)	74	3	13	2	1	0.19	—	0
Cereal, Product 19	1	cup(s)	100	2	25	1	0	0.00	0	0
Cereal, Raisin Bran	1	cup(s)	190	4	47	8	1	0.00	—	0
Cereal, Rice Chex	1	cup(s)	96	2	22	<1	0	0.00	0	0
Cereal, Rice Krispies	1	cup(s)	96	2	23	0	0	0.00	0	0
Cereal, Shredded Wheat	1	cup(s)	88	3	20	3	1	0.04	—	0
Cereal, Smacks	1	cup(s)	133	3	32	1	1	0.00	—	0
Cereal, Special K	1	cup(s)	110	7	22	1	0	0.00	0	0
Cereal, Total whole grain	1	cup(s)	146	3	31	4	1	0.00	—	0
Cereal, Wheaties	1	cup(s)	110	3	24	3	1	0.00	—	0
Cheese, American, processed	1	ounce(s)	106	6	<1	0	9	5.58	—	27
Cheese, blue, crumbled	1	ounce(s)	100	6	1	0	8	5.29	—	21
Cheese, cheddar, shredded	¼	cup(s)	114	7	<1	0	9	5.96	—	30
Cheese, feta	1	ounce(s)	74	4	1	0	6	4.18	—	25
Cheese, Monterey jack	1	ounce(s)	104	7	<1	0	8	5.34	—	25
Cheese, mozzarella, part skim milk	1	ounce(s)	71	7	1	0	4	2.83	—	18
Cheese, Parmesan, grated	1	tablespoon(s)	22	2	<1	0	1	0.87	—	4
Cheese, ricotta, part skim milk	¼	cup(s)	85	7	3	0	5	3.03	—	19
Cheese, Swiss	1	ounce(s)	106	8	2	0	8	4.98	—	26
Cherries, sweet, raw	½	cup(s)	46	1	12	2	<1	0.03	—	0

Food Description	Qty	Measure	Energy (cal)	Protein (g)	Carb (g)	Dietary Fiber (g)	Fat (g)	Sat Fat (g)	Trans Fat (g)	Cholesterol (mg)
Chicken, broiler breast, meat & skin, flour coated, fried	3	ounce(s)	189	27	1	<.1	8	2.08	–	76
Chicken, broiler drumstick, meat & skin, flour coated, fried	3	ounce(s)	208	23	1	<.1	12	3.11	–	77
Chicken, light meat, roasted	3	ounce(s)	130	23	0	0	3	0.92	–	64
Chicken, roasted (meat only)	3	ounce(s)	142	21	0	0	6	1.54	–	64
Chickpeas or bengal gram, garbanzo beans, boiled	½	cup(s)	134	7	22	6	2	0.22	–	0
Chocolate milk, low fat	1	cup(s)	158	8	26	1	3	1.54	–	8
Cilantro	1	teaspoon(s)	<1	<.1	<.1	<.1	<.1	0.00	–	0
Cocoa, hot, prepared w/milk	1	cup(s)	193	9	27	3	6	3.58	0.18	20
Coconut, dried, not sweetened	¼	cup(s)	393	4	14	10	38	34.06	–	0
Cod, Atlantic cod or scrod, baked or broiled	3	ounce(s)	46	10	0	0	<1	0.07	–	24
Coffee, brewed	8	fluid ounce(s)	9	<1	0	0	0	0.00	0	0
Collard greens, boiled, drained	½	cup(s)	25	2	5	3	<1	0.04	–	0
Cookies, animal crackers	12	piece(s)	134	2	22	<1	4	1.03	–	0
Cookies, chocolate chip	1	item(s)	140	2	16	1	8	2.09	0	13
Cookies, chocolate sandwich, extra crème filling	1	item(s)	65	<1	9	<1	3	0.50	1.10	0
Cookies, Fig Newtons	1	item(s)	55	1	10	1	1	0.50	0.50	0
Cookies, oatmeal	1	item(s)	234	6	45	3	4	0.70	0	<.1
Cookies, peanut butter	1	item(s)	163	4	17	1	9	1.65	0	13
Cookies, sugar	1	item(s)	61	1	7	<1	3	0.63	0	18
Corn, yellow sweet, frozen, boiled, drained	½	cup(s)	66	2	16	2	1	0.08	–	0
Cornbread	1	piece(s)	141	5	18	1	5	2.09	0	21
Cornmeal, yellow whole grain	½	cup(s)	221	5	47	4	2	0.31	–	0
Cottage cheese, low fat, 1% fat	½	cup(s)	81	14	3	0	1	0.73	–	5
Cottage cheese, low fat, 2% fat	½	cup(s)	102	16	4	0	2	1.38	–	9
Crab, blue, canned	2	ounce(s)	56	12	0	0	1	0.14	–	50
Crackers, cheese (mini)	30	item(s)	151	3	17	1	8	2.81	–	4
Crackers, honey graham	4	item(s)	118	2	22	1	3	0.43	–	0
Crackers, matzo, plain	1	item(s)	112	3	24	1	<1	0.06	–	0
Crackers, Ritz	5	item(s)	80	1	10	1	4	0.50	–	0
Crackers, rye crispbread	1	item(s)	37	1	8	2	<1	0.01	–	0
Crackers, saltine	5	item(s)	65	1	11	<1	2	0.44	0.54	0
Crackers, wheat	10	item(s)	142	3	19	1	6	1.55	–	0
Cranberry juice cocktail	½	cup(s)	72	0	18	<1	<1	0.01	–	0
Cream cheese	2	tablespoon(s)	101	2	1	0	10	6.37	–	32
Cream, heavy whipping, liquid	1	tablespoon(s)	52	<1	<1	0	6	3.45	–	21
Cream, light whipping, liquid	1	tablespoon(s)	44	.1	.1	0	5	2.90	–	17
Croissant, butter	1	item(s)	231	5	26	1	12	6.59	–	38
Cucumber	¼	item(s)	11	<1	3	<1	<.1	0.03	–	0
Danish pastry, nut	1	item(s)	280	5	30	1	16	3.78	–	30
Dates, domestic, whole	¼	cup(s)	126	1	33	4	<1	0.01	–	0

Food Description	Qty	Measure	Energy (cal)	Protein (g)	Carb (g)	Dietary Fiber (g)	Fat (g)	Sat Fat (g)	Trans Fat (g)	Cholesterol (mg)
Distilled alcohol, 90 proof	1	fluid ounce(s)	73	0	0	0	0	0.00	0	0
Doughnut, cake	1	item(s)	198	2	23	1	11	1.70	—	17
Doughnut, glazed	1	item(s)	242	4	27	1	14	3.49	—	4
Egg substitute, Egg Beaters	¼	cup(s)	30	6	1	0	0	0.00	0	0
Eggs, fried	1	item(s)	92	6	<1	0	7	1.98	—	210
Eggs, hard boiled	1	item(s)	78	6	1	0	5	1.63	—	212
Eggs, poached	1	item(s)	74	6	<1	0	5	1.54	—	211
Eggs, raw, white	1	item(s)	17	4	<1	0	<.1	0.00	—	0
Eggs, raw, whole	1	item(s)	74	6	<1	0	5	1.55	—	212
Eggs, raw, yolk	1	item(s)	53	3	1	0	4	1.59	—	205
Eggs, scrambled, prepared w/milk & butter	2	item(s)	203	14	3	0	15	4.49	—	429
Figs, raw, medium	2	item(s)	74	1	19	3	<1	0.06	—	0
Fish fillets, batter coated or breaded, fried	3	ounce(s)	197.19	12.46	14.42	0.42	10.44	2.39	—	28.89
Flounder, baked	3	ounce(s)	114	15	<1	<.1	6	1.15	0	44
Flour, all purpose, white, bleached, enriched	½	cup(s)	228	6	48	2	1	0.10	—	0
Flour, whole wheat	½	cup(s)	203	8	44	7	1	0.19	—	0
Frankfurter, beef & pork	1	item(s)	174	7	1	1	16	6.14	—	29
Frankfurter, beef	1	item(s)	149	5	2	0	13	5.26	—	24
Frankfurter, turkey	1	item(s)	102	6	1	0	8	2.65	—	48
Frozen yogurt, chocolate, soft serve	½	cup(s)	115	3	18	2	4	2.61	—	4
Frozen yogurt, vanilla, soft serve	½	cup(s)	117	3	17	0	4	2.46	—	1
Fruit cocktail, canned in heavy syrup	½	cup(s)	91	<1	23	1	<.1	0.01	—	0
Fruit cocktail, canned in juice	½	cup(s)	55	1	14	1	<.1	0.00	—	0
Granola bar, plain, hard	1	item(s)	115	2	16	1	5	0.58	—	0
Grape juice, sweetened, added vitamin C, from frozen concentrate	½	cup(s)	64	<1	16	<1	<1	0.04	—	0
Grapefruit juice, pink, sweetened, canned	½	cup(s)	58	1	14	<1	<1	0.02	—	0
Grapefruit juice, white	½	cup(s)	48	1	11	<1	<1	0.02	—	0
Grapefruit, raw, pink or red	½	cup(s)	48	1	12	2	<1	0.02	—	0
Grapes, European, red or green, adherent skin	½	cup(s)	55	1	14	1	<1	0.04	—	0
Haddock, baked or broiled	3	ounce(s)	50	11	0	0	<1	0.07	—	33
Halibut, Atlantic & Pacific, cooked, dry heat	3	ounce(s)	119	23	0	0	2	0.35	—	35
Ham, cured, boneless, 11% fat, roasted	3	ounce(s)	151	19	0	0	8	2.65	—	50
Ham, deli sliced, cooked	1	slice(s)	30	5	1	0	1	0.50	—	15
Honey	1	tablespoon(s)	64	<.1	17	<.1	0	0.00	0	0
Honeydew melon	½	cup(s)	32	<1	8	1	<1	0.03	—	0

Food Description	Qty	Measure	Energy (cal)	Protein (g)	Carb (g)	Dietary Fiber (g)	Fat (g)	Sat Fat (g)	Trans Fat (g)	Cholesterol (mg)
Ice cream, chocolate	½	cup(s)	143	3	19	1	7	4.49	–	22
Ice cream, chocolate, soft serve	½	cup(s)	177	3	24	1	8	5.17	–	22
Ice cream, light vanilla	½	cup(s)	109	4	18	<1	3	1.71	–	17
Jams, jellies, preserves, all flavors	1	tablespoon(s)	56	<.1	14	<1	<.1	0.00	–	0
Jams, jellies, preserves, all flavors, low sugar	1	tablespoon(s)	25	<.1	6	<1	<.1	0.00	–	0
Kale, frozen, chopped, boiled, drained	½	cup(s)	20	2	3	1	<1	0.04	–	0
Kiwifruit	1	item(s)	53	1	11	3	1	0.02	–	0
Lamb, chop, loin, domestic, lean & fat, ¼" fat, broiled	3	ounce(s)	269	21	0	0	20	8.36	–	85
Lamb, leg, domestic, lean & fat, ¼" fat, cooked	3	ounce(s)	250	21	0	0	18	7.51	–	82
Lemon juice	1	tablespoon(s)	4	<.1	1	<.1	0	0.00	–	0
Lemonade, from frozen concentrate	8	fluid ounce(s)	131	<1	34	<1	<1	0.02	–	0
Lentils, boiled	½	cup(s)	115	9	20	8	<1	0.05	–	0
Lentils, sprouted	1	cup(s)	82	7	17	0	<1	0.04	–	0
Lettuce, butterhead, Boston, or bibb	1	cup(s)	7	1	1	1	<1	0.02	–	0
Lettuce, romaine, shredded	1	cup(s)	10	1	2	1	<1	0.02	–	0
Lobster, northern, cooked, moist heat	3	ounce(s)	83	17	1	0	1	0.09	–	61
Macadamias, dry roasted, no salt added	¼	cup(s)	241	3	4	3	25	4.00	–	0
Mayonnaise w/soybean oil	1	tablespoon(s)	99	<1	1	0	11	1.64	0.04	5
Mayonnaise, low calorie	1	tablespoon(s)	37	<.1	3	0	3	0.53	–	4
Milk, fat free, nonfat, or skim	1	cup(s)	83	8	12	0	<1	0.29	–	5
Milk, fat free, nonfat, or skim, w/nonfat milk solids	1	cup(s)	91	9	12	0	1	0.40	–	5
Milk, low fat, 1%	1	cup(s)	102	8	12	0	2	1.54	–	12
Milk, low fat, 1%, w/nonfat milk solids	1	cup(s)	105	9	12	0	2	1.48	–	10
Milk, reduced fat, 2%	1	cup(s)	122	8	11	0	5	2.35	–	20
Milk, reduced fat, 2%, w/nonfat milk solids	1	cup(s)	125	9	12	0	5	2.93	–	20
Milk, whole, 3.3%	1	cup(s)	146	8	11	0	8	4.55	–	24
Milk, whole, evaporated, canned	2	tablespoon(s)	42	2	3	0	2	1.45	–	9
Milkshakes, chocolate	1	cup(s)	270	7	48	1	6	3.81	–	25
Muffin, English, plain, enriched	1	item(s)	134	4	26	2	1	0.15	–	0
Muffin, English, wheat	1	item(s)	127	5	26	3	1	0.16	–	0
Muffins, blueberry	1	item(s)	160	3	23	1	6	0.87	0	20
Mushrooms, raw	½	cup(s)	8	1	1	<1	<1	0.02	–	0
Mustard greens, frozen, boiled, drained	½	cup(s)	14	2	2	2	<1	0.01	–	0
Oil, canola	1	tablespoon(s)	120	0	0	0	14	0.97	–	0
Oil, corn	1	tablespoon(s)	120	0	0	0	14	1.73	0.04	0

Food Description	Qty	Measure	Energy (cal)	Protein (g)	Carb (g)	Dietary Fiber (g)	Fat (g)	Sat Fat (g)	Trans Fat (g)	Cholesterol (mg)
Oil, olive	1	tablespoon(s)	119	0	0	0	14	1.82	–	0
Oil, peanut	1	tablespoon(s)	119	0	0	0	14	2.28	–	0
Oil, safflower	1	tablespoon(s)	120	0	0	0	14	0.84	–	0
Oil, soybean w/cottonseed oil	1	tablespoon(s)	120	0	0	0	14	2.45	–	0
Okra, sliced, boiled, drained	½	cup(s)	18	1	4	2	<1	0.04	–	0
Onions, chopped, boiled, drained	½	cup(s)	47	1	11	1	<1	0.03	–	0
Orange juice, unsweetened, from frozen concentrate	½	cup(s)	56	1	13	<1	<.1	0.01	–	0
Orange, raw	1	item(s)	62	1	15	3	<1	0.02	–	0
Oysters, eastern, farmed, raw	3	ounce(s)	50	4	5	0	1	0.38	–	21
Oysters, eastern, wild, cooked, moist heat	3	ounce(s)	116	12	7	0	4	1.31	–	89
Pancakes, blueberry, from recipe	3	item(s)	253	7	33	1	10	2.26	–	64
Pancakes, from mix w/egg & milk	3	item(s)	249	9	33	2	9	2.33	–	81
Papaya, raw	½	cup(s)	27	<1	7	1	<.1	0.03	–	0
Pasta, egg noodles, enriched, cooked	½	cup(s)	106	4	20	1	1	0.25	0.02	26
Pasta, macaroni, enriched, cooked	½	cup(s)	99	3	20	1	<1	0.07	–	0
Pasta, spaghetti, al dente, cooked	½	cup(s)	95	4	20	1	1	0.05	–	0
Pasta, spaghetti, whole wheat, cooked	½	cup(s)	87	4	19	3	<1	0.07	–	0
Pasta, tricolor vegetable macaroni, enriched, cooked	½	cup(s)	86	3	18	3	<.1	0.01	–	0
Peach, halves, canned in heavy syrup	½	cup(s)	97	1	26	2	<1	0.01	–	0
Peach, halves, canned in water	½	cup(s)	29	1	7	2	<.1	0.01	–	0
Peach, raw, medium	1	item(s)	38	1	9	1	<1	0.02	–	0
Peanut butter, smooth	1	tablespoon(s)	96	4	3	1	8	1.60	–	0
Peanuts, oil roasted, salted	¼	cup(s)	216	10	5	3	19	3.12	–	0
Pear, halves, canned in heavy syrup	½	cup(s)	98	<1	25	2	<1	0.01	–	0
Pear, raw	1	item(s)	96	1	26	5	<1	0.01	–	0
Peas, green, canned, drained	½	cup(s)	59	4	11	3	<1	0.05	–	0
Peas, green, frozen, boiled, drained	½	cup(s)	62	4	11	4	<1	0.04	–	0
Pecans, dry roasted, no salt added	¼	cup(s)	403	5	8	5	42	3.56	–	0
Pepperoni, beef & pork	1	slice(s)	55	2	<1	0	5	1.77	–	9
Peppers, green bell or sweet, raw	½	cup(s)	15	1	3	1	<1	0.04	–	0
Pickle relish, sweet	1	tablespoon(s)	20	<.1	5	<1	<.1	0.01	–	0
Pickle, dill	1	ounce(s)	5	<1	1	<1	<.1	0.01	–	0
Pie crust, frozen, ready to bake, enriched, baked	1	slice(s)	82	1	8	<1	5	1.69	–	0

Food Description	Qty	Measure	Energy (cal)	Protein (g)	Carb (g)	Dietary Fiber (g)	Fat (g)	Sat Fat (g)	Trans Fat (g)	Cholesterol (mg)
Pie crust, prepared w/water, baked	1	slice(s)	100	1	10	<1	6	1.54	—	0
Pie, apple, from home recipe	1	slice(s)	411	4	58	2	19	4.73	—	0
Pie, pecan, from home recipe	1	slice(s)	503	6	64	0	27	4.87	—	106
Pie, pumpkin, from home recipe	1	slice(s)	316	7	41	0	14	4.92	—	65
Pineapple, canned in extra heavy syrup	½	cup(s)	108	<1	28	1	<1	0.01	—	0
Pineapple, canned in juice	½	cup(s)	75	1	20	1	<.1	0.01	—	0
Pineapple, raw, diced	½	cup(s)	37	<1	10	1	<.1	0.01	—	0
Pinto beans, boiled, drained, no salt added	½	cup(s)	25	2	5	0	<1	0.04	—	0
Pomegranate	1	item(s)	105	1	26	1	<1	0.06	—	0
Popcorn, air popped	1	cup(s)	31	1	6	1	<1	0.05	—	0
Popcorn, popped in oil	1	cup(s)	165	3	19	3	9	1.61	—	0
Pork, ribs, loin, country style, lean & fat, roasted	3	ounce(s)	279	20	0	0	22	7.83	—	78
Potato chips, salted	20	item(s)	152	2	15	1	10	3.11	—	0
Potatoes, au gratin mix, prepared w/water, whole milk, & butter	½	cup(s)	106	3	15	1	5	2.94	—	17
Potatoes, baked, flesh & skin	1	item(s)	220	5	51	4	<1	0.05	—	0
Potatoes, baked, flesh only	½	cup(s)	57	1	13	1	<.1	0.02	—	0
Potatoes, hashed brown	½	cup(s)	207	2	27	2	10	1.11	—	0
Potatoes, mashed, from dehydrated granules w/milk, water, & margarine	½	cup(s)	122	2	17	1	5	1.27	—	2
Pretzels, plain, hard, twists	5	item(s)	114	3	24	1	1	0.23	—	0
Prune juice, canned	1	cup(s)	182	2	45	3	<.1	0.01	—	0
Prunes, dried	2	item(s)	40	<1	11	1	<.1	0.01	—	0
Pudding, chocolate	½	cup(s)	154	5	23	1	5	2.78	0	35
Pudding, tapioca, ready to eat	1	item(s)	169	3	28	<1	5	0.85	—	1
Pudding, vanilla	½	cup(s)	116	5	17	<.1	3	1.31	0	35
Quinoa, dry	½	cup(s)	318	11	59	5	5	0.50	—	0
Raisins, seeded, packed	¼	cup(s)	122	1	32	3	<1	0.07	—	0
Raspberries, raw	½	cup(s)	32	1	7	4	<1	0.01	—	0
Raspberries, red, sweetened, frozen	½	cup(s)	129	1	33	6	<1	0.01	—	0
Rice, brown, long grain, cooked	½	cup(s)	108	3	22	2	1	0.18	—	0
Rice, white, long grain, boiled	½	cup(s)	103	2	22	<1	<1	0.06	—	0
Rice, wild brown, cooked	½	cup(s)	82.81	3.27	17.49	1.47	0.27	0.04	—	0
Roll, hard	1	item(s)	167	6	30	1	2	0.35	—	0
Salad dressing, blue cheese	2	tablespoon(s)	154	1	2	0	16	3.03	—	5
Salad dressing, French	2	tablespoon(s)	143	<1	5	0	14	1.76	—	0
Salad dressing, French, low fat	2	tablespoon(s)	76	<1	10	<1	4	0.36	—	0
Salad dressing, Italian	2	tablespoon(s)	86	<1	3	0	8	1.32	—	0
Salad dressing, Italian, diet	2	tablespoon(s)	23	<1	1	0	2	0.14	—	2
Salad dressing, ranch	2	tablespoon(s)	146	<1	2	<.1	16	2.32	—	1
Salad dressing, thousand island	2	tablespoon(s)	115	<1	5	<1	11	1.59	—	8
Salad dressing, thousand island, low calorie	2	tablespoon(s)	62	<1	7	<1	4	0.23	—	<1

Food Description	Qty	Measure	Energy (cal)	Protein (g)	Carb (g)	Dietary Fiber (g)	Fat (g)	Sat Fat (g)	Trans Fat (g)	Cholesterol (mg)
Salami, pork, dry or hard	1	slice(s)	52	3	<1	0	4	1.52	—	10
Salmon, broiled or baked w/ butter	3	ounce(s)	155	23	0	0	6	1.16	—	40
Salmon, smoked chinook (lox)	2	ounce(s)	66	10	0	0	2	0.52	—	13
Salsa	2	tablespoon(s)	4	<1	1	<1	<.1	0.00	—	0
Sardines, Atlantic, with bones, canned in oil	2	item(s)	50	6	0	0	3	0.36	—	34
Sauerkraut, canned	½	cup(s)	22	1	5	3	<1	0.04	—	0
Sausage, Italian, pork, cooked	1	item(s)	220	14	1	0	17	6.14	—	53
Sausage, smoked, pork link	1	piece(s)	295	17	2	—	24	8.58	—	52
Scallops, mixed species, breaded, fried	3	item(s)	100	8	5	0	5	1.24	—	28
Seaweed, spirulina, dried	½	cup(s)	22	4	2	<1	1	0.20	—	0
Shrimp, mixed species, breaded, fried	3	ounce(s)	205.69	18.18	9.74	0.34	10.43	1.77	—	150.44
Shrimp, mixed species, cooked, moist heat	3	ounce(s)	84	18	0	0	1	0.25	—	166
Soda, Coca-Cola Classic cola	12	fluid ounce(s)	146	0	41	0	0	0.00	0	0
Soda, Coke diet cola	12	fluid ounce(s)	2	0	<1	0	0	0.00	0	0
Soda, cola	12	fluid ounce(s)	179	<1	46	0	0	0.00	—	0
Soda, ginger ale	12	fluid ounce(s)	124	0	32	0	0	0.00	0	0
Soda, lemon lime	12	fluid ounce(s)	147	0	38	0	0	0.00	—	0
Soda, root beer	12	fluid ounce(s)	152	0	39	0	0	0.00	0	0
Sour cream	2	tablespoon(s)	51	1	1	0	5	3.13	—	11
Sour cream, fat free	2	tablespoon(s)	24	1	5	0	0	0.00	0	3
Soy sauce	1	tablespoon(s)	10	1	2	0	<.1	0.00	—	0
Spinach, canned, drained	½	cup(s)	25	3	4	3	1	0.09	—	0
Spinach, chopped, boiled, drained	½	cup(s)	21	3	3	2	<1	0.04	—	0
Spinach, raw, chopped	1	cup(s)	7	1	1	1	<1	0.02	—	0
Squash, acorn, baked	½	cup(s)	57	1	15	5	<1	0.03	—	0
Squash, summer, all varieties, sliced, boiled, drained	½	cup(s)	18	1	4	1	<1	0.06	—	0
Squash, winter, all varieties, baked, mashed	½	cup(s)	38	1	9	3	<1	0.13	—	0
Squid, mixed species, fried	3	ounce(s)	149	15	7	0	6	1.60	—	221
Strawberries, raw	½	cup(s)	23	<1	6	1	<1	0.01	—	0
Strawberries, sweetened, frozen, thawed	½	cup(s)	99	1	27	2	<1	0.01	—	0
Sugar, brown, packed	1	teaspoon(s)	17	0	4	0	0	0.00	0	0
Sugar, white, granulated	1	teaspoon(s)	15	0	4	0	0	0.00		
Sweet potatoes, baked, peeled	½	cup(s)	90	2	21	3	<1	0.03	—	0
Syrup, maple	¼	cup(s)	209	0	54	0	<1	0.03	—	0
Taco shell, hard	1	item(s)	62	1	8	1	3	0.43	—	0
Tangerine, raw	1	item(s)	37	1	9	2	<1	0.02	—	0
Tea, decaffeinated, prepared	8	fluid ounce(s)	2	0	1	0	0	0.00	0	0
Tea, herbal, prepared	8	fluid ounce(s)	2	0	<1	0	0	0.00	0	0
Tea, prepared	8	fluid ounce(s)	2	0	1	0	0	0.00	0	0
Teriyaki sauce	1	tablespoon(s)	15	1	3	<.1	0	0.00	0	0

Food Description	Qty	Measure	Energy (cal)	Protein (g)	Carb (g)	Dietary Fiber (g)	Fat (g)	Sat Fat (g)	Trans Fat (g)	Cholesterol (mg)
Tofu, firm	3	ounce(s)	80	8	2	1	4	0.50	—	0
Tomato juice, canned	½	cup(s)	21	1	5	<1	<.1	0.01	—	0
Tomato sauce	½	cup(s)	46	2	8	2	1	0.18	0	0
Tomatoes, fresh, ripe, red	1	item(s)	22.13	1.08	4.82	1.47	0.24	0.05	—	0
Tomatoes, stewed, canned, red	½	cup(s)	33	1	8	1	<1	0.03	—	0
Tortilla chips, plain	6	item(s)	142	2	18	2	7	1.43	—	0
Tortillas, corn, soft	1	item(s)	58	1	12	1	1	0.09	—	0
Tortillas, flour	1	item(s)	104	3	18	1	2	0.56	—	0
Tuna, light, canned in oil, drained	2	ounce(s)	113	17	0	0	5	0.87	—	10
Tuna, light, canned in water, drained	2	ounce(s)	66	14	0	0	<1	0.13	—	17
Turkey, breast, processed, oven roasted, fat free	1	slice(s)	25	4	1	0	0	0.00	0	10
Turkey, breast, processed, traditional carved	2	slice(s)	40	9	0	0	1	0.00	—	20
Turkey, roasted, dark meat, meat only	3	ounce(s)	159	24	0	0	6	2.06	—	72
Turkey, roasted, light meat, meat only	3	ounce(s)	133	25	0	0	3	0.88	—	59
Turnip greens, chopped, boiled, drained	½	cup(s)	14	1	3	3	<1	0.04	—	0
Turnips, cubed, boiled, drained	½	cup(s)	17	1	4	2	<.1	0.01	—	0
Vegetables, mixed, canned, drained	½	cup(s)	40	2	8	2	<1	0.04	—	0
Vinegar, balsamic	1	tablespoon(s)	10	0	2	0	0	0.00	0	0
Waffle, plain, frozen, toasted	2	item(s)	174	4	27	2	5	0.95	—	16
Walnuts, dried black, chopped	¼	cup(s)	193	8	3	2	18	1.05	—	0
Watermelon	½	cup(s)	23	<1	6	<1	<1	0.01	—	0
Wheat germ, crude	2	tablespoon(s)	52	3	7	2	1	0.24	—	0
Wine cooler	10	fluid ounce(s)	150	<1	18	<.1	<.1	0.01	—	0
Wine, red, California	5	fluid ounce(s)	125	<1	4	0	0	0.00	0	0
Wine, sparkling, domestic	5	fluid ounce(s)	105	<1	4	0	0	0.00	0	0
Wine, white	5	fluid ounce(s)	100	<1	1	0	0	0.00	0	0
Yogurt, custard style, fruit flavors	6	ounce(s)	190	7	32	0	4	2.00	—	15
Yogurt, fruit, low fat	1	cup(s)	243	10	46	0	3	1.82	—	12
Yogurt, fruit, nonfat, sweetened w/low calorie sweetener	1	cup(s)	122	11	19	1	<1	0.21	—	3
Yogurt, plain, low fat	1	cup(s)	154	13	17	0	4	2.45	—	15
VEGETARIAN FOODS										
Prepared										
Macaroni & cheese (lacto)	8	ounce(s)	181	8	17	<1	9	4.37	0	22
Steamed rice & vegetables (vegan)	8	ounce(s)	265	5	40	3	10	1.84	0	0
Vegan spinach enchiladas (vegan)	1	piece(s)	93	5	15	2	2	0.34	—	0
Vegetable chow mein (vegan)	8	ounce(s)	166	6	22	2	6	0.65	0	0
Vegetable lasagna (lacto)	8	ounce(s)	177	12	25	2	4	1.92	0	10

Food Description	Qty	Measure	Energy (cal)	Protein (g)	Carb (g)	Dietary Fiber (g)	Fat (g)	Sat Fat (g)	Trans Fat (g)	Cholesterol (mg)
VEGETARIAN FOODS (continued)										
Prepared (continued)										
Vegetarian chili (vegan)	8	ounce(s)	116	6	21	7	2	0.24	0	<1
Vegetarian vegetable soup (vegan)	8	ounce(s)	92	3	14	2	4	0.77	0	0
Boca burger										
All American flamed grilled patty	1	item(s)	110	14	6	4	4	1.00	0	3
Boca meatless ground burger	½	cup(s)	70	11	7	4	1	0.00	—	0
Breakfast links	2	item(s)	100	10	6	5	4	0.00	0	0
Breakfast patties	1	item(s)	80	8	5	3	4	0.00	0	0
Vegan original patty	1	item(s)	90	13	4	0	1	0.00	0	0
Gardenburger										
Black bean burger	1	item(s)	80	8	11	4	2	0.00	0	0
Chik'n grill	1	item(s)	100	13	5	3	3	0.00	0	0
Meatless breakfast sausage	1	item(s)	50	5	2	2	4	0.00	0	0
Meatless meatballs	6	item(s)	110	12	8	4	5	1.00	0	0
Original	3	ounce(s)	132	7	19	4	4	1.80	0	24
Morningstar Farms										
America's Original Veggie Dog links	1	item(s)	80	11	6	1	1	0.00	0	0
Better n Eggs egg substitute	¼	cup(s)	20	5	0	0	0	0.00	0	0
Breakfast links	2	item(s)	80	9	3	2	3	0.50	0	0
Breakfast strips	2	item(s)	60	2	2	1	5	0.50	0	0
Garden veggie patties	1	item(s)	100	10	9	4	3	0.50	0	0
Spicy black bean veggie burger	1	item(s)	150	11	16	5	5	0.50	0	0
MIXED FOODS, SOUPS, SANDWICHES										
Mixed Dishes										
Bean burrito	1	item(s)	327	17	33	6	15	8.30	0	38
Beef & vegetable fajita	1	item(s)	397	23	35	3	18	5.50	—	45
Chicken & vegetables w/broccoli, onion, bamboo shoots in soy based sauce	1	cup(s)	287	22	6	1	19	5.13	—	84
Chicken cacciatore	1	cup(s)	266	28	5	1	14	3.98	0	103
Chicken waldorf salad	½	cup(s)	178	14	6	1	11	1.76	0	42
Fettuccine alfredo	1	cup(s)	247	11	42	1	3	1.61	0	9
Hummus	½	cup(s)	218	6	25	5	11	1.38	—	0
Lasagna w/ground beef	1	cup(s)	288	18	22	2	15	7.47	0	68
Macaroni & cheese	1	cup(s)	393	15	40	1	19	8.18	—	30
Meat loaf	1	slice(s)	244	17	7	<1	16	6.15	0	85
Potato salad	½	cup(s)	179	3	14	2	10	1.79	—	85
Spaghetti & meatballs w/tomato sauce, prepared	1	cup(s)	330	19	39	3	12	3.90	—	89
Spicy thai noodles (pad thai)	8	ounce(s)	222	9	36	3	6	0.83	0	37
Sushi w/vegetables in seaweed	6	piece(s)	182	3	41	1	<1	0.10	—	0
Tuna salad	½	cup(s)	192	16	10	0	9	1.58	0	13

Food Description	Qty	Measure	Energy (cal)	Protein (g)	Carb (g)	Dietary Fiber (g)	Fat (g)	Sat Fat (g)	Trans Fat (g)	Cholesterol (mg)
MIXED FOODS, SOUPS, SANDWICHES (continued)										
Soups										
Chicken noodle, condensed, prepared w/water	1	cup(s)	75	4	9	1	2	0.65	–	7
Cream of chicken, condensed, prepared w/milk	1	cup(s)	191	7	15	<1	11	4.64	–	27
Cream of mushroom, condensed, prepared w/milk	1	cup(s)	203	6	15	<1	14	5.13	–	20
Manhattan clam chowder, condensed, prepared w/water	1	cup(s)	78	2	12	1	2	0.38	–	2
Minestrone, condensed, prepared w/water	1	cup(s)	82	4	11	1	3	0.55	–	2
New England clam chowder, condensed, prepared w/milk	1	cup(s)	164	9	17	1	7	2.95	–	22
Split pea	1	cup(s)	85	4	19	2	<1	0.07	0	0
Tomato, condensed, prepared w/milk	1	cup(s)	161	6	22	3	6	2.90	–	17
Tomato, condensed, prepared w/water	1	cup(s)	85	2	17	<1	2	0.37	–	0
Vegetable beef, condensed, prepared w/water	1	cup(s)	78	6	10	<1	2	0.85	–	5
Vegetarian vegetable, condensed, prepared w/water	1	cup(s)	72	2	12	–	2	0.29	–	0
Sandwiches										
Bacon, lettuce, & tomato w/ mayonnaise	1	item(s)	349	11	34	2	19	4.54	–	20
Cheeseburger, large, plain	1	item(s)	609	30	47	0	33	14.84	–	96
Cheeseburger, large, w/bacon, vegetables, & condiments	1	item(s)	608	32	37	2	37	16.24	–	111
Club w/bacon, chicken, tomato, lettuce, & mayonnaise	1	item(s)	555	31	48	3	26	5.94	–	72
Cold cut submarine w/cheese & vegetables	1	item(s)	456	22	51	2	19	6.81	–	36
Egg salad	1	item(s)	278	10	29	1	13	2.96	–	217
Hamburger, double patty, large, w/condiments & vegetables	1	item(s)	540	34	40	0	27	10.52	–	122
Hamburger, large, plain	1	item(s)	426	23	32	2	23	8.38	–	71
Hot dog w/bun, plain	1	item(s)	242	10	18	2	15	5.11	–	44
Pastrami	1	item(s)	331	14	27	2	18	6.18	–	51
Peanut butter & jelly	1	item(s)	330	11	42	3	15	3.00	–	1
FAST FOOD										
Arby's										
Au jus sauce	1	serving(s)	5	<1	1	<.1	<.1	0.02	–	0
Beef 'n cheddar sandwich	1	item(s)	480	23	43	2	24	8.00	–	90
Curly fries, medium	1	serving(s)	400	5	50	4	20	5.00	–	0
Market Fresh grilled chicken Caesar salad w/o dressing	1	serving(s)	230	33	8	3	8	3.50	–	80
Roast beef deluxe sandwich, light	1	item(s)	296	18	33	6	10	3.00	–	42

Food Description	Qty	Measure	Energy (cal)	Protein (g)	Carb (g)	Dietary Fiber (g)	Fat (g)	Sat Fat (g)	Trans Fat (g)	Cholesterol (mg)
FAST FOOD (continued)										
Arby's (continued)										
Roast beef sandwich, giant	1	item(s)	480	32	41	3	23	10.00	–	110
Roast beef sandwich, regular	1	item(s)	350	21	34	2	16	6.00	–	85
Roast chicken deluxe sandwich, light	1	item(s)	260	23	33	3	5	1.00	–	40
Burger King										
BK Broiler chicken sandwich	1	item(s)	550	30	52	3	25	5.00	–	105
Croissanwich w/sausage, egg, & cheese	1	item(s)	520	19	24	1	39	14.00	1.93	210
Fish Fillet sandwich	1	item(s)	520	18	44	2	30	8.00	1.12	55
French fries, medium, salted	1	item(s)	360	4	46	4	18	5.00	4.50	0
Onion rings, medium	1	serving(s)	320	4	40	3	16	4.00	3.50	0
Whopper	1	item(s)	710	31	52	4	43	13.00	1	85
Whopper w/cheese	1	item(s)	800	36	53	4	50	18.00	2	110
Chick-Fil-A										
Chargrilled chicken garden salad	1	item(s)	180	22	9	3	6	3.00	0	70
Chargrilled deluxe chicken sandwich	1	item(s)	290	27	31	2	7	1.50	0	70
Chicken biscuit w/cheese	1	item(s)	450	19	43	2	23	7.00	2.85	45
Chicken salad sandwich	1	item(s)	350	20	32	5	15	3.00	0	65
Chick-n-Strips	4	item(s)	290	29	14	1	13	2.50	0	65
Coleslaw	1	item(s)	210	1	14	2	17	2.50	0	20
Dairy Queen										
Banana split	1	item(s)	510	8	96	3	12	8.00	0	30
Chocolate chip cookie dough blizzard, small	1	item(s)	720	12	105	0	28	14.00	2.50	50
Chocolate malt, small	1	item(s)	650	15	111	0	16	10.00	0.50	55
Vanilla soft serve	½	cup(s)	140	3	22	0	5	3.00	0	15
Domino's										
Classic hand tossed pizza										
America's favorite feast, 12"	2	slice(s)	508	22	57	4	22	9.20	–	49
Pepperoni feast, extra pepperoni & cheese, 12"	2	slice(s)	534	24	56	3	25	10.92	–	57
Vegi feast, 12"	2	slice(s)	439	19	57	4	16	7.09	–	34
Thin crust pizza										
Extravaganzza, 12"	¼	item(s)	425	20	34	3	24	9.41	–	53
Pepperoni, extra pepperoni & cheese, 12"	¼	item(s)	420	20	32	2	24	10.46	–	54
Vegi, 12"	¼	item(s)	338	16	34	3	17	7.08	–	34
Ultimate deep dish pizza										
America's favorite, 12"	2	slice(s)	617	26	59	4	33	12.88	–	58
Pepperoni, extra pepperoni & cheese, 12"	2	slice(s)	629	26	57	4	34	13.57	–	61
Vegi, 12"	2	slice(s)	547	22	59	4	26	10.19	–	41
In-n-Out Burger										
Cheeseburger w/mustard & ketchup	1	item(s)	400	22	41	3	18	9.00	–	55

Food Description	Qty	Measure	Energy (cal)	Protein (g)	Carb (g)	Dietary Fiber (g)	Fat (g)	Sat Fat (g)	Trans Fat (g)	Cholesterol (mg)
FAST FOOD (continued)										
In-n-Out Burger (continued)										
Chocolate shake	1	item(s)	690	9	83	0	36	24.00	–	95
Double-Double cheeseburger w/mustard & ketchup	1	item(s)	590	37	42	3	32	17.00	–	115
French fries	1	item(s)	400	7	54	2	18	5.00	–	0
Hamburger w/mustard & ketchup	1	item(s)	310	16	41	3	10	4.00	–	35
Jack in the Box										
Chicken club salad	1	item(s)	310	28	15	5	16	6.00	0	65
Hamburger	1	item(s)	250	12	30	2	9	3.50	0.88	30
Jack's Spicy Chicken sandwich	1	item(s)	580	24	53	3	31	6.00	2.81	60
Jumbo Jack hamburger w/ cheese	1	item(s)	690	26	60	3	38	16.00	1.55	75
Sourdough Jack	1	item(s)	700	30	36	3	49	16.00	2.98	80
Jamba Juice										
Banana berry smoothie	24	fluid ounce(s)	470	5	112	5	2	0.50	–	5
Chocolate mood smoothie	24	fluid ounce(s)	690	16	142	2	8	4.50	–	25
Jamba powerboost smoothie	24	fluid ounce(s)	440	6	103	7	2	0.00	–	0
Orange juice, freshly squeezed	16	fluid ounce(s)	220	3	52	1	1	0.00	–	0
Protein berry pizzaz smoothie	24	fluid ounce(s)	440	20	92	6	2	0.00	–	0
Kentucky Fried Chicken (KFC)										
Extra Crispy chicken, breast	1	item(s)	470	34	19	0	28	8.00	4.50	135
Hot & spicy chicken, whole wing	1	item(s)	180	11	9	0	11	3.00	0	60
Original Recipe chicken, drum-stick	1	item(s)	140	14	4	0	8	2.00	1	75
Long John Silver's										
Baked cod	1	serving(s)	120	22	1	0	5	1.00	–	90
Batter dipped fish sandwich	1	item(s)	440	17	48	3	20	5.00	–	35
Clam chowder	1	item(s)	220	9	23	0	10	4.00	–	25
Crunchy shrimp basket	21	item(s)	340	12	32	2	19	5.00	–	105
McDonald's										
Big Mac hamburger	1	item(s)	590	24	47	3	34	11.00	1.48	85
Cheeseburger	1	item(s)	330	15	36	2	14	6.00	1.02	45
Chicken McNuggets	4	item(s)	210	10	12	1	13	2.50	1.13	35
Egg McMuffin	1	item(s)	300	18	29	2	12	4.50	0.42	235
Filet-o-fish sandwich	1	item(s)	470	15	45	1	26	5.00	1.11	50
French fries, small	1	serving(s)	210	3	26	2	10	1.50	2.30	0
Fruit 'n yogurt parfait	1	item(s)	380	10	76	2	5	2.00	0.18	15
Hash browns	1	item(s)	130	1	14	1	8	1.50	2	0
Honey sauce	1	item(s)	45	0	12	0	0	0.00	–	0
McSalad Shaker garden salad	1	item(s)	100	7	4	2	6	3.00	–	75
McSalad Shaker grilled chicken caesar salad	1	item(s)	100	17	3	2	3	1.50	–	40
Newman's Own creamy Cae-sar salad dressing	1	item(s)	190	2	4	0	18	3.50	0.29	20

Food Description	Qty	Measure	Energy (cal)	Protein (g)	Carb (g)	Dietary Fiber (g)	Fat (g)	Sat Fat (g)	Trans Fat (g)	Cholesterol (mg)
FAST FOOD (continued)										
McDonald's (continued)										
Plain hotcakes w/syrup & margarine	3	item(s)	600	9	104	0	17	3.00	4	20
Quarter Pounder hamburger	1	item(s)	430	23	37	2	21	8.00	1.01	70
Quarter Pounder hamburger w/cheese	1	item(s)	530	28	38	2	30	13.00	1.51	95
Sausage McMuffin w/egg	1	item(s)	450	20	29	2	28	10.00	0.59	255
Vanilla milkshake	8	fluid ounce(s)	254	9	40	0	7	4.28	–	27
Pizza Hut										
Pepperoni Lovers stuffed crust pizza	1	slice(s)	480	23	44	3	24	11.00	1.05	65
Pepperoni Lovers thin 'n crispy pizza	1	slice(s)	270	13	22	2	14	7.00	0.51	40
Personal Pan supreme pizza	1	slice(s)	170	8	19	1	7	3.00	0.95	15
Veggie Lovers stuffed crust pizza	1	slice(s)	370	17	45	3	14	7.00	0.53	35
Veggie Lovers thin 'n crispy pizza	1	slice(s)	190	8	23	2	7	3.00	0.54	15
Starbucks										
Cappuccino, tall	12	fluid ounce(s)	120	7	10	0	6	4.00	–	25
Cinnamon spice mocha, tall nonfat w/o whipped cream	12	fluid ounce(s)	170	11	32	0	0	0.50	0	5
Frappuccino, tall chocolate	12	fluid ounce(s)	290	13	52	1	5	1.00	–	3
Latte, tall w/nonfat milk	12	fluid ounce(s)	123	12	17	0	1	0.40	0	6
Latte, tall w/whole milk	12	fluid ounce(s)	212	11	17	0	11	6.90	–	46
Macchiato, tall caramel w/ whole milk	12	fluid ounce(s)	190	6	27	0	7	4.00	–	25
Tazo chai black tea, tall nonfat	12	fluid ounce(s)	170	6	37	0	0	0.00	0	5
Subway										
Chocolate chip cookie	1	item(s)	209	3	29	1	10	3.50	1.07	12
Classic Italian B.M.T. sandwich, 6", white bread	1	item(s)	453	21	40	3	24	8.00	0	56
Meatball sandwich, 6", white bread	1	item(s)	501	23	46	4	25	10.00	0.75	56
Roast beef sandwich, 6", white bread	1	item(s)	264	18	39	3	5	1.00	0	20
Roasted chicken breast sandwich, 6", white bread	1	item(s)	311	25	40	3	6	1.50	0	48
Tuna sandwich, 6", white bread	1	item(s)	419	18	39	3	21	5.00	–	42
Turkey breast sandwich, 6", white bread	1	item(s)	254	16	39	3	4	1.00	0	15
Taco Bell										
7-layer burrito	1	item(s)	530	18	67	10	22	8.00	3	25
Beef burrito supreme	1	item(s)	440	18	51	7	18	8.00	2	40
Grilled chicken burrito	1	item(s)	390	19	49	3	13	4.00	–	40
Taco	1	item(s)	170	8	13	3	10	4.00	0.50	25
Veggie fajita wrap supreme	1	item(s)	470	11	55	3	22	7.00	–	30

Food Description	Qty	Measure	Energy (cal)	Protein (g)	Carb (g)	Dietary Fiber (g)	Fat (g)	Sat Fat (g)	Trans Fat (g)	Cholesterol (mg)
CONVENIENCE MEALS										
Budget Gourmet										
Cheese manicotti w/meat sauce	1	item(s)	420	18	38	4	22	11.00	–	85
Chicken w/fettuccine	1	item(s)	380	20	33	3	19	10.00	–	85
Light beef stroganoff	1	item(s)	290	20	32	3	7	4.00	–	35
Light sirloin of beef in herb sauce	1	item(s)	260	19	30	5	7	4.00	–	30
Light vegetable lasagna	1	item(s)	290	15	36	5	9	1.79	–	15
Healthy Choice										
Chicken enchilada suprema meal	1	item(s)	360	13	59	8	7	3.00	–	30
Lemon pepper fish meal	1	item(s)	280	11	49	5	5	2.00	–	30
Traditional salisbury steak meal	1	item(s)	360	23	45	5	9	3.50	–	45
Traditional turkey breasts meal	1	item(s)	330	21	50	4	5	2.00	–	35
Zucchini lasagna	1	item(s)	280	13	47	5	4	2.50	–	10
Stouffers										
Cheese enchiladas with Mexican rice	1	serving(s)	370	12	48	5	14	5.00	–	25
Chicken pot pie	1	item(s)	740	23	56	4	47	18.00	–	65
Homestyle beef pot roast & potatoes	1	item(s)	270	16	25	3	12	4.50	–	35
Homestyle roast turkey breast w/stuffing & mashed potatoes	1	item(s)	300	16	34	2	11	3.00	–	35
Lean Cuisine Everyday Favorites chicken chow mein w/rice	1	item(s)	210	12	33	2	3	1.00	0	30
Lean Cuisine Everyday Favorites lasagna w/meat sauce	1	item(s)	300	19	41	3	8	4.00	0	30
Weight Watchers										
Smart Ones chicken enchiladas suiza entree	1	serving(s)	270	15	33	2	9	3.50	–	50
Smart Ones garden lasagna entree	1	item(s)	270	14	36	5	7	3.50	–	30
Smart Ones pepperoni pizza	1	item(s)	390	23	46	4	12	4.00	–	45
Smart Ones spicy penne pasta & ricotta	1	item(s)	280	11	45	4	6	2.00	–	5
Smart Ones spicy Szechuan style vegetables & chicken	1	item(s)	220	11	39	3	2	0.50	–	10

Chapter 1

1. W. M. Bortz II, "Disuse and Aging," *Journal of the American Medical Association*, 248 (1982): 1203–1208.
2. U.S. Department of Health and Human Services, Centers for Disease Control and Prevention, National Center for Health Statistics, *National Vital Statistics Reports, Deaths: Final Data for 2004*, 55:19 (August 21, 2007).
3. T. A. Murphy and D. Murphy, *The Wellness for Life Workbook* (San Diego: Fitness Publications, 1987).
4. W. L. Haskell et al., "Physical Activity and Public Health: Updated Recommendation for Adults from the American College of Sports Medicine and the American Heart Association," *Medicine and Science in Sports and Exercise* 39 (2007): 1423–1434.
5. U.S. Department of Health and Human Services, *Physical Activity and Health: A Report of the Surgeon General* (Atlanta: Centers for Disease Control and Prevention, National Center for Chronic Disease Prevention and Health Promotion, 1996).
6. American College of Sports Medicine, *ACSM's Guidelines for Exercise Testing and Prescription* (Baltimore: Williams & Wilkins, 2006).
7. National Academy of Sciences, Institute of Medicine, *Dietary Reference Intakes for Energy, Carbohydrates, Fiber, Fat, Protein and Amino Acids (Macronutrients)* (Washington, DC: National Academy Press, 2002).
8. U.S. Department of Health and Human Services and Department of Agriculture, *Dietary Guidelines for Americans, 2005* (Washington, DC: DHHS, 2005).
9. R. S. Paffenbarger, Jr., R. T. Hyde, A. L. Wing, and C. H. Steinmetz, "A Natural History of Athleticism and Cardiovascular Health," *Journal of the American Medical Association* 252 (1984): 491–495.
10. S. N. Blair, H. W. Kohl III, R. S. Paffenbarger, Jr., D. G. Clark, K. H. Cooper, and L. W. Gibbons, "Physical Fitness and All-Cause Mortality: A Prospective Study of Healthy Men and Women," *Journal of the American Medical Association* 262 (1989): 2395–2401.
11. S. N. Blair, H. W. Kohl III, C. E. Barlow, R. S. Paffenbarger, Jr., L. W. Gibbons, and C. A. Macera, "Changes in Physical Fitness and All-Cause Mortality: A Prospective Study of Healthy and Unhealthy Men," *Journal of the American Medical Association* 273 (1995): 1193–1198.
12. I. Lee, C. Hsieh, and R. S. Paffenbarger, Jr., "Exercise Intensity and Longevity in Men: The Harvard Alumni Health Study," *Journal of the American Medical Association* 273 (1995): 1179–1184.
13. U.S. Department of Health and Human Services, *Healthy People 2010 Objectives: Draft for Public Comment* (Washington, DC: Public Health Service, 1998).
14. J. O. Prochaska, J. C. Norcross, and C. C. DiClemente, *Changing for Good* (New York: William Morrow and Co., 1994).
15. See note 6.

Chapter 2

1. R. B. O'Hara et al., "Increased Volume Resistance Training: Effects upon Predicted Aerobic Fitness in a Select Group of Air Force Men," *ACSM's Health and Fitness Journal* 8, no. 4 (2004): 16–25.
2. W. L. Haskell et al., "Physical Activity and Public Health: Updated Recommendation for Adults from the American College of Sports Medicine and the American Heart Association," *Medicine and Science in Sports and Exercise* 39 (2007): 1423–1434.
3. American College of Sports Medicine, *Guidelines for Exercise Testing and Prescription* (Philadelphia: Lippincott Williams & Wilkins, 2006).
4. W. J. Evans, "Exercise Nutrition and Aging," *Journal of Nutrition* 122 (1992): 786–801.
5. R. Kjorstad, *Validity of Two Field Tests of Abdominal Strength and Muscular Endurance*, unpublished master's thesis, Boise State University, 1997.
6. G. L. Hall, R. K. Hetzler, D. Perrin, and A. Weltman, "Relationship of Timed Sit-Up Tests to Isokinetic Abdominal Strength," *Research Quarterly for Exercise and Sport* 63 (1992): 80–84.
7. American College of Obstetricians and Gynecologists, "Exercise During Pregnancy and the Postpartum Period," *Obstetrics and Gynecology* 99 (2002): 171–173.
8. "Stretch Yourself Younger," *Consumer Reports on Health* 11 (August 1999): 6–7.
9. J. H. Wilmore, *Exercise and Weight Control: Myths, Misconceptions, Gadgets, Gimmicks, and Quackery*, lecture given at annual meeting of American College of Sports Medicine, Indianapolis, June 1994.
10. K. M. Flegal, M. D. Carrol, R. J. Kuczmarski, and C. L. Johnson, "Overweight and Obesity in the United States: Prevalence and Trends, 1960–1994," *International Journal of Obesity and Related Metabolic Disorders* 22 (1998): 39–47.

Chapter 3

1. H. Atkinson, "Exercise for Longer Life: The Physician's Perspective," *Health News* 3:7 (1997): 3.
2. W. W. K. Hoeger, L. Bond, L. Ransdell, J. M. Shimon, and S. Merugu, "One-Mile Step Count at Walking and Running Speeds." *ACSM Health & Fitness Journal* 12, no. 1 (2008): 14–19.
3. American College of Sports Medicine, *Guidelines for Exercise Testing and Prescription* (Philadelphia: Lippincott Williams & Wilkins, 2006).
4. See note 3.
5. W. L. Haskell et al., "Physical Activity and Public Health: Updated Recommendation for Adults from the American College of Sports Medicine and the American Heart Association," *Medicine and Science in Sports and Exercise* 39 (2007): 1423–1434.
6. U.S. Department of Health and Human Services, *Physical Activity and Health: A Report of the Surgeon General* (Atlanta: Centers for Disease Control and Prevention, National Center for Chronic Disease Prevention and Health Promotion, 1996).
7. D. P. Swain, "Moderate- or Vigorous-Intensity Exercise: What Should We Prescribe?" *ACSM's Health & Fitness Journal* 10, no. 5 (2006): 7–11.
8. D. P. Swain and B. A. Franklin, "Comparative Cardioprotective Benefits of Vigorous vs. Moderate Intensity Aerobic Exercise," *American Journal of Cardiology* 97, no. 1 (2006): 141–147.

9. See note 5.

10. S. N. Blair, "Surgeon General's Report on Physical Fitness: The Inside Story," *ACSM's Health & Fitness Journal* 1 (1997): 14–18.

11. R. F. DeBusk, U. Stenestrand, M. Sheehan, and W. L. Haskell, "Training Effects of Long Versus Short Bouts of Exercise in Healthy Subjects," *American Journal of Cardiology* 65 (1990): 1010–1013.

12. National Academy of Sciences, Institute of Medicine, *Dietary Reference Intakes for Energy, Carbohydrates, Fiber, Fat, Protein and Amino Acids (Macronutrients)* (Washington, DC: National Academy Press, 2002).

13. U.S. Department of Health and Human Services, Department of Agriculture, *Dietary Guidelines for Americans 2005* (Washington, DC: DHHS, 2005).

14. W. W. K. Hoeger, D. R. Hopkins, S. L. Barette, and D. F. Hale, "Relationship Between Repetitions and Selected Percentages of One Repetition Maximum: A Comparison Between Untrained and Trained Males and Females," *Journal of Applied Sport Science Research* 4, no. 2 (1990): 47–51.

15. See note 3.

16. M. E. Nelson et al., "Physical Activity and Public Health in Older Adults: Recommendation from the American College of Sports Medicine and the American Heart Association," *Medicine and Science in Sports and Exercise* 39 (2007): 1435–1445.

17. See note 3.

18. Gatorade Sports Science Institute, "Core Strength Training," *Sports Science Exchange Roundtable* 13, no. 1 (2002): 1–4.

19. S. B. Thacker, J. Gilchrist, D. F. Stroup, and C. D. Kimsey, Jr., "The Impact of Stretching on Sports Injury Risk: A Systematic Review of the Literature," *Medicine and Science in Sports and Exercise* 36 (2004): 371–378.

20. "Should You Stretch Before Exercise?" *Gatorade Sports Science Institute: Sports Science Exchange* 30, no. 1 (2007).

21. R. Deyo, "Chiropractic Care for Back Pain: The Physician's Perspective," *HealthNews* 4 (September 10, 1998).

22. J. A. Hides, G. A. Jull, and C. A. Richardson, "Long-Term Effects of Specific Stabilizing Exercises for First-Episode Low Back Pain," *Spine* 26 (2001): E243–E248.

Chapter 4

1. J. L. Christi, L. M. Sheldahl, F. E. Tristani, L. S. Wann, K. B. Sagar, S. G. Levandoski, M. J. Ptacin, K. A. Sobocinski, and R. D. Morris, "Cardiovascular Regulation During Head-out Water Immersion Exercise," *Journal of Applied Physiology* 69 (1990): 657–664; L. M. Sheldahl, F. E. Tristani, P. S. Clifford, C. V. Hughes, K. A. Sobocinski, and R. D. Morris, "Effect of Head-out Water Immersion on Cardiorespiratory Response to Dynamic Exercise," *Journal of American College of Cardiology* 10 (1987): 1254–1258; J. Svedenhang and J. Seger, "Running on Land and in Water: Comparative Exercise Physiology," *Medicine and Science in Sports and Exercise* 24 (1992): 1155–1160.

2. W. W. K. Hoeger, D. Hopkins, and D. Barber, "Physiologic Responses to Maximal Treadmill Running and Water Aerobic Exercise," *National Aquatics Journal* 11 (1995): 4–7.

3. W. W. K. Hoeger, T. A. Spitzer-Gibson, N. Kaluhiokalani, R. K. M. Cardejon, and J. Kokkonen, "A Comparison of Physiological Responses to Self-Paced Water Aerobics and Self-Paced Treadmill Running," *International Council for Health, Physical Education, Recreation, Sport, and Dance Journal* 30, no. 4 (2004): 27–30.

4. W. W. K. Hoeger, T. S. Gibson, J. Moore, and D. R. Hopkins, "A Comparison of Selected Training Responses to Low Impact Aerobics and Water Aerobics," *National Aquatics Journal* 9 (1993): 13–16.

5. E. J. Marcinick, J. Potts, G. Schlabach, S. Will, P. Dawson, and B. F. Hurley, "Effects of Strength Training on Lactate Threshold and Endurance Performance," *Medicine and Science in Sports and Exercise* 23 (1991): 739–743.

Chapter 5

1. E. B. Rimm, A. Ascherio, E. Giovannucci, D. Spiegelman, M. J. Stampfer, and W. C. Willett, "Vegetable, Fruit, and Cereal Fiber Intake and Risk of Coronary Heart Disease Among Men," *Journal of the American Medical Association* 275 (1996): 447–451.

2. National Academy of Sciences, Institute of Medicine, *Dietary Reference Intakes for Energy, Carbohydrates, Fiber, Fat, Protein and Amino Acids (Macronutrients)* (Washington, DC: National Academy Press, 2002).

3. G. Bjelakovic et al., "Mortality in Randomized Trials of Antioxidant Supplements for Primary and Secondary Prevention," *Journal of the American Medical Association* 297 (2007): 842–857.

4. L. C. Clark et al., "Effects of Selenium Supplementation for Cancer Prevention in Patients with Carcinoma of the Skin: A Randomized Controlled Trial," *Journal of the American Medical Association* 276 (1996):1957–1963.

5. "Does This Mineral Prevent Cancer?" *University of California at Berkeley Wellness Letter* 16, no. 9 (2000): 1–2.

6. "The Merits of Multivitamins: EN's Guide to Choosing a Supplement," *Environmental Nutrition* 24, no. 6 (2001): 1.

7. "Vitamin D May Help You Dodge Cancer; How To Be Sure You Get Enough," *Environmental Nutrition* 30, no. 6 (2007): 1, 4.

8. "Ride the D Train: Research Finds Even More Reasons to Get Vitamin D," *Environmental Nutrition* 28, no. 9 (2005): 1, 4.

9. "Eating Fish: Rewards Outweigh Risks," *Tufts University Health & Nutrition Letter* (January 2007).

10. D. Mozaffarian and E. B. Rimm, "Fish Intake, Contaminants, and Human Health," *Journal of the American Medical Association* 296 (2006): 1885–1899.

11. American Psychiatric Association, *Diagnostic and Statistical Manual of Mental Disorders* (Washington, DC: APA, 1994).

12. See note 11.

13. U.S. Department of Health and Human Services, Department of Agriculture, *Dietary Guidelines for Americans 2005* (Washington, DC: DHHS, 2005).

Chapter 6

1. Centers for Disease Control and Prevention, "Fast Stats A to Z: Overweight," http://www.cdc.gov/nchs/faststats/overwt.htm (Atlanta: CDC). Accessed July 5, 2007.

2. A. H. Mokdad, J. S. Marks, D. F. Stroup, and J. L. Gerberding, "Actual Causes of Death in the United States, 2000," *Journal of the American Medical Association* 291 (2004): 1238–1241.

3. R. Sturm and K. B. Wells, "Does Obesity Contribute as Much to Morbidity as Poverty or Smoking?" *Public Health* 115 (2001): 229–235.

4. E. E. Calle et al., "Overweight, Obesity, and Mortality from Cancer in a Prospectively Studied Cohort of U.S. Adults," *New England Journal of Medicine* 348 (2003): 1625–1638.

5. S. Thomsen, "A Steady Diet of Images," *BYU Magazine* 57, no. 3 (2003): 20–21.

6. G. D. Foster et al., "A Randomized Trial of a Low-Carbohydrate Diet for Obesity," *New England Journal of Medicine* 348 (2003): 2082–2090; F. F. Samaha et al., "A Low-Carbohydrate as Compared with Low-Fat Diet in Severe Obesity," *New England Journal of Medicine* 348 (2003): 2074–2081.

7. R. L. Leibel, M. Rosenbaum, and J. Hirsh, "Changes in Energy Expenditure Resulting from Altered Body Weight," *New England Journal of Medicine* 332 (1995): 621–628.

8. American College of Sports Medicine, "Position Stand: Appropriate Intervention Strategies for Weight Loss and Prevention for Weight Regain for Adults," *Medicine and Science in Sports and Exercise* 33 (2001): 2145–2156.

9. J. H. Wilmore, "Exercise, Obesity, and Weight Control," *Physical Activity and Fitness Research Digest* (Washington, DC: President's Council on Physical Fitness & Sports, 1994).

10. National Academy of Sciences, Institute of Medicine, *Dietary Reference Intakes for Energy, Carbohydrates, Fiber, Fat, Protein and Amino Acids (Macronutrients)* (Washington, DC: National Academy Press, 2002).

11. M. K. Serdula et al., "Prevalence of Attempting Weight Loss and Strategies for Controlling Weight," *Journal of the American Medical Association* 282 (1999): 1353–1358.

12. E. T. Poehlman et al., "Effects of Endurance and Resistance Training on Total Daily Energy Expenditure in Young Women: A Controlled Randomized Trial," *Journal of Clinical Endocrinology and Metabolism* 87 (2002): 1004–1009; L. M. Van Etten et al., "Effect of an 18-wk Weight-Training Program on Energy Expenditure and Physical Activity," *Journal of Applied Physiology* 82 (1997): 298–304;. W. W. Campbell, M. C. Crim, V. R. Young, and W. J. Evans, "Increased Energy Requirements and Changes in Body Composition with Resistance Training in Older Adults," *American Journal of Clinical Nutrition* 60 (1994): 167–175; Z. Wang et al., "Resting Energy Expenditure: Systematic Organization and Critique of Prediction Methods," *Obesity Research* 9 (2001): 331–336.

13. J. R. Karp and W. L. Wescott, "The Resting Metabolic Rate Debate," *Fitness Management* 23, no. 1 (2007): 44–47.

14. American College of Sports Medicine, *ACSM's Guidelines for Exercise Testing and Prescription* (Baltimore: Williams & Wilkins, 2006).

15. A. Tremblay, J. A. Simoneau, and C. Bouchard, "Impact of Exercise Intensity on Body Fatness and Skeletal Muscle Metabolism," *Metabolism* 43 (1994): 814–818.

16. W. W. K. Hoeger, C. Harris, E. M. Long, and D. R. Hopkins, "Four-Week Supplementation with a Natural Dietary Compound Produces Favorable Changes in Body Composition," *Advances in Therapy* 15, no. 5 (1998): 305–313; W. W. K. Hoeger, C. Harris, E. M. Long, R. L. Kjorstad, M. Welch, T. L. Hafner, D. R. Hopkins, "Dietary Supplementation with Chromium Picolinate/L-Carnitine Complex in Combination with Diet and Exercise Enhances Body Composition," *Journal of the American Nutraceutical Association* 2, no. 2 (1999): 40–45.

Chapter 7

1. H. E. Selye, *Stress Without Distress* (New York: Signet, 1974).

2. See Ray Rosenman, "Do You Have Type 'A' Behavior?" *Health and Fitness* (supplement): 1987; Redford Williams, *The Trusting Heart: Great News About Type A Behavior* (New York: Times Books, 1989): 120; Howard Friedman, *The Self-Healing Personality* (New York: Henry Holt & Co., 1991).

3. See note 2, Williams.

4. D. A. Girdano, D. E. Dusek, and G. S. Everly, *Controlling Stress and Tension* (San Francisco: Benjamin Cummings, 2005); W. Schafer, *Stress Management for Wellness* (Ft. Worth: HBJ College Publishers, 1995).

5. S. Bodian, "Meditate Your Way to Much Better Health," *Bottom Line Health* 18 (June 2004): 11–13.

6. D. Mueller, "Yoga Therapy," *ACSM's Health & Fitness Journal* 6, no. 1 (2002): 18–24.

7. S. C. Manchanda et al., "Retardation of Coronary Atherosclerosis with Yoga Lifestyle Intervention," *Journal of the Association of Physicians of India* 48 (2000): 687–694.

8. M. Samuels, "Use Your Mind to Heal Your Body," *Bottom Line/Health* 19 (February 2005): 13–14.

Chapter 8

1. E. R. Growald and A. Lusks, "Beyond Self," *American Health* (March 1988): 51–53.

2. U.S. Department of Health and Human Services, Centers for Disease Control and Prevention, National Center for Health Statistics, National Vital Statistics Reports, *Deaths: Final Data for 2004*, 55:19 (August 21, 2007).

3. See note 2.

4. American Heart Association, *Heart Disease and Stroke Statistics–2007 Update At-a-Glance* (Dallas: AHA, 2007).

5. S. N. Blair, H. W. Kohl III, R. S. Paffenbarger, Jr., D. G. Clark, K. H. Cooper, and L. W. Gibbons, "Physical Fitness and All-Cause Mortality: A Prospective Study of Healthy Men and Women," *Journal of the American Medical Association* 262 (1989): 2395–2401.

6. "Water, Sodium, Potassium: The Verdict Is In," *University of California at Berkeley Wellness Letter* (Palm Coast, FL: The Editors, May 2004).

7. G. A. Kelley and Z. Tran, "Aerobic Exercise and Normotensive Adults: A Meta-analysis," *Medicine and Science in Sports and Exercise* 27 (1995): 1371–1377.

8. R. Collins et al., "Blood Pressure, Stroke, and Coronary Heart Disease: Part 2, Short-term Reductions in Blood Pressure: Overview of Randomized Drug Trials in Their Epidemiological Context," *Lancet* 335 (1990): 827–838.

9. S. N. Blair et al., "Influences of Cardiorespiratory Fitness and Other Precursors on Cardiovascular Disease and All-Ccause Mortality in Men and Women," *Journal of the American Medical Association* 276 (1996): 205–210.

10. G. A. Kelley and K. S. Kelley, "Progressive Resistance Exercise and Resting Blood Pressure: A Meta-Analysis of Randomized Controlled Trials," *Hypertension* 35 (2000): 838–843.

11. "Lipid Research Clinics Program: The Lipid Research Clinic Coronary Primary Prevention Trial Results," *Journal of the American Medical Association* 251 (1984): 351–364.

12. See note 4.

13. American Heart Association, *Heart and Stroke Facts* (Dallas: AHA, 1999).

14. "From Starring Role to Bit Part: Has the Curtain Come Down on Vitamin E?" *Environmental Nutrition* 25, no. 5 (May 2002): 1, 4.

15. A. H. Lichtenstein et al., "Diet and Lifestyle Recommendations Revision 2006: A Scientific Statement from the American Heart Association Nutrition Committee," *Circulation* 114 (2006): 82–96.

16. E. B. Rimm, A. Ascherio, E. Giovannucci, D. Spiegelman, M. J. Stampfer, and W. C. Willett, "Vegetable, Fruit, and Cereal Fiber Intake and Risk for Coronary Heart Disease Among Men," *Journal of the American Medical Association* 275 (1996): 447–451.

17. "The Homocysteine-CVD Connection," *HealthNews* (October 25, 1999).

18. "Inflammation May Be Key Cause of Heart Disease and More: Diet's Role," *Environmental Nutrition* 27, no. 7 (July 2004): 1, 4.

19. G. M. Reaven, T. K. Strom, and B. Fox, *Syndrome X: Overcoming the Silent Killer That Can Give You a Heart Attack* (New York: Simon & Schuster, 2000).

20. See note 4.

21. American Cancer Society, *2008 Cancer Facts and Figures* (New York: ACS, 2008).

22. N. Ahmad et al., "Green Tea Constituent Epigallocatechin-3-Gallate and Induction of Apoptosis and Cell Cycle Arrest in Human Carcinoma Cells," *Journal of the National Cancer Institute* 89 (1997): 1881–1886.

23. C. W. Matthews et al., "Physical Activity and Risk for Endometrial Cancer: A Report from the Shanghai Endometrial Cancer Study," *Cancer Epidemiology Biomarkers & Prevention* 14 (2005): 779–785.

24. M. D. Holmes et al., "Physical Activity and Survival After Breast Cancer Diagnosis," *Journal of the American Medical Association* 293 (2005): 2479–2486.

25. E. L. Giovannucci, "A Prospective Study of Physical Activity and Incident and Fatal Prostate Cancer," *Archives of Internal Medicine* 165 (2005): 1005–1010.

26. H. Weinstock, S. Berman, and W. Cates, "Sexually Transmitted Diseases Among American Youth: Incidence and Prevalence Estimates, 2000," *Perspectives on Sexual and Reproductive Health* 36 (2004): 6–10.

Chapter 9

1. R. S. Paffenbarger, Jr., R. T. Hyde, A. L. Wing, and C. H. Steinmetz, "A Natural History of Athleticism and Cardiovascular Health," *Journal of the American Medical Association* 252 (1984): 491–495.

2. S. N. Blair, H. W. Kohl III, R. S. Paffenbarger, Jr., D. G. Clark, K. H. Cooper, and L. W. Gibbons, "Physical Fitness and All-Cause Mortality: A Prospective Study of Healthy Men and Women," *Journal of the American Medical Association* 262 (1989): 2395–2401.

3. R. Hambrecht et al., "Various Intensities of Leisure Time Physical Activity in Patients with Coronary Artery Disease: Effects on Cardiorespiratory Fitness and Progression of Coronary Atherosclerotic Lesions," *Journal of the American College of Cardiology* 22 (1993): 468–477.

4. C. L. Otis, B. Drinkwater, M. Johnson, A. Loucks, and J. Wilmore, "The Female Athlete Triad," *Medicine and Science in Sports and Exercise* 29 (1997): i–ix.

5. American College of Obstetricians and Gynecologists, "Exercise During Pregnancy and the Postpartum Period," ACOG Committee Opinion No. 267, *International Journal of Gynecology and Obstetrics* 77 (2002): 79–81.

6. "New Advice About Bone Density Tests," *University of California at Berkeley Wellness Letter* 18, no. 10 (2002): 1–2.

7. M. T. Goodman et al., "Association of Dairy Products, Lactose, and Calcium with the Risk of Ovarian Cancer," *American Journal of Epidemiology* 156 (2002): 148–157.

8. Writing Group for the Women's Health Initiative, "Risks and Benefits of Combined Estrogen and Progestin in Healthy Postmenopausal Women: Principal Results from the Women's Health Initiative Randomized Controlled Trial," *Journal of the American Medical Association* 288 (2002): 321–333.

9. "Are Fruits and Vegetables Less Nutritious Today?" *University of California Berkeley Wellness Letter* 14:8 (1998): 1.

10. American College of Sports Medicine, "Position Stand: Exercise and Physical Activity for Older Adults," *Medicine and Science in Sports and Exercise* 30 (1998): 992–1008.

11. F. W. Kash, J. L. Boyer, S. P. Van Camp, L. S. Verity, and J. P. Wallace, "The Effect of Physical Activity on Aerobic Power in Older Men (A Longitudinal Study)," *Physician and Sports Medicine* 18:4 (1990): 73–83.

12. See note 10.

Chapter 1
1. a   2. e   3. d   4. c   5. c   6. b   7. b   8. d   9. a   10. e

Chapter 2
1. e   2. a   3. e   4. e   5. c   6. b   7. b   8. a   9. d   10. c

Chapter 3
1. d   2. c   3. c   4. d   5. a   6. c   7. b   8. c   9. e   10. e

Chapter 4
1. d   2. a   3. c   4. d   5. c   6. a   7. e   8. d   9. a   10. b

Chapter 5
1. b   2. e   3. c   4. d   5. d   6. a   7. a   8. c   9. a   10. e

Chapter 6
1. c   2. d   3. e   4. a   5. b   6. c   7. a   8. c   9. d   10. e

Chapter 7
1. a   2. c   3. c   4. e   5. b   6. e   7. e   8. a   9. e   10. c

Chapter 8
1. e   2. a   3. b   4. e   5. b   6. e   7. e   8. b   9. d   10. c

Chapter 9
1. b   2. e   3. e   4. d   5. d   6. e   7. b   8. a   9. e   10. c

A

Acquired immunodeficiency syndrome (AIDS) End stage of HIV infection, manifested by any of a number of diseases that arise when the body's immune system is compromised by HIV.

Action stage Stage of change in which people are actively changing a negative behavior or adopting a new, healthy behavior.

Activities of daily living Everyday behaviors that people normally do to function in life (cross the street, carry groceries, lift objects, do laundry, sweep floors).

Adequate Intake (AI) The recommended amount of a nutrient intake when sufficient evidence is not available to calculate the EAR and subsequent RDA.

Aerobic dance A series of exercise routines performed to music; more commonly termed "aerobics" now.

Aerobic exercise Activity that requires oxygen to produce the necessary energy to carry out the activity.

Alcoholism Disease in which an individual loses control over drinking alcoholic beverages.

Altruism True concern for and action on behalf of others (opposite of egoism); a sincere desire to serve others above one's personal needs.

Amenorrhea Absence (primary amenorrhea) or cessation (secondary amenorrhea) of normal menstrual function.

Amino acids The basic building blocks of proteins.

Anabolic steroids A synthetic version of the male sex hormone testosterone, which promotes muscle development and hypertrophy through intense strength training.

Android obesity Obesity pattern seen in individuals who tend to store fat in the trunk or abdominal area.

Angiogenesis Capillary (blood vessel) formation into a tumor.

Anorexia nervosa An eating disorder characterized by self-imposed starvation to lose and then maintain very low body weight.

Antibodies Substances produced by the white blood cells in response to an invading agent.

Antioxidants Compounds that prevent oxygen from combining with other substances it might damage.

Arrhythmias Irregular heart rhythms.

Atherosclerosis Fatty/cholesterol deposits in the walls of the arteries, leading to formation of plaque.

B

Ballistic (or dynamic) stretching Exercises performed using jerky, rapid, and bouncy movements.

Basal metabolic rate (BMR) Lowest level of caloric intake necessary to sustain life.

Behavior modification The process used to permanently change negative behaviors in favor of positive behaviors that will lead to better health and well-being.

Benign Noncancerous.

Binge eating An eating disorder characterized by uncontrollable episodes of eating excessive amounts of food within a relatively short time.

Blood lipids Cholesterol and triglycerides.

Blood pressure A measure of the force exerted against the walls of the vessels by the blood flowing through them.

Body composition The fat and nonfat components of the human body.

Body mass index (BMI) Incorporates height and weight to estimate critical fat values at which risk for disease increases.

Bulimia nervosa An eating disorder characterized by a pattern of binge eating and purging.

C

Calorie The amount of heat necessary to raise the temperature of 1 gram of water 1 degree centigrade; used to measure the energy value of food and the cost of physical activity.

Cancer Group of diseases characterized by uncontrolled growth and spread of abnormal cells into malignant tumors.

Carbohydrates Compounds composed of carbon, hydrogen, and oxygen that the body uses as its major source of energy.

Carcinogens Substances that contribute to the formation of cancers.

Carcinoma in situ Encapsulated malignant tumor that is found at an early stage and has not spread.

Cardiomyopathy A disease affecting the heart muscle.

Cardiorespiratory endurance Ability of the lungs, heart, and blood vessels to deliver adequate amounts of oxygen to the cells to meet the demands of prolonged physical activity.

Cardiorespiratory training zone The range of intensity at which a person should exercise to develop the cardiorespiratory system.

Cardiovascular diseases The array of conditions that affect the heart and blood vessels.

Carotenoids Pigment substances (more than 600) in plants, about 50 of which are precursors to vitamin A; the most potent carotenoid is beta-carotene.

Cholesterol A waxy substance, technically a steroid alcohol, found only in animal fats and oil; used in making cell membranes, as a building block for some hormones, in the fatty sheath around nerve fibers, and in other necessary substances.

Chronic diseases Illnesses that develop and last over a long time.

Chronic lower respiratory disease (CLRD) A group of diseases that limit air flow, such as chronic obstructive pulmonary disease, emphysema, and chronic bronchitis (all diseases of the respiratory system).

Chronological age Calendar age.

Chronotropic incompetence A condition in which the heart rate increases slowly during exercise and never reaches maximum.

Chylomicrons Molecules that transport triglycerides in the blood.

Cirrhosis A disease characterized by scarring of the liver.

Concentric Shortening of a muscle during muscle contraction.

Concentric muscle contraction A dynamic contraction in which the muscle shortens as it develops tension.

Contemplation stage Stage of change in which people are considering changing behavior in the next six months.

Contraindicated exercises Exercises that are not recommended because they pose potentially high risk for injury.

Cool-down A period at the end of an exercise session when exercise is tapered off.

Coronary heart disease (CHD) Condition in which the arteries that supply the heart muscle with oxygen and nutrients are narrowed by fatty deposits such as cholesterol and triglycerides.

C-reactive protein (CPR) A protein whose level in the blood increases with inflammation (which may be hidden deep in the body); elevation of this protein is an indicator of potential cardiovascular events.

Cross-training Using a combination of different aerobic activities to develop or maintain cardiorespiratory endurance.

Cruciferous vegetables Plants that produce cross-shaped leaves (cauliflower, broccoli, cabbage, Brussels sprouts, kohlrabi); these seem to have a protective effect against cancer.

D

Daily Values (DVs) Reference values for nutrients and food components used in food labels.

Deoxyribonucleic acid (DNA) Genetic substance of which genes are made; molecule that bears a cell's genetic code.

Diabetes mellitus A condition in which blood glucose is unable to enter the cells because the pancreas either totally stops producing insulin, does not produce enough to meet the body's needs, or the cells become insulin resistant.

Diastolic blood pressure Pressure exerted by the blood against the walls of the arteries during the relaxation phase (diastole) of the heart.

Dietary Reference Intakes (DRIs) Four types of nutrient standards that are used to establish adequate amounts and maximum safe nutrient intakes in the diet: Estimated Average Requirements (EARs), Recommended Dietary Allowances (RDAs), Adequate Intakes (AIs), and Tolerable Upper Intake Levels (ULs).

Distress Negative or harmful stress under which health and performance begin to deteriorate.

Duration of exercise Time exercising per session.

Dynamic exercise Strength training with muscle contraction that produces movement.

Dysmenorrhea Painful menstruation.

E

Eccentric Lengthening of a muscle during muscle contraction.

Eccentric muscle contraction A dynamic contraction in which the muscle lengthens as it develops tension.

Electrocardiogram (ECG or EKG) A recording of the electrical activity of the heart.

Energy-balancing equation A body weight formula stating that when caloric intake equals caloric output, weight remains unchanged.

Epidemiological Related to the study of epidemic diseases.

Essential fat Body fat needed for normal physiological functions.

Essential nutrients Carbohydrates, fats, proteins, vitamins, minerals, and water—the nutrients the human body requires for survival.

Estimated Average Requirement (EAR) The amount of a nutrient that meets the dietary needs in half the people.

Estimated energy requirement (EER) The average dietary energy (caloric) intake that is predicted to maintain energy balance in a healthy adult of defined age, gender, weight, height, and level of physical activity, consistent with good health.

Estrogen Female sex hormone; essential for bone formation and conservation of bone density.

Eustress Positive stress.

Exercise A type of physical activity that requires planned, structured, and repetitive bodily movement done to improve or maintain one or more components of physical fitness.

F

Fats (lipids) A class of nutrients that the body uses as a source of energy.

Female athlete triad Three interrelated disorders—disordered eating, amenorrhea, and bone mineral disorders—seen in some highly trained female athletes.

Ferritin Iron stored in the body.

Fiber Plant material that human digestive enzymes cannot digest.

Fight or flight Physiological response of the body to stress that prepares the individual to take action by stimulating the vital defense systems.

Fixed-resistance training Exercise with strength-training equipment that provides a constant amount of resistance through the range of motion.

Flexibility The achievable range of motion at a joint or group of joints without causing injury.

Free radicals Oxygen compounds produced in normal metabolism.

Free weights Barbells and dumbbells.

Frequency of exercise How often a person engages in an exercise session.

Functional fitness The physical capacity of the individual to meet ordinary and unexpected demands of daily life safely and effectively.

Functional independence Ability to carry out activities of daily living without assistance from other individuals.

G

General adaptation syndrome (GAS) A theoretical model that explains the body's adaptation to sustained stress which includes three stages: alarm reaction, resistance, and exhaustion/recovery.

Goal The ultimate aim toward which effort is directed.

Gynoid obesity Obesity pattern seen in people who store fat primarily around the hips and thighs.

H

Hatha yoga A yoga style that incorporates a series of static-stretching postures performed in specific sequences.

Health fitness standard The lowest fitness requirements for maintaining good health, decreasing the risk for chronic diseases, and lowering the incidence of musculoskeletal injuries.

Health-related fitness A physical state encompassing cardiorespiratory endurance, muscular strength and endurance, muscular flexibility, and body composition.

Healthy life expectancy (HLE) Number of years a person is expected to live in good health; this number is obtained by subtracting ill-health years from overall life expectancy.

Heart rate reserve The difference between the maximal heart rate (MHR) and resting heart rate (RHR).

Hemoglobin Protein-iron compound in red blood cells that transports oxygen in the blood.

High-density lipoprotein (HDL) Cholesterol-transporting molecules in the blood (good cholesterol).

High-impact aerobics (HIA) Exercises incorporating movements in which both feet are off the ground at the same time momentarily.

Homeostasis A natural state of equilibrium. The body attempts to maintain this equilibrium by constantly reacting to external forces that attempt to disrupt this fine balance.

Homocysteine Intermediate amino acid in the interconversion of two other amino acids: methionine and cysteine.

Human immunodeficiency virus (HIV) Virus that leads to acquired immunodeficiency syndrome (AIDS).

Hypertension Chronically elevated blood pressure.

Hypokinetic diseases Diseases related to a lack of physical activity.

Hypothermia A breakdown in the body's ability to generate heat, resulting in body temperature below 95°F.

I

Imagery Mental visualization of relaxing images and scenes to induce body relaxation in times of stress or as an aid in the treatment of certain medical conditions, such as cancer, hypertension, asthma, chronic pain, and obesity.

Insulin-dependent diabetes mellitus (IDDM or Type 1) A form of diabetes in which the pancreas produces little or no insulin.

Intensity (in flexibility exercise) Degree of stretch.

Intensity of exercise How hard a person has to exercise to improve cardiorespiratory endurance.

Interval training A repeated series of exercise work bouts (intervals) interspersed with low-intensity or rest intervals.

Isokinetic exercise Strength training method in which the speed of the muscle contraction is kept constant because the equipment (machine) provides an accommodating resistance to match the user's force through the full range of motion.

Isometric exercise Strength training with muscle contraction that produces little or no movement.

Isotonic exercise See *Dynamic exercise.*

L

Lean body mass Nonfat component of the body.

Life expectancy Number of years a person is expected to live based on the person's birth year.

Lipoproteins Complex molecules that transport cholesterol in the bloodstream.

Locus of control The extent to which a person believes that he or she can influence the external environment.

Low-density lipoprotein (LDL) Cholesterol-transporting molecules in the blood (bad cholesterol).

Low-impact aerobics (LIA) Exercises in which at least one foot is in contact with the ground or floor at all times.

Lymphocytes Immune system cells responsible for waging war against disease or infection.

M

Macronutrients The nutrients the body needs in proportionately large amounts: Carbohydrates, fats, proteins, and water.

Maintenance stage Stage of change in which people maintain behavioral change for up to five years.

Malignant Cancerous.

Maximal oxygen uptake (VO$_{2max}$) Maximum amount of oxygen the human body is able to utilize per minute of physical activity.

Meditation A mental exercise in which the objective is to gain control over one's attention, clearing the mind and blocking out stressors.

Megadoses For most vitamins, 10 times the RDA or more; for vitamins A and D, 5 and 2 times the RDA, respectively.

Melanoma The most virulent, rapidly spreading form of skin cancer.

MET One "MET," short for *metabolic equivalent,* represents the rate of energy expenditure while sitting quietly at rest. This energy expenditure is approximately 3.5 milliliters of oxygen per kilogram of body weight per minute (mL/kg/min) or 1.2 calories per minute for a 70-kilogram person. A 3 MET activity requires three times the energy expenditure of sitting quietly at rest.

Metabolic fitness Denotes improvements in the metabolic profile through a moderate-intensity exercise program in spite of little or no improvement in health-related fitness.

Metabolic profile Result of the assessment of diabetes and cardiovascular disease risk through plasma insulin, glucose, lipid, and lipoprotein levels.

Metabolic syndrome An array of metabolic abnormalities that contribute to the development of atherosclerosis triggered by resistance to insulin; these conditions include low HDL cholesterol, high triglycerides, high blood pressure, and an increased blood clotting mechanism.

Metastasis Movement of bacteria or body cells from one part of the body to another.

Micronutrients The nutrients the body needs in small quantities—vitamins and minerals—that serve specific roles in transformation of energy and body tissue synthesis.

Minerals Inorganic elements needed by the body.

Mode of exercise Form of exercise (e.g., aerobic).

Moderate-impact aerobics (MIA) Aerobics that include plyometric training.

Moderate-intensity aerobic physical activity Defined as the equivalent of a brisk walk that noticeably increases the heart rate.

Motivation The desire and will to do something.

Muscular endurance Ability of a muscle to exert submaximal force repeatedly over a period of time.

Muscular fitness A term that is used to define good levels of both muscular strength and muscular endurance.

Muscular hypertrophy An increase in muscle mass or size.

Muscular strength Ability to exert maximum force against resistance.

Myocardial infarction Heart attack; damage or death of an area of the heart muscle as a result of an obstructed artery to that area.

N

Negative resistance The lowering or eccentric phase of a repetition during the performance of a strength-training exercise.

Nitrosamines Potentially cancer-causing compounds formed when nitrites and nitrates—which are used to prevent the growth of harmful bacteria in processed meats—combine with other chemicals in the stomach.

Non-insulin-dependent diabetes mellitus (NIDDM or Type 2) A form of diabetes in which the pancreas either does not produce sufficient insulin or it produces adequate amounts but the cells become insulin-resistant, keeping glucose from entering the cell.

Nonresponders Individuals who exhibit small or no improvements in fitness as compared with others who undergo the same training program.

Nutrients Substances found in food that provide energy, regulate metabolism, and help with growth and repair of body tissues.

Nutrition The science that studies the relationship of foods to optimal health and performance.

O

Obesity A chronic disease characterized by an excessively high amount of body fat (about 20 percent above recommended weight or a BMI of 30 or above).

Objectives Steps required to reach a goal.

Oligomenorrhea Irregular menstrual cycles.

One repetition maximum (1 RM) The maximal amount of resistance a person is able to lift in a single effort.

Opportunistic infections Diseases that arise in the absence of a healthy immune system that would fight them off in healthy people.

Osteopenia Low bone mass.

Osteoporosis Softening, deterioration, or loss of bone.

Overload principle Training concept holding that the demands placed on a body system must be increased systematically and progressively over time to cause physiological adaptation.

Overweight Excess body weight when compared with a given standard such as height or recommended percent body fat.

P

Pedometer An electronic device that senses body motion and counts footsteps. Some pedometers also record distance, calories burned, speeds, and time spent being physically active.

Percent body fat (fat mass) Fat component of the body.

Personal trainer An exercise specialist who works one-on-one with an individual and is typically paid by the hour or exercise session.

Physical activity Bodily movement produced by skeletal muscles that requires energy expenditure and produces progressive health benefits.

Physical fitness The general capacity to adapt and respond favorably to physical effort.

Physical fitness standard Required criteria to achieve a high level of physical fitness; ability to do moderate to vigorous physical activity without undue fatigue.

Physiological age Age based on the individual's functional and physical capacity.

Physiological fitness Biological systems that are affected by physical activity; also the role of activity in disease prevention.

Phytonutrients Compounds found in fruits and vegetables that block formation of cancerous tumors and disrupt the process of cancer.

Pilates Exercises that help strengthen the body's core by developing pelvic stability and abdominal control coupled with focused breathing patterns.

Plyometric training A form of exercise that requires forceful jumps or springing off the ground immediately after landing from a previous jump.

Positive resistance The lifting, pushing, or concentric phase of a repetition during the performance of a strength-training exercise.

Precontemplation stage Stage of change in which people are unwilling to change their behavior.

Preparation stage Stage of change in which people are getting ready to make a change within the coming month.

Principle of individuality Training concept stating that genetics plays a major role in individual responses to exercise training and that these differences must be considered when designing exercise programs for different people.

Progressive muscle relaxation A relaxation technique that involves contracting, then relaxing muscle groups in the body in succession.

Progressive resistance training A gradual increase of resistance over a period of time.

Proprioceptive neuromuscular facilitation (PNF) A stretching technique in which muscles are stretched out progressively with intermittent isometric contractions.

Proteins A class of nutrients that the body uses to build and repair body tissues.

Q

Quackery/fraud The conscious promotion of unproven claims for profit.

R

Recommended body weight The weight at which there appears to be no harm to human health.

Recommended Dietary Allowance (RDA) The daily amount of a nutrient (statistically determined from the EARs) considered adequate to meet the known nutrient needs of almost 98 percent of all healthy people in the United States.

Registered dietitian (RD) A person with a college degree in dietetics who meets all certification and continuing education requirements of the American Dietetic Association or Dietitians of Canada.

Relapse Slipping or falling back into unhealthy behavior(s) or failing to maintain healthy behaviors.

Repetitions The number of times a movement is performed.

Resistance Amount of weight lifted.

Responders Individuals who exhibit improvements in fitness as a result of exercise training.

Resting metabolism The energy requirement to maintain the body's vital processes in the resting state.

Ribonucleic acid (RNA) Genetic material involved in the formation of cell proteins.

Risk factors Lifestyle and genetic variables that may lead to disease.

RM zone A range of repetitions that are to be performed maximally during one set. For example, an 8 to 12 RM zone implies that the individual will perform anywhere from 8 to 12 repetitions but cannot perform any more (e.g., 9 RM and could not perform a 10th repetition).

S

Sedentary Death Syndrome (SeDS) Cause of death due to a lack of regular physical activity.

Set The number of repetitions performed for a given exercise.

Setpoint Body weight and body fat percentage unique to each person that are regulated by genetic and environmental factors.

Sexually transmitted infections (STIs) Communicable infections spread through sexual contact.

Shin splint Injury to the lower leg characterized by pain and irritation at the front of the leg.

Skill-related fitness Components of fitness important for successful motor performance in athletic events and in lifetime sports and activities.

Slow-sustained stretching Technique whereby the muscles are lengthened gradually through a joint's complete range of motion and the final position is held for several seconds.

SMART An acronym for *s*pecific, *m*easurable, *a*cceptable, *r*ealistic, and *t*imely.

Specificity of training A principle holding that for a muscle to increase in strength or endurance, the training program must be specific.

Spirituality A sense of meaning and direction in life, a relationship to a higher being; encompasses freedom, prayer, faith, love, closeness to others, peace, joy, fulfillment, and altruism.

Step aerobics (SA) A form of exercise that combines stepping up and down from a bench with arm movements.

Storage fat Body fat stored in adipose tissue.

Stress The mental, emotional, and physiological response of the body to any situation that is new, threatening, frightening, or exciting.

Stress electrocardiogram (stress ECG) An exercise test during which the workload is gradually increased (until the subject reaches maximal fatigue), with blood pressure and electrocardiographic monitoring throughout the test.

Stressor Stress-causing agent.

Stretching Moving the joints beyond the accustomed range of motion.

Substrates Foods that are used as energy sources (carbohydrates, fats, proteins).

Sun protection factor (SPF) Degree of protection offered by ingredients in sunscreen lotion; at least SPF 15 is recommended.

Supplements Tablets, pills, capsules, liquids, or powders that contain vitamins, minerals, amino acids, herbs, or fiber that are taken to increase the intake of these substances.

Synergistic action The effect of mixing two or more drugs, the effects of which can be much greater than the sum of two or more drugs acting by themselves.

Synergy A reaction in which the result is greater than the sum of its two parts.

Systolic blood pressure Pressure exerted by the blood against the walls of the arteries during the forceful contraction (systole) of the heart.

T

Termination/adoption stage Stage of change in which people have eliminated an undesirable behavior or maintained a positive behavior for more than five years.

Tolerable Upper Intake Level (UL) The highest level of nutrient intake that appears to be safe for most healthy people without an increased risk for adverse effects.

Tolerable weight A realistic body weight that is close to the health fitness percent body fat standard.

Trans fatty acid Solidified fat formed by adding hydrogen to monounsaturated and polyunsaturated fats to increase shelf life.

Triglycerides Fats formed by glycerol and three fatty acids.

Type A Behavior pattern characteristic of a hard-driving, overly ambitious, aggressive, at times hostile and overly competitive person.

Type B Behavior pattern characteristic of a calm, casual, relaxed, and easygoing individual.

V

Variable-resistance training Exercise that utilizes special equipment with mechanical devices that provide differing amounts of resistance through the range of motion.

Vegetarians Individuals whose diet is of vegetable or plant origin.

Vigorous exercise An exercise intensity that is either above 6 metabolic equivalents (METs) or 60 percent of maximal oxygen uptake or that provides a "substantial" challenge to the individual.

Vigorous-intensity aerobic physical activity Defined as an activity similar to jogging that causes rapid breathing and a substantial increase in heart rate.

Vitamins Organic substances essential for normal bodily metabolism, growth, and development.

W

Waist circumference (WC) A waist girth measurement to assess potential risk for disease based on intra-abdominal fat content.

Warm-up A preliminary period when exercise begins slowly.

Wellness The constant and deliberate effort to stay healthy and achieve the highest potential for well-being.

Y

Yoga A school of thought in the Hindu religion that seeks to help the individual attain a higher level of spirituality and peace of mind.